Find surgical technique videos and animations for *Moyamoya Disease* online at MediaCenter.thieme.com!

Surgical videos and animations available online:

1. Animation of Arterial Wall Pathology in Moyamoya Disease
2. Animation of Collateral Circulation Development in Moyamoya Disease
3. Parietal Branch STA Harvest
4. EDAS without Pial Sutures
5. EDAS with Pial Sutures
6. EDAS with Rotated MMA and Dural inversion
7. Direct STA-MCA Bypass with Continuous Sutures
8. Direct STA-MCA Bypass with Interrupted Sutures
9. ICG Angiography of STA-MCA bypass
10. EEG Changes During Direct Bypass
11. EDMAPS Combined Direct and Indirect Bypass
12. OA-PCA Anastomosis for Pediatric Moyamoya Disease

Total length of videos: approximately 40 minutes

Simply visit MediaCenter.thieme.com and, when prompted during the registration process, enter the scratch-off code below to get started today.

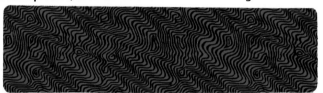

This book cannot be returned once this panel has been scratched off.

	WINDOWS	MAC	TABLET
Recommended Browser(s)**	Microsoft Internet Explorer 8.0 or later, Firefox 3.x	Firefox 3.x, Safari 4.x	HTML5 mobile browser. iPad — Safari. Opera Mobile — Tablet PCs referred.
	** all browsers should have JavaScript enabled		
Flash Player Plug-in	Flash Player 9 or Higher* ** Mac users: ATI Rage 128 GPU does not support full-screen mode with hardware scaling*		Tablet PCs with Android OS support Flash 10.1
Minimum Hardware Configurations	Intel® Pentium® II 450 MHz, AMD Athlon™ 600 MHz or faster processor (or equivalent) 512 MB of RAM	PowerPC® G3 500 MHz or faster processor Intel Core™ Duo 1.33 GHz or faster processor 512MB of RAM	Minimum CPU powered at 800MHz 256MB DDR2 of RAM
Recommended for optimal usage experience	Monitor resolutions: • Normal (4:3) 1024×768 or Higher • Widescreen (16:9) 1280×720 or Higher • Widescreen (16:10) 1440×900 or Higher DSL/Cable internet connection at a minimum speed of 384.0 Kbps or faster WiFi 802.11 b/g preferred.		7-inch and 10-inch tablets on maximum resolution. WiFi connection is required.

Moyamoya Disease

Diagnosis and Treatment

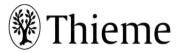

Moyamoya Disease

Diagnosis and Treatment

John E. Wanebo, MD, FACS
Director, Barrow Moyamoya Center
Barrow Neurological Institute
St. Joseph's Hospital and Medical Center
Phoenix, Arizona

Assistant Clinical Professor of Neurosurgery
University of Arizona
Phoenix, Arizona

Head, Division of Neurosurgery
Scottsdale Healthcare
Scottsdale, Arizona

Associate Professor of Surgery
Uniformed Services University of the Health Sciences
Bethesda, Maryland

Nadia Khan, MD
Associate Professor and Head of Moyamoya Center
Division of Pediatric Neurosurgery
Department of Surgery
University Children's Hospital Zurich
Zurich, Switzerland

Joseph M. Zabramski, MD
Professor of Neurological Surgery and Chief of Cerebrovascular Surgery
Barrow Neurological Institute
St. Joseph's Hospital and Medical Center
Phoenix, Arizona

Chairman, Department of Surgery
Scottsdale Healthcare
Scottsdale, Arizona

Robert F. Spetzler, MD
Director and J.N. Harber Chair of Neurological Surgery
Barrow Neurological Institute
St. Joseph's Hospital and Medical Center
Phoenix, Arizona

Professor, Department of Surgery
Section of Neurosurgery
University of Arizona College of Medicine
Tucson, Arizona

Thieme
New York • Stuttgart

Thieme Medical Publishers, Inc.
333 Seventh Ave.
New York, NY 10001

Executive Editor: Kay Conerly
Managing Editor: Judith Tomat
Senior Vice President, Editorial and Electronic Product Development: Cornelia Schulze
Production Editor: Teresa Exley
International Production Director: Andreas Schabert
Vice President, Finance and Accounts: Sarah Vanderbilt
President: Brian D. Scanlan
Compositor: Maryland Composition
Printer: Everbest Printing Co.

Library of Congress Cataloging-in-Publication Data

Moyamoya disease (Wanebo)
  Moyamoya disease : diagnosis and treatment / [edited by] John E. Wanebo, Nadia Khan, Joseph M. Zabramski, Robert F. Spetzler.
      p. ; cm.
  Includes bibliographical references and index.
    ISBN 978-1-60406-730-9 (hardback)
    I. Wanebo, John E., editor of compilation. II. Khan, Nadia, editor of compilation. III. Zabramski, Joseph M., editor of compilation. IV. Spetzler, Robert F. (Robert Friedrich), 1944- editor of compilation. V. Title.
    [DNLM: 1. Moyamoya Disease—diagnosis. 2. Moyamoya Disease—therapy. WL 357]
    RC388.5
    616.8'1—dc23
                                                                                        2013025185

Important note: Medical knowledge is ever-changing. As new research and clinical experience broaden our knowledge, changes in treatment and drug therapy may be required. The authors and editors of the material herein have consulted sources believed to be reliable in their efforts to provide information that is complete and in accord with the standards accepted at the time of publication. However, in view of the possibility of human error by the authors, editors, or publisher of the work herein or changes in medical knowledge, neither the authors, editors, nor publisher, nor any other party who has been involved in the preparation of this work, warrants that the information contained herein is in every respect accurate or complete, and they are not responsible for any errors or omissions or for the results obtained from use of such information. Readers are encouraged to confirm the information contained herein with other sources. For example, readers are advised to check the product information sheet included in the package of each drug they plan to administer to be certain that the information contained in this publication is accurate and that changes have not been made in the recommended dose or in the contraindications for administration. This recommendation is of particular importance in connection with new or infrequently used drugs.

Some of the product names, patents, and registered designs referred to in this book are in fact registered trademarks or proprietary names even though specific reference to this fact is not always made in the text. Therefore, the appearance of a name without designation as proprietary is not to be construed as a representation by the publisher that it is in the public domain.

Printed in China

ISBN 978-1-60406-730-9

Also available as an e-book:
eISBN 978-1-60406-732-3

To my parents, Harold and Claire, for showing me the way; to my children, Oliver, Grace, and Ella; and to my lovely wife, Sonja, for her inspiration and support.

John E. Wanebo, MD, FACS

To all of the children and their parents managed at the Moyamoya Center in Zurich, hoping that this will be yet another important and additional step in increasing awareness for the disease. Also to our team of physicians, nurses, and OR staff for continuously setting high standards for support and quality of care.

Nadia Khan, MD

My special gratitude to the many contributing authors and to the dedicated editorial staff involved in preparing this text. It is my sincere hope that it might improve the treatment of patients everywhere suffering from moyamoya and encourage further research into the etiology and management of this disease.

Joseph M. Zabramski, MD

For the many lessons I have learned from my patients, I dedicate this book to them and hope that future patients will benefit from the collective knowledge presented in these pages.

Robert F. Spetzler, MD

Contents

Contents

List of Videos

Contents

Foreword

The time is ripe for a new book on moyamoya disease. Much has been learned since Jiro Suzuki and Akira Takaku in Japan first described this "orphan" disease in 1969. The very first case of moyamoya that I saw as a resident in the late 1960s was not recognized as such, because the description of the condition had not yet reached the shores of North America; it took another 20 years before an accurate diagnosis was made in that particular patient's case after she had suffered two additional strokes. I was not aware of the pediatric presentation of this condition until the work of Harold Hoffman and his colleagues in Toronto in the late 1970s, and my first operation on a pediatric patient took place in 1982. Much information on the condition has been discovered since then, and this new volume, edited by John E. Wanebo, Nadia Khan, Joseph M. Zabramski, and Robert F. Spetzler, updates us on the latest information regarding this condition. The first section of their monograph contains an essential chapter from Kiyohiro Houkin and Takeshi Mikami in Japan on the definitions of the "syndrome" versus the "disease"—a distinction commonly made only in the past several decades, a chapter from Toronto on the codification of the various imaging findings that are so typical of this condition, and a review of its natural history from the group at the Columbia Neurological Surgery Department. Many of us are intrigued by the genetics of moyamoya, and the chapter of Constantin Roder and Boris Krischek reviews what we presently know about this topic. One of the more difficult aspects of moyamoya management has been the interpretation of cerebral perfusion studies in moyamoya diagnosis to determine treatment, and this issue is addressed by authors from the very experienced imaging group at Washington University in St. Louis. As many of us know, moyamoya disease has now been reported virtually worldwide, and the editors have included a chapter from the Cincinnati group on its epidemiology throughout the globe. One of the least understood aspects of moyamoya disease has been the role played by the cortical microvasculature, and a chapter from the Berlin Neurosurgical Department addresses this subject matter. Completing this first section of chapters is a contribution by the neurology and neuropsychology group from Phoenix describing how psychological testing can be used to assess patients with moyamoya.

The second section of the book discusses the various treatment options available for patients with this condition. Groups from London and Stanford review medical and endovascular treatments. The endovascular chapter frankly discusses the limitations of such therapy for this condition, and provides effective argument against the use of endovascular techniques in this patient population. This section of the book closes with descriptions of a number of surgical procedures developed to carry out cortical revascularization in these patients, with contributions from neurosurgical groups in Boston, Phoenix, Zurich, and Japan. The Stanford anesthesia group completes the section with a review of anesthetic and perioperative patient management strategies in the moyamoya patient.

The third section of the book discusses one of the most interesting and important aspects of the condition—what happens over the long term to patients with moyamoya—utilizing contributions from well-established groups in Stanford, Japan, and Korea about the long-term surgical outcomes of moyamoya patients treated at their institutions. These chapters will be important to all physicians treating moyamoya patients, because this issue is one of the most common concerns of patients and families during late follow-up, a concern that continues to be studied in patient cohorts throughout the world.

This book will be of a great benefit to neurologists and neurosurgeons who treat patients with stroke and TIA both in the adult and pediatric age groups. The information provided in this monograph will allow the interested physician to diagnose the condition, and employ and interpret the appropriate diagnostic tests as they manage their patients. Neurosurgeons will appreciate the very thorough descriptions of the various surgical techniques that have been developed to treat this condition, and all will benefit from learning about the long-term experience after treatment has been carried out. I hope that as the years progress after this book's publication, these same authors can be recruited again for a second edition to provide the interested physician with continuing updates on this fascinating condition, about which we are all continuing to learn.

R. Michael Scott, MD
Fellows Family Chair in Pediatric Neurosurgery
Professor of Surgery (Neurosurgery)
Harvard Medical School
Boston Children's Hospital
Boston, Massachusetts

Foreword

Moyamoya disease was recognized as a single clinical entity in 1960s as the term *moyamoya* first appeared in Jiro Suzuki's English article in 1969. Since then clinical and basic research has been conducted mostly by such Japanese groups as the Research Committee on Spontaneous Occlusion of the Circle of Willis, because of the relatively high incidence of this disease in Asia. As interest and reports increased, Suzuki's monograph of this disease first appeared in English in 1986 and the first International Symposium on Moyamoya Disease in 1996 was organized by Professor Masashi Fukui. Since then, international awareness of this disease has spread all over the world and several comprehensive reviews of this disease have been released periodically, mostly from Asian authors. John E. Wanebo, Nadia Khan, Joseph M. Zabramski, and Robert F. Spetzler have brought together world-leading physicians in this field whose years of experience in moyamoya disease shows in this book.

This multi-authored, well-organized monograph is a must read for any physician involved in the care of patients with moyamoya disease. It is moderately short and very easy to read but still provides a state-of-the-art review of the disease with updated aspects, especially in its etiology and pathogenesis, epidemiology, and long-term results.

The book is divided into three parts. The first chapters provide important background information about moyamoya disease and discuss the diagnostic evaluation of moyamoya. It will be of most interest and use to neurologists and neuroradiologists. The second set of chapters focus on patient care and cover medical, endovascular, and all of the different revascularization procedures used to treat patients with moyamoya disease. It concludes with a short chapter about anesthetic management of patients with moyamoya disease. The third section compares the long-term outcome after bypass surgery between the United States, Japan, and Korea.

Although this book was primarily intended for a neurosurgical audience, it can be recommended for purchase by institutional libraries and by clinicians (not only by neurosurgeons, but neurologists, neuroradiologists, pediatricians, and anesthesiologists) and allied researchers who frequently study moyamoya disease in their practice.

The authors can be confident that there will be many grateful readers worldwide who are challenged to treat their patients with moyamoya disease. As a result of the editors' efforts, I sincerely hope that moyamoya disease will be recognized more correctly, studied collaboratively in the world, and that this book will help elucidate a cause and establish a complete cure of this disease.

Kiyonobu Ikezaki, MD, PhD
International University of Health and Welfare
Fukuoka, Japan

Preface

Moyamoya Angiopathy: Diagnosis and Treatment is primarily geared toward neurologists and neurosurgeons involved in the firsthand care of moyamoya patients. Understanding and treating moyamoya angiopathy requires a multidisciplinary approach, with close collaboration of several specialists managing both adults and children diagnosed with this disease. Hence, a wide range of caretakers—including pediatricians, neuropsychologists, child development specialists, nurses, rehabilitation physicians, anesthesiologists, and radiologists—would benefit equally from this information.

Although rare, moyamoya has become more widely recognized and should be treated aggressively. An explosion of information on the topic has occurred in the literature, with more than 2,000 publications since 1970; half of these have been published in the past 10 years. The current moyamoya texts are becoming outdated with the most recent two books on the subject being published in English in 2001 and 2010.

Conceptualized and edited by neurosurgeons, this book is organized into three sections. The first section provides up-to-date knowledge on the definition and characterization of moyamoya; the second provides correct indications for cerebral revascularization; and the third elaborates on surgical techniques for moyamoya and their outcomes.

Advances in the understanding of the pathophysiology and natural history of moyamoya angiopathy are presented. Important diagnostic tools such as neurocognitive batteries and cerebral blood flow testing are clarified by experts in the field. Dynamic topics not covered in prior moyamoya texts are addressed by chapters on cortical microvasculature, genetics, neuropsychiatric evaluation, and endovascular therapy. Technical aspects of treatment are elaborated, with a range of excellent descriptions and detailed illustrations of both the direct and indirect methods of revascularization, along with lessons learned from decades of medical and surgical management of these patients.

Moyamoya Angiopathy: Diagnosis and Treatment has benefitted from significant international input, reflecting ideas and long-term treatment experience from leading authorities in eight countries from Asia to North America to Europe.

We hope to have provided a practical, clinically oriented reference that will assist clinicians and neurosurgeons alike in their day-to-day practice and training.

John E. Wanebo, MD, FACS
Nadia Khan, MD
Joseph M. Zabramski, MD
Robert F. Spetzler, MD

Acknowledgments

The completion of this work was made possible by the exceptional team efforts from the Neuroscience Publication office at Barrow Neurological Institute. We would like to thank editors Shelley Kick and Dawn Mutchler, and editorial assistants Clare Prendergast, Talisa Umfress, and Mandi Leite, for their large time investment and diligence in working with the text. Clare Prendergast deserves our special thanks for keeping us on track. We are also indebted to our illustrators, Mark Schornak and Kristen Larson, whose artwork brought to life the anatomical and surgical concepts, and to our animator, Michael Hickman, who created the outstanding animations. We also thank Jaime-Lynn Canales, who formatted and managed the many figures. In addition, our thanks go to Marie Clarkson, who expertly edited and prepared the video and corresponding audio in the dozen videos included with the book.

John E. Wanebo
Nadia Khan
Joseph M. Zabramski
Robert F. Spetzler

Contributors

Hiroshi Abe, MD, PhD
Assistant Professor of Neurosurgery
Department of Neurosurgery
Faculty of Medicine, Fukuoka University
Fukuoka, Japan

Norberto Andaluz, MD
Associate Professor of Neurosurgery
Department of Neurosurgery
University of Cincinnati College of Medicine
UC Neuroscience Institute
Mayfield Clinic
Cincinnati, Ohio

Terry C. Burns, MD, PhD
Neurosurgery Resident
Department of Neurosurgery
Stanford University School of Medicine
Stanford, California

E. Sander Connolly Jr., MD
Professor of Neurological Surgery
Vice Chairman of Neurosurgery
Director, Cerebrovascular Research Laboratory
Surgical Director, Neuro-Intensive Care Unit
Neurological Surgery
Columbia University
New York, New York

Douglas J. Cook, MD, FRCS(C)
Assistant Professor
Department of Neurosurgery
Queen's University
Ontario, Canada

Marcus Czabanka, MD
Department of Neurosurgery
University Medicine Charité, Berlin
Berlin, Germany

Colin P. Derdeyn, MD
Professor of Radiology, Neurology, and
   Neurological Surgery
Mallinckrodt Institute of Radiology
Washington University School of Medicine
St. Louis, Missouri

Andrew J. Duren, BA
Department of Neurosurgery
Columbia University College of Physicians
   and Surgeons
New York, New York

Vijeya Ganesan, MB ChB, MD
Senior Lecturer Paediatric Neurology
Neurosciences Unit
UCL Institute of Child Health
London, United Kingdom

Peter A. Gooderham, MD
Cerebrovascular Surgery Fellow
Department of Neurosurgery
Stanford University School of Medicine
Stanford, California

Toshiaki Hayashi, MD, PhD
Department of Neurosurgery
Miyagi Children's Hospital
Sendai, Japan

Toshio Higashi, MD, PhD
Associate Professor of Neurosurgery
Department of Neurosurgery
Faculty of Medicine, Fukuoka University
Fukuoka, Japan

Kiyohiro Houkin, MD, PhD
Professor
Department of Neurosurgery
Hokkaido University
Sapporo, Japan

Kiyonobu Ikezaki, MD, PhD
Professor of Medicine
Neuroscience Center
Fukuoka Sanno Hospital
International University of Health and
   Welfare
Fukuoka, Japan

Tooru Inoue, MD, PhD
Professor of Neurosurgery
Department of Neurosurgery
Faculty of Medicine, Fukuoka University
Fukuoka, Japan

Richard A. Jaffe, MD, PhD
Professor of Anesthesia
Department of Anesthesia
Stanford University School of Medicine
Stanford, California

Nadia Khan, MD
Associate Professor and Head of Moyamoya
   Center
Division of Pediatric Neurosurgery
Department of Surgery
University Children's Hospital Zurich
Zurich, Switzerland

Tomomi Kimiwada, MD, PhD
Department of Neurosurgery
Miyagi Children's Hospital
Sendai, Japan

Boris Krischek, MD, PhD
Professor of Neurosurgery
Department of Neurosurgery
University Hospital of Cologne
Cologne, Germany

Jaime R. López, MD
Associate Professor
Department of Neurology and Neurological
   Sciences
Department of Neurosurgery
Stanford University School of Medicine
Stanford, California

Michael P. Marks, MD
Professor of Radiology and Neurosurgery
Chief of Interventional Neuroradiology
Department of Radiology
Stanford University School of Medicine
Stanford University Medical Center
Stanford, California

Diana G. McGregor, MB, BCh
Clinical Associate Professor of Anesthesia
Department of Anesthesia
Stanford University School of Medicine
Stanford, California

Takeshi Mikami, MD, PhD
Associate Professor
Department of Neurosurgery
Sapporo Medical University
Sapporo, Japan

Jeannine V. Morrone-Strupinsky, PhD
Arizona Neuropsychological Services
Chandler, Arizona

Peter Nakaji, MD, FACS, FAANS
Professor of Neurosurgery
Director, Neurosurgery Residency Program
Director, Minimally Invasive Neurosurgery
Division of Neurological Surgery
Barrow Neurological Institute
Phoenix, Arizona

Ramon L. Navarro, MD
Cerebrovascular Surgery Fellow
Department of Neurosurgery
Stanford University School of Medicine
Stanford, California

Joanne Ng, MB ChB
Clinical Research Fellow
Neurosciences Unit
UCL Institute of Child Health
London, United Kingdom

George P. Prigatano, PhD, ABPP-CN
Newsome Chair, Department of Clinical
  Neuropsychology
Barrow Neurological Institute
St. Joseph's Hospital and Medical Center
Phoenix, Arizona

Hyoung Kyun Rha, MD, PhD
Professor
Department of Neurosurgery
St. Mary's Hospital
Catholic University
Seoul, Korea

Constantin Roder, MD
Department of Neurosurgery
University of Tübingen
Tübingen, Germany

James R. Sagar, MD
Stroke Research Fellow
Mallinckrodt Institute of Radiology
Washington University School of Medicine
St. Louis, Missouri

Reizo Shirane, MD, PhD
Professor of Pediatric Neurosurgery
Departments of Pediatric Neurosurgery
Miyagi Children's Hospital
Tohoku University
Sendai, Japan

Edward R. Smith, MD
Associate Professor of Surgery (Neurosurgery),
  Harvard Medical School
Department of Neurosurgery
Boston Children's Hospital
Boston, Massachusetts

Robert F. Spetzler, MD
Director and J.N. Harber Chair of Neurological
  Surgery
Barrow Neurological Institute
St. Joseph's Hospital and Medical Center
Phoenix, Arizona

Professor, Department of Surgery
Section of Neurosurgery
University of Arizona College of Medicine
Tucson, Arizona

Robert M. Starke, MD, MSc
Resident in Neurological Surgery
Department of Neurological Surgery
University of Virginia
Charlottesville, Virginia

Gary K. Steinberg, MD, PhD
Bernard and Ronni Lacroute-
  William Randolph Hearst Professor of
  Neurosurgery and the Neurosciences
Department of Neurosurgery
Stanford University School of Medicine
Stanford, California

Teiji Tominaga, MD, PhD
Department of Neurosurgery
Tohoku University Graduates School of
  Medicine
Sendai, Japan

Michael Tymianski, MD, PhD, FRCS(C)
Professor of Surgery
Division of Neurosurgery
University of Toronto
Ontario, Canada

Peter Vajkoczy, MD
Professor
Department of Neurosurgery
Charite Universitaetsmedizin Berlin
Berlin, Germany

Gregory J. Velat, MD
Division of Neurological Surgery
Barrow Neurological Institute
St. Joseph's Hospital and Medical Center
Phoenix, Arizona

John E. Wanebo, MD, FACS
Director, Barrow Moyamoya Center
Barrow Neurological Institute
St. Joseph's Hospital and Medical Center
Phoenix, Arizona

Assistant Clinical Professor of Neurosurgery
University of Arizona
Phoenix, Arizona

Head, Division of Neurosurgery
Scottsdale Healthcare
Scottsdale, Arizona

Associate Professor of Surgery
Uniformed Services University of the
  Health Sciences
Bethesda, Maryland

Yasuhiro Yonekawa, MD
Professor Emeritus
University of Zurich
Zurich, Switzerland

Joseph M. Zabramski, MD
Professor of Neurological Surgery and Chief of
    Cerebrovascular Surgery
Barrow Neurological Institute
St. Joseph's Hospital and Medical Center
Phoenix, Arizona

Chairman, Department of Surgery
Scottsdale Healthcare
Scottsdale, Arizona

Mario Zuccarello, MD
Professor and Frank H. Mayfield Chair for
    Neurological Surgery
Chairman
Department of Neurosurgery
University of Cincinnati College of Medicine
Cincinnati, Ohio

I

Diagnosing Moyamoya Angiopathy: Definition, Classifications, Symptomatology

1

Moyamoya Disease and Moyamoya Syndrome

Kiyohiro Houkin and Takeshi Mikami

◆ Introduction

Moyamoya disease is a unique cerebrovascular disease characterized by the primary chronic progressive stenotic change of the terminal portion of the internal carotid arteries (ICAs) bilaterally. These changes induce the formation of an abnormal vascular network composed of collateral pathways at the base of the brain to compensate for the cerebral ischemia related to the primary pathological change. The term for this vascular network is "moyamoya vessels." Moyamoya is the Japanese term for a "puff of smoke," which has been used to describe the appearance of these collateral vessels on cerebral angiography.[1] The concept of moyamoya disease was established in the 1960s.[2,3] The angiography of this disease shows unique longitudinal changes from the very early stage with an equivocal minimum stenotic change of the terminal portion of the ICA to the final stage with bilateral occlusion of the ICAs. In the final stage of the disease, the entire brain is perfused by the external carotid system and the vertebrobasilar system.[1–4]

Another unique feature of this disease is its clinical presentation. Most pediatric patients have ischemic episodes that range from transient ischemic attacks (TIAs) to completed infarction. In pediatric cases, TIAs and completed infarction can be induced by hyperventilation from activities such as blowing hot food to cool it and blowing a wind musical instrument. In adults, half of the cases suffer from intracranial bleeding. Many patients also complain of migrainelike headache. Some pediatric patients show involuntary movement similar to chorea.

◆ Epidemiology

The incidence of moyamoya disease appears to have a unique ethnic bias. It predominantly occurs in eastern Asians, although its distribution is worldwide. In a Japanese epidemiological survey conducted by Wakai et al[5] in 1994, the prevalence was supposed to be 3.16 people per 100,000 persons with an incidence of 0.35 people per 100,000 persons. Survey studies from the United States suggest that the incidence is 0.086 people per 100,000 persons. Compared with Caucasians, the ethnicity-specific incidence rate ratios were 4.6 (95% confidence interval [CI], 3.4–6.3) for Asian Americans, 2.2 (95% CI, 1.3–2.4) for African Americans, and 0.5 (95% CI, 0.3–0.8) for Hispanics.[6] According to a recent survey in Japan (Hokkaido area), the number of patients with moyamoya disease markedly increased compared with a previous national survey.[7,8] This increase may reflect the increased awareness of this disease and its familial occurrence.

In particular, magnetic resonance imaging (MRI) and magnetic resonance angiography (MRA) offer noninvasive screening for adults and asymptomatic people with a familial history of moyamoya disease. In recent years, asymptomatic cases of moyamoya disease and moyamoya disease manifesting with only nonspecific symptoms such as headache have drawn attention.[9,10] The increase in the number of such patients could be attributable, at least partially, to the current widespread availability of MRI and the increase in the number of people undergoing medical check-up procedures for the brain. Indeed, in the contemporary Japanese survey, the familial occurrence ranged between 10 and 16%, and the rate of asymptomatic registered moyamoya patients in some areas in Japan was 17%. The male-to-female ratio of occurrence of moyamoya disease is well established at 1:2.[5] There has been no reasonable explanation for this female dominancy in moyamoya disease.

Moyamoya syndrome is not a well-defined entity. The associated angiographic changes are similar to those associated with moyamoya disease, but there are differences in other features. The clinical symptoms are similar to those of moyamoya disease. There has been no systematic study of the epidemiology of moyamoya syndrome.

◆ Diagnostic Criteria

Moyamoya disease is defined by its characteristic angiographic findings; there are no specific laboratory findings in patients with moyamoya disease. In 1977, a research committee supported by the Japanese Ministry of Health and Welfare started basic and clinical research on this disease. In 1995, this committee proposed guidelines for the diagnosis (**Table 1.1**) and treatment of moyamoya disease.[11]

Although cerebral angiography has been essential for the diagnosis of this disease, MRA and MRI clearly show the major intracranial arteries and have become indispensable modalities for the management of moyamoya disease (**Figs. 1.1** and **1.2**). Based on this dramatic technical evolution, the diagnostic guidelines for moyamoya disease have included MRA and MRI as the definitive diagnostic techniques since 1994.[12,13] MRA is an acceptable alternative to the use of conventional angiography for diagnosing moyamoya disease and has

been acknowledged as a reliable diagnostic tool with high sensitivity and specificity as a result of the remarkable developments in MRI technology.[14–17]

However, in typical pediatric cases, the diagnosis can be confirmed only by MRI. In elderly adults, the disease is not always clearly differentiated from other atherosclerotic diseases despite the high resolution of MRI. In such cases, conventional angiography is indispensable.

◆ Disease Type Manifested at Initial Attack

As mentioned, moyamoya disease can occur at any age from childhood to adulthood. Interestingly, however, it has two peaks: one in the first decade of childhood and one in the middle-aged population. Symptoms vary according to the age and disease type. In children, the disease often first manifests with cerebral ischemic symptoms, particularly after hyperventilation caused by crying, playing a wind instrument, and eating a hot meal. Symptoms such as motor weakness (quadriplegia, hemiplegia, and monoplegia), sensory disturbance, disturbance in consciousness, seizure, and headache occur in a paroxysmal and recurrent manner. In many patients, the symptoms always appear on the same side. Occasionally, the affected side fluctuates between the right and left. Some patients develop involuntary movements such as chorea[18] and limb shaking. In patients with repeated cerebral ischemic attacks, the serious cerebral atrophy that occurs induces mental dysfunction or diminished intelligence, or attention deficit hyperactivity disorder in pediatric patients.

In moyamoya disease, the posterior cerebral arteries often remain patent until the advanced stage of the disease.[2] However, in some patients, posterior cerebral artery disorder may result in visual impairment or a visual field defect.[19] In pediatric patients, particularly those younger than 5 years old, intracranial bleeding is rare, unlike in adult patients. In adults, especially those 25 years or older, moyamoya disease frequently manifests with the sudden onset of intracranial hemorrhage (intraventricular, subarachnoid, or intracerebral) and causes symptoms such as a disturbance in consciousness, headache, muscle

Table 1.1 Diagnostic Criteria of Moyamoya Disease

A. Cerebral angiography is indispensable for diagnosis and should show at least the following findings:

1. Stenosis or occlusion at terminal portion of the ICA and/or at proximal portion of ACAs and/or MCAs.

2. Abnormal vascular networks in the vicinity of the occlusive or stenotic lesions in arterial phase.

3. Findings should appear bilaterally.

B. When MRI and MRA demonstrate all subsequently described findings, conventional cerebral angiography is not mandatory:

1. Stenosis or occlusion at terminal portion of ICA and at the proximal portion of ACAs and MCAs on MRA.

2. An abnormal vascular network in the basal ganglia on MRA. An abnormal vascular network can be diagnosed when more than two apparent flow voids are observed in one side of the basal ganglia on MRI.

3. (1) and (2) observed bilaterally.

C. Because the origin of this disease is unknown, cerebrovascular disease with the following basic diseases or conditions should be eliminated:

1. Arteriosclerosis	6. Recklinghausen disease
2. Autoimmune disease	7. Head trauma
3. Meningitis	8. Irradiation to the head
4. Brain neoplasm	9. Others (e.g., sickle cell disease, tuberous sclerosis)
5. Down syndrome	

D. Instructive pathological findings:

1. Intimal thickening and resulting stenosis or occlusion of lumen observed in and around terminal portion of ICA, usually on both sides. Lipid deposits occasionally noted in proliferating intima.

2. Arteries constituting the circle of Willis such as the ACAs, MCAs, and posterior communicating arteries often show stenosis of various degrees or occlusion associated with fibrocellular thickening of intima, waving of the internal elastic lamina, and attenuation of media.

3. Numerous small vascular channels (perforators and anastomotic branches) observed around circle of Willis.

4. Reticular conglomerates of small vessels often noted in pia mater.

Diagnosis: In reference to A to D, the diagnostic criteria are classified as follows (autopsy cases not undergoing cerebral angiography should be investigated separately while referring to D):

1. Definite case: Fulfills criteria A or B, and C. Pediatric case that fulfills A-1 and A-2 (or B-1 and B-2) on one side. Remarkable stenosis at terminal portion of ICA on opposite side also included.

2. Probable case: Fulfills criteria A-1 and A-2 (or B-1 and B-2) and C (unilateral involvement).

Abbreviations: ACA, anterior cerebral artery; ICA, interior carotid artery; MCA, middle cerebral artery; MRA, magnetic resonance angiography; MRI, magnetic resonance imaging.

Source: Text used with permission from Elsevier. From Fukui M, Members of the Research Committee on Spontaneous Occlusion of the Circle of the Willis (Moyamoya Disease) of the Ministry of Health and Welfare. Guidelines for the diagnosis and treatment of spontaneous occlusion of the circle of Willis ('Moyamoya disease'). Clin Neurol Neurosurg 1997;99(Suppl 2):S238–S240.[11]

weakness, and speech disorder, depending on the site of hemorrhage.

Histologically, bleeding has been attributed to the rupture of fragile collateral vessels associated with moyamoya vessels as progressive stenosis of the ICA.[20] Shifting circulatory patterns at the base of the brain have also been implicated in cerebral microaneurysms.[21] Intracranial hemorrhage often manifests as small intraventricular hemorrhage, so the symptoms are mild. If, however, a serious intracerebral hemorrhage occurs, it can cause fixed neurological deficits or progress to a more serious condition and lead to death. Furthermore, the patients are at a high risk of rebleeding, and approximately half die as a result of bleeding.

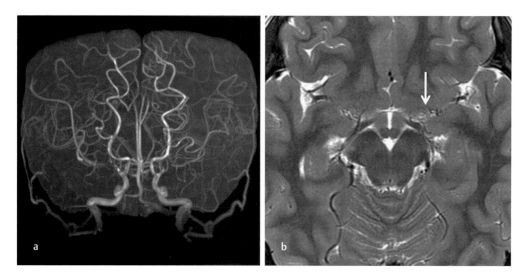

Fig. 1.1a, b (**a**) Magnetic resonance angiography reveals steno-occlusive change at the terminal portion of the bilateral carotid artery. (**b**) T2-weighted magnetic resonance imaging at the level of basal cistern shows small characteristic signal voids suggesting moyamoya vessels (*arrow*).

◆ Moyamoya Syndrome

The term moyamoya syndrome refers to the presence of stenosis or occlusion of the terminal portion of the ICA or proximal portion of the anterior and/or middle cerebral arteries accompanied by an abnormal vascular network detected in association with an underlying disease. Even in cases with unilateral lesions, if an underlying disease is present, the condition is considered moyamoya syndrome. This condition is also called "rui-moyamoya disease" in Japanese and "quasi-moyamoya disease" in English. Various clinical conditions or systemic disorders have been reported in conjunction with moyamoya syndrome (**Table 1.2**).[22,23]

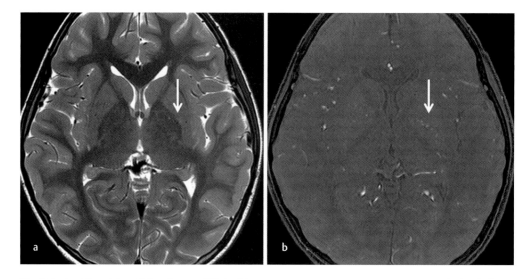

Fig. 1.2a, b T2-weighted (**a**) and time-of-flight (**b**) magnetic resonance imaging sequences at the level of basal ganglia show small signal voids (*arrows*).

Table 1.2 Moyamoya Syndrome and Associated Disorders

Congenital Disorders	Acquired Disorders
Hematological disorders	*Autoimmune disorders*
Anaplastic anemia	Systemic lupus erythematosus
Fanconi anemia	Antiphospholipid antibody syndrome
Sickle cell anemia	Thrombotic thrombocytopenic purpura
Thalassemia	Periarteritis nodusa
Spherocytosis	Sjögren syndrome
Protein C deficiency	Hyperthyroidism
Protein S deficiency	
	Neoplasm
Congenital anomalies	Parasellar tumor
Down syndrome	
Neurofibromatosis-I	*Infectious diseases*
Tuberous sclerosis	Leptospirosis
Marfan syndrome	Tuberculosis
Coarctation of aorta	Meningitis
Fibromuscular dysplasia	
Osteogenesis imperfecta	*Others*
Turner syndrome	Traumatic brain injury
Hirschsprung disease	Cranial irradiation
Wilms tumor	Oral contraceptive
Polycystic kidney	Drug abuse (cocaine, etc.)
Prader Willi syndrome	
Apert syndrome	*Vascular disorders*
Alagille syndrome	Cerebral aneurysm
Williams syndrome	Arteriovenous malformation
Noonan syndrome	Venous angioma
	Cavernous angioma
Metabolic disorders	Atherosclerotic disease
Hyperlipoproteinemia	Renovascular hypertension
Glycogen storage disease	Unclassified disorders
Lipohyalinosis	
NADH-CoQ reductase activity	
Pyruvate kinase deficiency	
Homocystinuria	

Abbreviations: CoQ, coenzyme Q10; NADH, nicotinamide adenine dinucleotide.

Moyamoya syndrome can affect people of all ethnic backgrounds. It often occurs concurrently with an underlying congenital disease in children, whereas in adults an acquired underlying disease is common.[24,25] Moyamoya syndrome can manifest as epilepsy or headache, or it can be asymptomatic.[24,25] The copresence of symptoms associated with mental retardation related to an underlying disease and those associated with cerebrovascular disorder results in a complicated clinical condition.[25]

The treatment of moyamoya syndrome is considered to be similar to that of definitive moyamoya disease. Interestingly, however, for moyamoya syndrome associated with hormonal abnormalities, such as hyperthyroidism, or with an autoimmune disorder, correction of the hormonal abnormality and immunosuppressive therapy, respectively, are reported to be effective.[26,27] Revascularization (direct and indirect) has been demonstrated to be effective for moyamoya syndrome associated with von Recklinghausen disease, Down syndrome, or irradiation.[28–30] The nature of the underlying diseases influences the prognosis of patients with moyamoya syndrome.[31]

◆ Unilateral Cases

The term unilateral moyamoya disease is also referred to as probable moyamoya disease and indicates the presence of unilateral stenosis or occlusion of the terminal portion of the ICAs accompanied by the formation of moyamoya vessels. These unilateral changes may occur concurrently with other underlying diseases, such as hyperthyroidism, intracranial arteriovenous malformations, Down syndrome, Apert syndrome, von Recklinghausen disease, radiation-induced angiopathy, systemic lupus erythematosus, and Sjögren syndrome. When these diseases are also present, the condition is still classified as moyamoya syndrome. In pediatric patients with stenosis of the terminal portion of the ICAs with moyamoya vessels and very mild changes involving the other side of the ICA, it can be considered definitive moyamoya disease. These changes are only seen in moyamoya disease, and most cases eventually progress to typical bilateral moyamoya disease.[11] With the availability of MRI, the number of asymptomatic cases of moyamoya disease has been increasing. Consequently, the real incidence is thought to be higher than currently reported.

The frequency of progression from unilateral to bilateral moyamoya disease has varied from 10 to 39%.[32,33] A more rapid rate of progression was presumed to be associated with a younger age at diagnosis.[34] However, adult cases also progress from unilateral to bilateral.[35]

References

1. Suzuki J, Takaku A. Cerebrovascular "moyamoya" disease. Disease showing abnormal net-like vessels in base of brain. Arch Neurol 1969;20(3):288–299
2. Kudo T. Spontaneous occlusion of the circle of Willis. A disease apparently confined to Japanese. Neurology 1968;18(5):485–496
3. Nishimoto A, Takeuchi S. Abnormal cerebrovascular network related to the internal cartoid arteries. J Neurosurg 1968;29(3):255–260
4. Suzuki J, Kodama N. Cerebrovascular "Moyamoya" disease. 2. Collateral routes to forebrain via ethmoid sinus and superior nasal meatus. Angiology 1971;22(4):223–236
5. Wakai K, Tamakoshi A, Ikezaki K, et al. Epidemiological features of moyamoya disease in Japan: findings from a nationwide survey. Clin Neurol Neurosurg 1997;99(Suppl 2):S1–S5
6. Uchino K, Johnston SC, Becker KJ, Tirschwell DL. Moyamoya disease in Washington State and California. Neurology 2005;65(6):956–958
7. Baba T, Houkin K, Kuroda S. Novel epidemiological features of moyamoya disease. J Neurol Neurosurg Psychiatry 2008;79(8):900–904
8. Kuriyama S, Kusaka Y, Fujimura M, et al. Prevalence and clinicoepidemiological features of moyamoya disease in Japan: findings from a nationwide epidemiological survey. Stroke 2008;39(1):42–47
9. Kuroda S, Hashimoto N, Yoshimoto T, Iwasaki Y; Research Committee on Moyamoya Disease in Japan. Radiological findings, clinical course, and outcome in asymptomatic moyamoya disease: results of multicenter survey in Japan. Stroke 2007;38(5):1430–1435
10. Ikeda K, Iwasaki Y, Kashihara H, et al. Adult moyamoya disease in the asymptomatic Japanese population. J Clin Neurosci 2006;13(3):334–338
11. Fukui M. Guidelines for the diagnosis and treatment of spontaneous occlusion of the circle of Willis ('moyamoya' disease). Research Committee on Spontaneous Occlusion of the Circle of Willis (Moyamoya Disease) of the Ministry of Health and Welfare, Japan. Clin Neurol Neurosurg 1997;99(Suppl 2):S238–S240
12. Houkin K, Aoki T, Takahashi A, Abe H. Diagnosis of moyamoya disease with magnetic resonance angiography. Stroke 1994;25(11):2159–2164
13. Yamada I, Matsushima Y, Suzuki S. Moyamoya disease: diagnosis with three-dimensional time-of-flight MR angiography. Radiology 1992;184(3):773–778
14. Yamada I, Suzuki S, Matsushima Y. Moyamoya disease: comparison of assessment with MR angiography and MR imaging versus conventional angiography. Radiology 1995;196(1):211–218
15. Hasuo K, Mihara F, Matsushima T. MRI and MR angiography in moyamoya disease. J Magn Reson Imaging 1998;8(4):762–766
16. Takanashi JI, Sugita K, Niimi H. Evaluation of magnetic resonance angiography with selective maximum intensity projection in patients with childhood moyamoya disease. Eur J Paediatr Neurol 1998;2(2):83–89
17. Kuroda S, Houkin K. Moyamoya disease: current concepts and future perspectives. Lancet Neurol 2008;7(11):1056–1066
18. Lyoo CH, Oh SH, Joo JY, Chung TS, Lee MS. Hemidystonia and hemichoreoathetosis as an initial manifestation of moyamoya disease. Arch Neurol 2000;57(10):1510–1512

19. Miyamoto S, Kikuchi H, Karasawa J, Nagata I, Ikota T, Takeuchi S. Study of the posterior circulation in moyamoya disease. Clinical and neuroradiological evaluation. J Neurosurg 1984;61(6):1032–1037

20. Iwama T, Hashimoto N, Murai BN, Tsukahara T, Yonekawa Y. Intracranial rebleeding in moyamoya disease. J Clin Neurosci 1997;4(2):169–172

21. Kawaguchi S, Sakaki T, Morimoto T, Kakizaki T, Kamada K. Characteristics of intracranial aneurysms associated with moyamoya disease. A review of 111 cases. Acta Neurochir (Wien) 1996;138(11):1287–1294

22. Scott RM, Smith ER. Moyamoya disease and moyamoya syndrome. N Engl J Med 2009;360(12):1226–1237

23. Roach ES, Golomb MR, Adams R, et al; American Heart Association Stroke Council; Council on Cardiovascular Disease in the Young. Management of stroke in infants and children: a scientific statement from a Special Writing Group of the American Heart Association Stroke Council and the Council on Cardiovascular Disease in the Young. Stroke 2008;39(9):2644–2691

24. Rosser TL, Vezina G, Packer RJ. Cerebrovascular abnormalities in a population of children with neurofibromatosis type 1. Neurology 2005;64(3):553–555

25. Inoue T, Matsushima T, Fujii K, Fukui M, Hasuo K, Matsuo H. [Akin moyamoya disease in children]. No Shinkei Geka 1993;21(1):59–65

26. Czartoski T, Hallam D, Lacy JM, Chun MR, Becker K. Postinfectious vasculopathy with evolution to moyamoya syndrome. J Neurol Neurosurg Psychiatry 2005; 76(2):256–259

27. Im SH, Oh CW, Kwon OK, Kim JE, Han DH. Moyamoya disease associated with Graves disease: special considerations regarding clinical significance and management. J Neurosurg 2005;102(6):1013–1017

28. Ishikawa T, Houkin K, Yoshimoto T, Abe H. Vasoreconstructive surgery for radiation-induced vasculopathy in childhood. Surg Neurol 1997;48(6): 620–626

29. Jea A, Smith ER, Robertson R, Scott RM. Moyamoya syndrome associated with Down syndrome: outcome after surgical revascularization. Pediatrics 2005;116(5):e694–e701

30. Scott RM, Smith JL, Robertson RL et al. Long-term outcome in children with moyamoya syndrome after cranial revascularization by pial synangiosis. J Neurosurg 2004;100(2 Suppl Pediatrics):142–149

31. Kestle JR, Hoffman HJ, Mock AR. Moyamoya phenomenon after radiation for optic glioma. J Neurosurg 1993;79(1):32–35

32. Houkin K, Abe H, Yoshimoto T, Takahashi A. Is "unilateral" moyamoya disease different from moyamoya disease? J Neurosurg 1996;85(5):772–776

33. Hirotsune N, Meguro T, Kawada S, Nakashima H, Ohmoto T. Long-term follow-up study of patients with unilateral moyamoya disease. Clin Neurol Neurosurg 1997;99(Suppl 2):S178–S181

34. Kawano T, Fukui M, Hashimoto N, Yonekawa Y. Follow-up study of patients with "unilateral" moyamoya disease. Neurol Med Chir (Tokyo) 1994;34(11): 744–747

35. Kuroda S, Ishikawa T, Houkin K, Nanba R, Hokari M, Iwasaki Y. Incidence and clinical features of disease progression in adult moyamoya disease. Stroke 2005; 36(10):2148–2153

2

Classification and Imaging of Moyamoya Phenomena

Douglas J. Cook and Michael Tymianski

◆ Introduction

Moyamoya disease was originally described in 1957 as an idiopathic steno-occlusive disorder of the carotid arteries.[1] The name "moyamoya" comes from the Japanese word meaning "hazy" or "puff of smoke," and describes the angiographic appearance of both dilated collateral vessels and new vessels that form to supply ischemic regions of the brain resulting from progressive carotid stenosis.[2–4]

◆ Classification of Moyamoya

The classification of moyamoya is based on angiographic anatomy and clinical history of associated diseases. Specific angiographic findings include bilateral or unilateral involvement, absence or presence of a systemic or local condition associated with moyamoya, and involvement of the supraclinoid carotid artery (C1-C2 segment) or distal anterior circulation or posterior circulation vessels (**Fig. 2.1** and **Table 2.1**).

The term *moyamoya disease* is specifically used to describe idiopathic, bilateral steno-occlusive carotid disease in the supraclinoid division of the carotid artery.[2,5] *Moyamoya syndrome* is used to describe the appearance of bilateral or unilateral moyamoya vessels in the setting of an associated, underlying disease state (**Table 2.2**) or in the case of unilateral idiopathic carotid disease.[3] *Atypical moyamoya* is a term used by many authors to describe moyamoya vessel formation related to noncarotid steno-occlusive disease or in cases with associated aneurysms or pseudoaneurysms.[6,7] Suggesting that this classification system generates confusion, some authors propose using the term *moyamoya disease* for the idiopathic, bilateral disease state and *angiographic moyamoya* for all other cases of moyamoya associated with another disease state, isolated unilateral disease, and disease within other vascular distributions.[8] However, this simplified categorization has not yet been widely adopted.

◆ Staging of Moyamoya

Moyamoya is a progressive disease that begins with narrowing of the carotid artery and progresses to occlusion and exuberant formation of moyamoya vessels supplied by dural-pial and ethmoidal collaterals to the affected hemisphere. The condition is ultimately limited by the gradual obliteration of moyamoya vessels as an exclusive external carotid arterial supply of the hemisphere is established. The Suzuki staging system (**Fig. 2.2** and **Table 2.3**) is a useful grading system for moyamoya, dividing the disease state into six stages from initiation to resolution.[2,9]

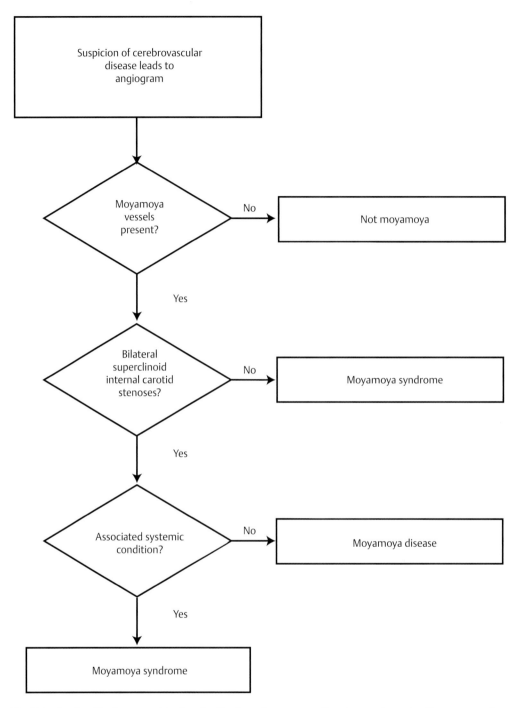

Fig. 2.1 An algorithmic approach to the classification of moyamoya. Based on angiography, the presence of moyamoya vessels, bilaterality versus unilaterality, and finally the clinical history of associated diseases are used to determine whether a case fits the definition of moyamoya disease or syndrome.

Table 2.1 Conditions Associated with Moyamoya Syndrome[*]

Differential Diagnosis

Vascular disorders

  Atherosclerosis[†]

  Cranial trauma dissection/skull base fracture

  Hypertension

  Fibromuscular dysplasia

  Renal artery stenosis

  Giant cervicofacial hemangioma

  Coarctation of the aorta

Infectious disease

  Tuberculosis

  Leptospirosis

Neoplastic

  Craniocervical radiotherapy[†]

  Tuberous sclerosis

  Parasellar tumor

Developmental disorders

  Neurofibromatosis[†]

  Down syndrome[†]

  Apert syndrome

  Marfan syndrome

  Turner syndrome

  von Recklinghausen disease

  Hirschsprung disease

  Congenital cardiac anomaly

Hematological/inflammatory/endocrine disorders

  Sickle cell disease

  Hyperthyroidism

  Aplastic anemia

  Fanconi anemia

  Lupus erythematous

[*]Lists compiled from Scott and Smith[3] and Natori et al.[8]

[†]Commonly associated with moyamoya syndrome.

Table 2.2 Classification of Moyamoya

Moyamoya disease

  Bilateral, idiopathic steno-occlusive supraclinoid carotid disease

  Bimodal age of diagnosis: 5 and 40 years old

  Predominantly Asian heritage

  Twice as common in females as in males

Moyamoya syndrome

  Associated disease state (see **Table 2.1**)

  Unilateral carotid disease (even if idiopathic)

  Variable epidemiology

Atypical moyamoya

  Moyamoya vessels in noncarotid distribution

  Associated aneurysm or pseudoaneurysms

  Associated arteriovenous malformation

Imaging of Moyamoya

The choice and order of imaging modalities in the evaluation of moyamoya disease depend on the patient's presentation. In the case of a hemorrhagic presentation, an anatomical imaging protocol using computed tomography (CT) followed by digital subtraction angiography helps diagnose and characterize the location and grade of disease, and can be used to help plan acute treatment if needed (**Fig. 2.3**). Patients with ischemic symptoms, including stroke and transient ischemic attacks, may initially be imaged with diffusion-weighted magnetic resonance imaging (MRI) to define regions of infarction sequences and to determine the anatomical localization of moyamoya vessels and magnetic resonance angiography of carotid stenosis (**Fig. 2.4**). If, based on anatomical imaging, the cause of strokes is consistent with flow-related ischemia (e.g., infarction in watershed distributions) or if the source of ischemic symptoms cannot be determined, functional imaging measures of cerebral blood flow (CBF) and cerebrovascular reserve may be appropriate to identify brain regions at risk of stroke (**Fig. 2.5**). Some groups consider impaired cerebrovascular reserve to be an indication for intervention with revascularization procedures.[10,11]

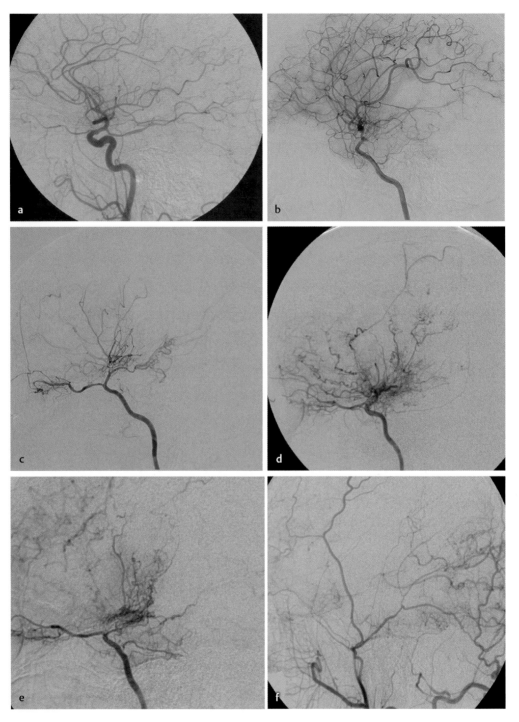

Fig. 2.2a–f Representative internal carotid (**a–e**) and external carotid (**f**) artery angiograms demonstrate Suzuki staging of moyamoya. (**a**) Stage I disease with narrowing of the supraclinoid internal carotid artery. (**b**) Stage II disease with dilatation of the middle cerebral artery and early formation of basal moyamoya vessels. (**c**) Stage III disease with occlusion of the middle and anterior cerebral arteries but patent posterior communicating artery and further formation of moyamoya vessels. (**d**) Stage IV disease with intensification of moyamoya vessels and loss of the posterior communicating artery. (**e**) Stage V disease with diminishing moyamoya vessels as prominence of external collaterals increases. (**f**) External carotid artery angiogram demonstrates Stage VI disease: the loss of moyamoya vessels and collateral supply via the external carotid artery.

Table 2.3 Suzuki Staging of Moyamoya[a]

Suzuki Stage	Angiographic Description (Based on Carotid Angiography)
I	Isolated narrowing of supraclinoid carotid (C1-C2 segment)
II	Progressive narrowing of carotid, dilatation of native cerebral arteries, early formation of moyamoya vessels in basal carotid circulation
III	Intensification of moyamoya vasculature in basal regions, exuberant moyamoya vessel formation, severe carotid stenosis with decreased flow in middle and anterior cerebral arteries
IV	Minimization of moyamoya vessels, severe carotid stenosis with impaired filling of middle, anterior, and posterior cerebral arteries
V	Further minimization of moyamoya vessels, complete cessation of flow in ipsilateral middle, anterior, and posterior cerebral arteries
VI	Disappearance of moyamoya vessels, filling of cerebral vasculature by external carotid supply via leptomeningeal anastomoses

[a]Data from Suzuki and Takaku.[2]

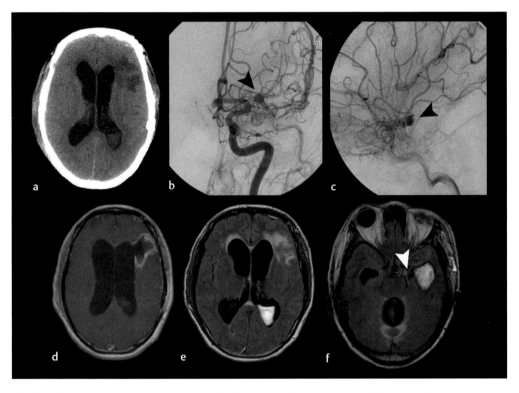

Fig. 2.3a–f Atypical moyamoya presenting with intraventricular hemorrhage. (**a**) Computed tomography acquired 1 week after ictus demonstrates old stroke in the left frontal region (*asterisk*) and subacute hematoma in the left occipital horn. Anteroposterior (**b**) and lateral angiograms (**c**) demonstrate occlusion of the middle cerebral artery with reconstitution of the artery via moyamoya collaterals. *Arrowheads* demonstrate an aneurysm, another atypical feature, that has formed on the reconstituted middle cerebral artery perforators distal to the moyamoya vessels. The aneurysm is the likely source of hemorrhage. (**d**) Enhanced T1-weighted magnetic resonance imaging demonstrates a subacute or chronic stroke with enhancement that correlates to computed tomography (*asterisk*). (**e, f**) Axial fluid-attenuation inversion recovery magnetic resonance imaging demonstrates chronic changes in the left frontal lobe related to prior stroke and subacute hematoma in the occipital and temporal horns of the left lateral ventricle with evidence of ventriculomegaly.

2 Classification and Imaging of Moyamoya Phenomena

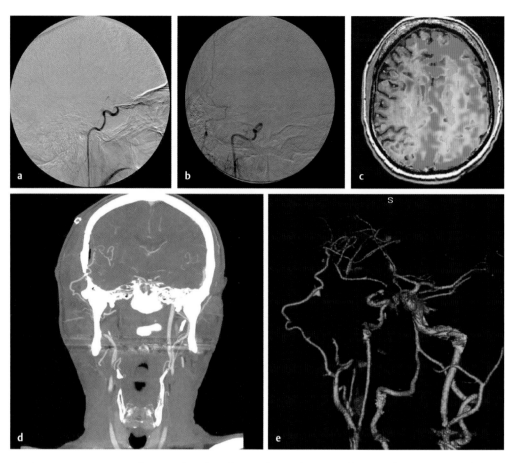

Fig. 2.4a–e Moyamoya syndrome with unilateral internal carotid artery occlusion and reconstitution of cerebral flow via external carotid collaterals. (**a, b**) Angiograms demonstrate occlusion of the supraclinoid internal carotid artery. The patient was symptomatic with transient motor ischemic attacks and had impaired cerebrovascular reactivity (**c**). The patient underwent a superficial temporal artery-to-middle cerebral artery bypass on the right side and symptoms resolved. (**d**) Postoperative computed tomography angiography used to follow graft patency shows blood flow through the superficial temporal artery graft. (**e**) Three-dimensional computed tomography angiography demonstrates the patent superficial temporal artery graft.

Computed Tomography

In the acute setting of stroke or hemorrhage, CT is usually the first imaging modality used (see **Fig. 2.3**). Intraventricular, intraparenchymal, and subarachnoid hemorrhage are readily demonstrated with CT and can guide the emergent treatment of the patient (e.g., by guiding cerebrospinal fluid diversion or clot evacuation). In addition to these acute findings, CT can demonstrate chronic ischemic changes, which appear as hypodensities in both subcortical and cortical regions, pointing to prior or ongoing flow-related versus embolic ischemic insults.

Computed Tomographic Angiography

Modern CT angiography (CTA) provides high-resolution images of the cerebral vasculature and is best for imaging larger parent arteries. Carotid stenosis and occlusion can be readily visualized. In stage II disease, dilated parent vessels and leptomeningeal collaterals become apparent on CTA. Prominent moyamoya vessels may be visualized in the basal ganglia and cortex; however, they are not always visible with this study. In late-stage disease (stages V and VI), CTA shows the prominent external carotid collateral circulation and loss of flow, stenosis, and/or loss of major cerebral artery divisions.

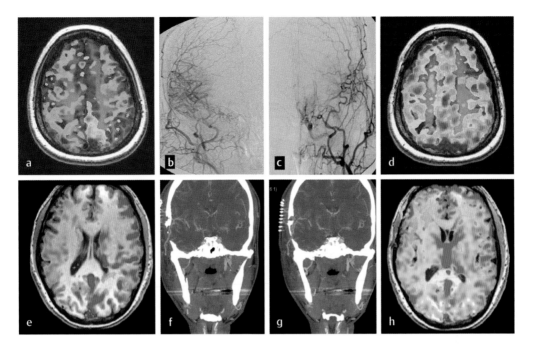

Fig. 2.5a–h Cerebrovascular reserve studies (magnetic resonance imaging–blood oxygen level dependent with a hypercapnic challenge) are useful for diagnosing chronic ischemia in moyamoya and for following treatment effect. (**a**) Patient 1 (upper row) was diagnosed with moyamoya disease with impaired cerebrovascular reserve (*blue*) in both hemispheres. The patient underwent bilateral encephaloduroarteriosynagiosis to treat the disease. Postoperative right (**b**) and left (**c**) external carotid artery angiograms. (**d**) One year after surgery, a follow-up study showed that the patient's cerebrovascular reserve was normal. (**e**) Patient 2 (lower row), who was diagnosed with moyamoya and impaired cerebrovascular reserve in the right hemisphere, underwent a right superficial temporal artery-to-middle cerebral artery anastomosis with good reconstitution of blood flow in the right middle cerebral artery (**f, g**). (**h**) On a delayed study, the patient's cerebrovascular reserve was normal.

CTA provides excellent three-dimensional imaging of the cerebral vasculature and can reveal small aneurysms or pseudoaneurysms in patients with atypical moyamoya.[12] The lack of temporal resolution with CTA results in a "snapshot" of the vasculature and can be biased toward the arterial or venous phase of cranial circulation. That is, the extent of moyamoya may be under- or overestimated based on the scan acquisition time relative to the mean transit time of contrast through the affected area.[13] During the postoperative period, CTA can be used to determine bypass patency (**Figs. 2.4d, e** and **2.5f, g**).

Magnetic Resonance Imaging

MRI is a powerful modality for visualizing both the vascular and parenchymal sequelae of moyamoya disease. Typical MRI studies include multiple sequence acquisitions that are specific to the various features of moyamoya. On T2-weighted imaging, carotid stenosis and occlusion may appear as a change in caliber of vessels or as a loss of the carotid flow void. Furthermore, magnetic resonance angiography using gadolinium or arterial spin labeling techniques can detect carotid stenosis or occlusion. Moyamoya vessels are apparent as flow voids in the basal cisterns and basal ganglia. They represent dilated vessels of the anastomotic networks that evolve from dural-pial connections and dilated lenticulostriate vessels, respectively. Contrast-enhanced T1-weighted and fluid-attenuation inversion recovery (FLAIR) sequences can demonstrate leptomeningeal enhancement, termed the "ivy sign," which represents pial collaterals, congestion of the leptomeninges, or both (see **Fig. 2.3f**).[14]

Both acute and chronic signs of ischemia and stroke are best imaged with MRI. In the

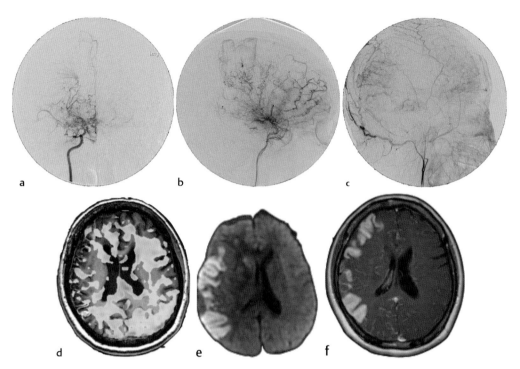

Fig. 2.6a–f This case of moyamoya disease was discovered due to transient ischemic attacks resulting in left motor weakness. Right anteroposterior (**a**) and lateral internal (**b**) carotid artery angiograms demonstrate Stage III moyamoya disease. (**c**) Right external carotid artery angiogram demonstrates partial reconstitution of cortical flow. (**d**) Hypercapnic cerebrovascular reactivity study performed with blood oxygen level–dependent magnetic resonance imaging (MRI) shows bilateral impairment of cerebrovascular reactivity (*blue*), which was worse in the right hemisphere than in the left. Later, the patient suffered a retroperitoneal hematoma and hypovolemic shock, after which she experienced fixed arm and leg weakness. (**e**) Diffusion MRI shows a right cortical stroke that enhances with gadolinium on T1-weighted MRI (**f**). The right hemisphere also exhibited the "ivy" sign on gadolinium-enhanced T1-weighted MRI.

acute setting, diffusion-restriction or diffusion-weighted imaging indicates stroke (**Fig. 2.6**). On T1-weighted MRI, gadolinium enhancement is commonly observed during the subacute progression of stroke. In the chronic stage stroke can appear as regions of cortical and subcortical atrophy and as *ex vacuo* ventricular dilatation on T2-weighted images. FLAIR images demonstrate hyperintensities in regions of chronic stroke where atrophy and gliosis occur in both cortical regions and white matter.

Stroke identified in "watershed" regions between vascular distributions indicates insufficient flow in the distal vasculature, whereas embolic strokes are visible in parent vessel and end artery distributions. Differentiating the etiology of ischemic injury in moyamoya is critical in selecting the appropriate diagnostic tests and ultimately in determining therapy. In this regard, MRI is an important early modality in the evaluation of ischemic presentations of moyamoya.

During the long-term follow-up of patients with moyamoya disease, MRI is an important modality because it permits surveillance of carotid steno-occlusive disease in the ipsilateral and contralateral sides. MRI also can show bypass patency and allows surveillance of the parenchyma to judge the effect on tissue and to identify new or evolving infarcts. In a recent study on follow-up MRI, patients with effective revascularization via a superficial temporal artery-to-middle cerebral artery bypass had increased cortical thickness, a feature that may serve as a potential imaging biomarker for therapeutic effect.[10]

Catheter Angiography

The "puff of smoke" appearance from which the name moyamoya is derived was originally observed on carotid angiography. Moreover, the Suzuki staging system was based on this modality (see **Fig. 2.2**).[2] Hence, angiographic imaging remains the diagnostic gold standard for moyamoya. However, some authors have suggested that a combination of noninvasive tests may be adequate to make the diagnosis and to plan treatment.[15]

Modern catheter-based angiographic techniques provide high-spatial resolution images through the arterial and venous phases of contrast injection, as well as three-dimensional imaging. Catheter angiography permits selective imaging of the distributions of the internal carotid, vertebral, and external carotid arteries so the extent of carotid occlusion and the origin of the collateral supply can be characterized in moyamoya. Atypical features of moyamoya, such as aneurysms and, rarely, arteriovenous malformations, are best visualized on catheter angiography because the images are high quality and magnified views of suspicious regions are possible.[6,12,16]

Imaging of Cerebral Blood Flow and Cerebrovascular Reserve

Functional vascular imaging modalities give indirect and direct measures of both cerebral blood flow (CBF) and metabolic function in the brain. In moyamoya, these data drive treatment decisions for revascularization therapy in both symptomatic ischemic patients and in asymptomatic patients because impaired hemodynamics are predictive of stroke risk.[17,18]

Blood flow is measured by introducing a tracer (usually a contrast agent) that can be tracked through the cerebral circulation serially over time. The mean transit time and an estimation of cerebral blood volume can be derived from the curve defining tracer concentration in a region of interest over time.[19] Relative CBF can be calculated using the central volume theorem (CBF = CBV/MTT) and quantitatively expressed as mL/100 g tissue/min based on estimations from known blood flow values. Blood flow maps are generated by applying this method to each pixel in an axial image and assigning color values from reference tables. Diminished CBF is thought to correlate to parent vessel stenosis in moyamoya and may be apparent in ischemic regions, indicating a need for treatment using revascularization techniques.[20]

Both direct measures of tissue metabolism and measures of vascular autoregulatory function (indirect measure of metabolic demand) are useful in guiding treatment decisions for patients with early ischemic symptoms or in predicting the course of asymptomatic cases. Metabolic demand in the brain is measured noninvasively as the oxygen extraction fraction using positron emission tomography (PET). The oxygen extraction fraction is derived by injecting radio-labeled oxygen ($^{15}O_2$) intravenously and measuring the proportion of oxygen that is extracted from the blood by the tissue. In ischemic tissue, the oxygen extraction fraction increases as more oxygen is extracted from red blood cells to meet equivalent metabolic demands in the setting of decreased CBF.

Vascular autoregulation in the brain occurs at the level of the arterioles where tissue demand for oxygen is detected as local changes in pH, nitric-oxide signaling, and other paracrine mediators. This autoregulation results in changes in smooth muscle contraction and relaxation with a resultant increase or decrease in vascular resistance and blood flow. Under normal conditions, arterioles can either contract or relax in response to a stimulus to alter CBF as required. This process is known as cerebrovascular reactivity. However, in the case of moyamoya, if persistent oligemia occurs, the arterioles are persistently, maximally dilated to maximize blood flow. They cannot react to further hypoxic or hypercarbic stimuli, a condition known as "exhaustion of cerebrovascular reserve." Patients in this state are at higher risk for ischemic symptoms and may develop a stroke.[18]

To test cerebrovascular reactivity, CBF is measured before and after a hypercapnic challenge induced by a dose of acetazolamide, a carbonic anhydrase inhibitor, by adjusting end-tidal PCO_2,[21] or by breath holding. In normal patients, CBF increases to the hypercarbic challenge compared with baseline. In patients with exhausted cerebrovascular reserve, there is either no change or a reduction between baseline and the challenge CBF. Under these conditions, the reduction in CBF has been labeled as "steal phenomenon" and is believed to be associated with an increased risk of stroke.

Computed Tomography Perfusion and Magnetic Resonance Imaging Perfusion

CT perfusion uses an iodinated contrast agent to track the transit of blood through the cerebral vasculature. MRI perfusion uses gadolinium contrast or endogenous contrast generated by arterial spin labeling to do the same. CBF is derived from the mean transit time and cerebral blood volume, which are derived from the perfusion curve, as discussed previously. These methods suffer from variability related to changes in blood pressure, hematocrit, and motion and susceptibility artifacts. The selection of arterial input function is difficult in patients with bilateral stenoses. An acetazolamide challenge can be used during CT perfusion or MRI perfusion to estimate cerebrovascular reactivity and to detect steal phenomenon (**Fig. 2.7**).

Xenon Computed Tomography

Xenon is a radiopaque, diffusible gas. Patients inhale a gas mixture of oxygen and stable xenon, which then enters brain tissue by diffusion. The accumulation of xenon correlates to blood flow and is used to derive estimates of CBF. Xenon CT can be undertaken at baseline and with acetazolamide or breath holding challenges to calculate cerebrovascular reactivity (**Fig. 2.8**). However, xenon is associated with several potential side effects, including vomiting, headache, convulsions, and respiratory failure, and may present difficulties in some patients.

Positron Emission Tomography

As described previously, PET scanning uses $^{15}O_2$ to measure the oxygen extraction fraction. This method also can provide direct, quantitative measures of CBF using $H_2^{15}O$ and of cerebral blood volume using $C^{15}O$. These capabilities make PET a powerful tool. PET is limited by its availability and by the short half-life of ^{15}O. However, a cyclotron or high-energy linear accelerator is needed on site to generate the necessary radiopharmaceuticals.

Single-Photon Emission Computed Tomography

In this methodology, a radioactive tracer such as [^{123}I] *N*-isopropyl-*p*-iodoamphetamine autoradiography (^{123}I-IMP-ARG) or technetium hexamethylpropylene amine oxide (^{99m}Tc-HMPAO) is injected intravenously. The contrast agent crosses the blood–brain barrier and is temporarily fixed in the tissue. The amount of fixed tracer correlates with blood flow. During this interval, gamma emissions are measured and used to approximate blood flow. In moyamoya, two sets of measurements are made to calculate cerebral reactivity. First, baseline CBF is measured. CBF is then measured under an acetazolamide challenge. The two tests are separated by a sufficient time interval to allow washout of the tracer.

Blood Oxygen Level–Dependent Magnetic Resonance Imaging

Blood oxygen level–dependent (BOLD) MRI is a functional technique based on detecting the difference between the field inhomogeneity

---

Fig. 2.7a–f Computed tomography perfusion imaging can be used to determine cerebral blood flow (CBF), mean transit time, and cerebral blood volume. With an acetazolamide challenge, cerebrovascular reserve and steal phenomenon can be imaged. In this case of bilateral moyamoya, right (**a**) and left (**b**) anteroposterior catheter angiograms show carotid occlusion with collateralization reconstituting blood flow in the middle cerebral artery. Baseline computed tomography perfusion images of CBF (**c**) and mean transit time (**d**) demonstrate relative elevation of blood flow (**c**, *arrowhead*) with delayed mean transit time (**d**, *arrowhead*) in the middle cerebral artery territory through collateral supply on the right side. (**e, f**) After acetazolamide was administered, (**e**) CBF increased asymmetrically. The relatively lower CBF in the left hemisphere suggests decreased cerebrovascular reserve in that hemisphere. After acetazolamide was administered, (**f**) mean transit time was delayed in the right middle cerebral artery territory (*large arrowhead*) and bilaterally in the anterior cerebral artery territories (*small arrowheads*). The delay represents delayed blood flow through moyamoya collaterals in these areas. (Used with permission from Barrow Neurological Institute.)

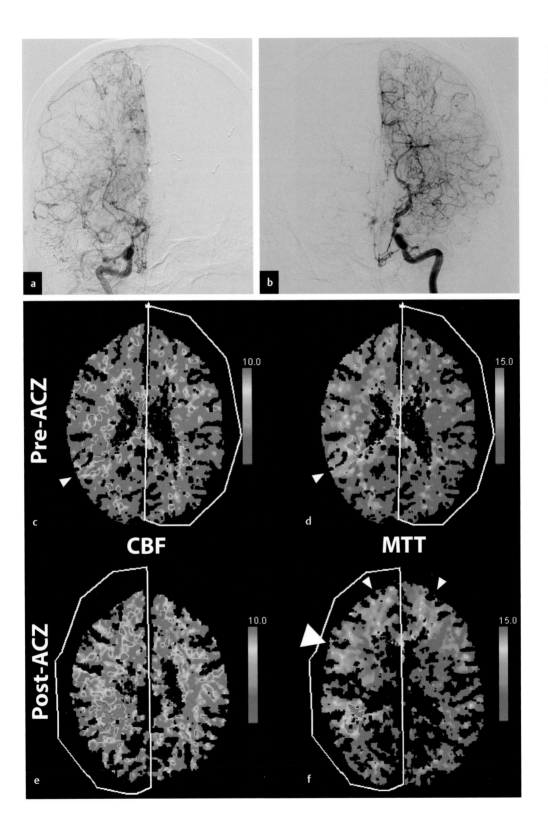

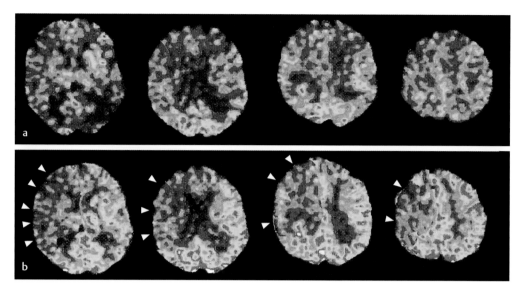

Fig. 2.8a, b Xenon computed tomography perfusion study provides an estimate of cerebral blood flow. Measurements before and after an acetazolamide challenge provide an estimate of cerebrovascular reserve. In this case of right internal carotid artery occlusion, (**a**) cerebral blood flow is symmetric between hemispheres at baseline. After acetazolamide was administered, (**b**) a relative increase in blood flow was absent in the right middle cerebral artery territory (*arrowheads*). This pattern suggests an exhausted cerebrovascular reserve in the oligemic right middle cerebral artery territory where arterioles are maximally dilated at baseline to maximize collateral flow. (Used with permission from Barrow Neurological Institute.)

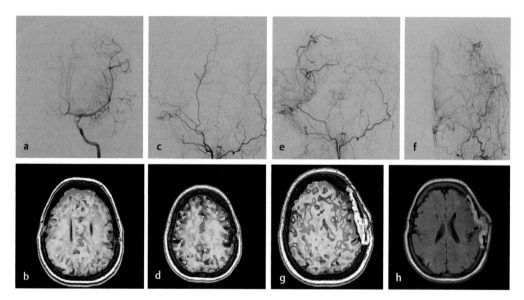

Fig. 2.9a–h This patient underwent bilateral encephaloduroarteriosynangiosis (EDAS) for early-stage moyamoya disease. (**a**) Early moyamoya demonstrated on left internal carotid artery angiogram. (**b**) Hypercapnic cerebrovascular reactivity map performed 1 year after EDAS demonstrates good cerebrovascular reserve. (**c**) Left external carotid artery angiogram demonstrates minimal reconstitution of cerebral blood flow after EDAS. The patient experienced intermittent episodes of speech stalling and word-finding difficulty. (**d**) Repeat cerebrovascular reactivity demonstrates impaired cerebrovascular reserve in the left hemisphere. Because the superficial temporal artery was used for the prior EDAS, an external carotid artery–supplied omental flap was laid on the left hemisphere. Lateral (**e**) and anteroposterior (**f**) external carotid artery angiograms of omental flap in place show reconstitution of blood flow to the left hemisphere. (**g**) Cerebrovascular reactivity study demonstrates normal cerebrovascular reserve after omental flap placement. (**h**) T1-weighted magnetic resonance imaging demonstrates fat within the omental flap laid on the left cerebral hemisphere.

created by deoxyhemoglobin (dHb) contained within red blood cells in the microvasculature and the relatively homogenous field of adjacent parenchyma.[22] The BOLD sequence detects susceptibility caused by dHb; hence, signal intensity decreases when dHb concentrations increase. After neuronal firing, there is a brief drop in BOLD signal related to increased oxygen extraction and elevated dHb. Seconds later, there is an autoregulatory elevation in local CBF and the BOLD signal increases. In this way, BOLD detects neuronal activity indirectly.

The BOLD technique has been adapted for cerebrovascular reactivity imaging by acquiring images before and after a hypercapnic challenge using a rebreathing circuit designed to adjust and maintain specific end tidal CO_2.[21,23,24] In response to a hypercapnic challenge, regions of the brain with normal cerebrovascular reactivity induce a regional increase in blood flow and a resultant increase in BOLD. Regions with exhausted cerebrovascular reactivity and chronic, maximal vascular dilatation cannot respond with an elevation in CBF, and the BOLD signal decreases due to a relative increase in dHb.[25,26] Under these conditions, CBF in these regions may drop due to the steal phenomenon where blood flow is shunted away from the oligemic regions toward adjacent, dilated vascular beds. This method provides a noninvasive, nonradioactive methodology to diagnose, grade, and follow patients undergoing revascularization therapy (see **Figs. 2.4, 2.5, and 2.9**).[10]

◆ Conclusion

The classification of moyamoya is based on angiographic appearance and clinical history. The classification assigned to a given patient is pertinent to the surveillance of moyamoya, a progressive disease with the potential for clinical decline from stroke and hemorrhage. Cases of unilateral disease have a high likelihood of involving the contralateral side on follow-up imaging.

Imaging in moyamoya encompasses both anatomical imaging for grading and classification and functional imaging that guides treatment decisions in ischemic and asymptomatic cases.

Imaging is also a critical component of patient follow-up because evidence of disease progression may trigger a treatment decision.

References

1. Takeuchi KS, Shimizu K. Hypoplasia of the bilateral internal carotid arteries. Brain Nerve 1957;9:37–43
2. Suzuki J, Takaku A. Cerebrovascular "moyamoya" disease. Disease showing abnormal net-like vessels in base of brain. Arch Neurol 1969;20(3):288–299
3. Scott RM, Smith ER. Moyamoya disease and moyamoya syndrome. N Engl J Med 2009;360(12):1226–1237
4. Kono S, Oka K, Sueishi K. Histopathologic and morphometric studies of leptomeningeal vessels in moyamoya disease. Stroke 1990;21(7):1044–1050
5. Fukui M. Guidelines for the diagnosis and treatment of spontaneous occlusion of the circle of Willis ('moyamoya' disease). Research Committee on Spontaneous Occlusion of the Circle of Willis (Moyamoya Disease) of the Ministry of Health and Welfare, Japan. Clin Neurol Neurosurg 1997;99(Suppl 2):S238–S240
6. Grabel JC, Levine M, Hollis P, Ragland R. Moyamoya-like disease associated with a lenticulostriate region aneurysm. Case report. J Neurosurg 1989;70(5):802–803
7. Adams HP Jr, Kassell NF, Wisoff HS, Drake CG. Intracranial saccular aneurysm and moyamoya disease. Stroke 1979;10(2):174–179
8. Natori Y, Ikezaki K, Matsushima T, Fukui M. 'Angiographic moyamoya' its definition, classification, and therapy. Clin Neurol Neurosurg 1997;99(Suppl 2):S168–S172
9. Suzuki J, Kodama N. Moyamoya disease—a review. Stroke 1983;14(1):104–109
10. Fierstra J, Maclean DB, Fisher JA, et al. Surgical revascularization reverses cerebral cortical thinning in patients with severe cerebrovascular steno-occlusive disease. Stroke 2011;42(6):1631–1637
11. Mikulis DJ, Krolczyk G, Desal H, et al. Preoperative and postoperative mapping of cerebrovascular reactivity in moyamoya disease by using blood oxygen level-dependent magnetic resonance imaging. J Neurosurg 2005;103(2):347–355
12. Kawaguchi S, Sakaki T, Morimoto T, Kakizaki T, Kamada K. Characteristics of intracranial aneurysms associated with moyamoya disease. A review of 111 cases. Acta Neurochir (Wien) 1996;138(11):1287–1294
13. Romero JR, Pikula A, Nguyen TN, Nien YL, Norbash A, Babikian VL. Cerebral collateral circulation in carotid artery disease. Curr Cardiol Rev 2009;5(4):279–288
14. Maeda M, Tsuchida C. "Ivy sign" on fluid-attenuated inversion-recovery images in childhood moyamoya disease. AJNR Am J Neuroradiol 1999;20(10):1836–1838
15. Bacigaluppi S, Dehdashti AR, Agid R, Krings T, Tymianski M, Mikulis DJ. The contribution of imaging in diagnosis, preoperative assessment, and follow-up of moyamoya disease: a review. Neurosurg Focus 2009;26(4):E3
16. Nakashima T, Nakayama N, Furuichi M, Kokuzawa J, Murakawa T, Sakai N. Arteriovenous malformation in association with moyamoya disease. Report of two cases. Neurosurg Focus 1998;5(5):e6
17. Lee M, Zaharchuk G, Guzman R, Achrol A, Bell-Stephens T, Steinberg GK. Quantitative hemodynamic

studies in moyamoya disease: a review. Neurosurg Focus 2009;26(4):E5

18. Ogasawara K, Ogawa A, Yoshimoto T. Cerebrovascular reactivity to acetazolamide and outcome in patients with symptomatic internal carotid or middle cerebral artery occlusion: a xenon-133 single-photon emission computed tomography study. Stroke 2002;33(7): 1857–1862

19. Jackson A. Analysis of dynamic contrast enhanced MRI. Br J Radiol 2004;77(Spec No 2):S154–S166

20. Neff KW, Horn P, Schmiedek P, Düber C, Dinter DJ. 2D cine phase-contrast MRI for volume flow evaluation of the brain-supplying circulation in moyamoya disease. AJR Am J Roentgenol 2006;187(1):W107-15

21. Mandell DM, Han JS, Poublanc J, et al. Mapping cerebrovascular reactivity using blood oxygen level-dependent MRI in Patients with arterial steno-occlusive disease: comparison with arterial spin labeling MRI. Stroke 2008;39(7):2021–2028

22. Logothetis NK, Pfeuffer J. On the nature of the BOLD fMRI contrast mechanism. Magn Reson Imaging 2004; 22(10):1517–1531

23. Blockley NP, Driver ID, Francis ST, Fisher JA, Gowland PA. An improved method for acquiring cerebrovascular reactivity maps. Magn Reson Med 2011;65(5):1278–1286

24. Vesely A, Sasano H, Volgyesi G, et al. MRI mapping of cerebrovascular reactivity using square wave changes in end-tidal PCO2. Magn Reson Med 2001;45(6): 1011–1013

25. Conklin J, Fierstra J, Crawley AP, et al. Impaired cerebrovascular reactivity with steal phenomenon is associated with increased diffusion in white matter of patients with Moyamoya disease. Stroke 2010;41(8):1610–1616

26. Heyn C, Poublanc J, Crawley A, et al. Quantification of cerebrovascular reactivity by blood oxygen level-dependent MR imaging and correlation with conventional angiography in patients with Moyamoya disease. AJNR Am J Neuroradiol 2010;31(5):862–867

3

The Natural History of Moyamoya Disease

Robert M. Starke, Andrew J. Duren, and E. Sander Connolly Jr.

◆ Introduction

Moyamoya phenomena represent a chronic vascular disorder that causes progressive occlusion of the intracranial vessels. As these arteries gradually stenose, small collateral capillaries form, resulting in the characteristic "puff of smoke" on angiography. The natural history of moyamoya phenomena is difficult to assess and quite variable. Progression may follow several different routes, including latency, slow indolent course, intermittent symptom occurrence, or rapid progression.

Aside from the variable nature of the disease, the natural history of moyamoya phenomena is difficult to assess because there is considerable disease heterogeneity. Unlike moyamoya disease, moyamoya phenomena represent the presence of moyamoya collateralization thought to arise from a known primary condition. The outcomes of moyamoya disease and syndrome are often not distinguished in the literature, and the two conditions often have a significantly different courses. Both children and adults experience different forms of the disease with variable outcomes. In Asians, moyamoya disease has a well-defined phenotype. The age of presentation follows a bimodal distribution. Children usually manifest with ischemic symptoms related to inadequate collaterals, and adults often have intracranial hemorrhages related to rupture of fragile collateral vessels.[1,2] Many studies have suggested

that moyamoya phenomena in Europe and the United States may be distinct entities with a different prognosis.[3-13] Patient ethnicities reflect the local ethnic demographics, and both children and adults more often become symptomatic with ischemic rather than hemorrhagic events.

Aside from significant disease heterogeneity, overall outcomes reflect differences in both selection and treatment bias. Inclusion of patients in a study is often marked by a disease event, and disease severity varies across reports. The Ministry of Health and Welfare of Japan has defined four types of moyamoya phenomena according to presentation: ischemic (63.4%), hemorrhagic (21.6%), epileptic (7.6%), and "other" (7.5%).[14,15] Asymptomatic or incidental cases and unilateral versus bilateral forms of disease may represent further categories.

Medical therapy is distrusted and unevenly incorporated, and it is likely that patients with the most severe disease undergo surgical therapy. Even among surgically treated patients, there are numerous treatment options and variations in reported outcomes. No randomized clinical trials have been conducted to assess the efficacy of various interventions. Finally, outcome measures differ across studies. Although numerous studies have demonstrated that significant neurocognitive declines parallel the course of moyamoya phenomena, overall functional outcome measures and assessment of neurocognitive alterations have seldom been reported. Despite the wide range of factors affecting reports of the natural history of moyamoya phenomena and its varied course, the disease progresses in most patients and is usually associated with poor outcomes.[7,16–18] Similarly, asymptomatic patients still develop symptoms and experience disease progression.[16,17] Medical therapy has not been demonstrated to decrease disease progression, but numerous studies have demonstrated improved outcomes after surgical therapy in select patients.[5,7,12,19–33] The best predictor of the course of the disease is the patient's neurological status at presentation.[32] Early diagnosis, close monitoring, and intervention when appropriate are the major determinants of a favorable outcome. A better understanding of the natural history of moyamoya phenomena is thus needed to improve early outcomes and to identify which patients can benefit from intervention.

◆ Natural History of Pediatric Patients with Moyamoya Phenomena

Moyamoya phenomena are an uncommon cause of stroke in children, occurring in ~6% of cases.[34–36] In Asians, the peak age of presentation is in the first decade of life.[1,2,13,15,37] In North Americans younger than 18 years, the mean age at most hospital admissions is 10 years old.[13] As in adults, the cause of the disease varies, but most children continue to experience both transient ischemic attacks (TIAs), ischemic strokes, or both. Ischemic strokes are often multiple and usually involve watershed areas. Ischemic events may follow periods of sickness, fever, crying, coughing, or hyperventilation.[35] Diagnosis and treatment in children may be delayed because TIAs and strokes are difficult to diagnose depending on the child's age at presentation and on language and motor development.

Although the natural history of moyamoya phenomena is difficult to predict, some researchers have estimated that more than 50% of untreated patients have progressive neurological dysfunction and poor outcomes.[5,7,16,35,39,40] The overall disease progression and outcome depend on the degree of vascular stenosis and

occlusion, on the development of collateral vessels, on the severity of neurological deficits at presentation, and on the degree of infarction and vascular reserve on imaging.[41] Moyamoya phenomena often lead to a low intelligence quotient and mental retardation.[6,42–44]

There is a general notion that pediatric moyamoya phenomena progress more quickly than adult phenomena, although children often initially present with less devastating phenomena.[45,46] Pediatric cases tend to progress into adult cases. Children younger than 2 years old tend to have a particularly poor prognosis. In one study, the majority of children with moyamoya disease developed more severe angiographic grades of disease within 5 to 10 years, and some had angiographic worsening after adolescence.[46]

Most children and adults become symptomatic, although "asymptomatic" cases have been reported. Asymptomatic cases may represent earlier forms of the disease.[47] In a study by Kuroda et al,[48] 20% of patients had a silent infarction and 40% demonstrated impaired vascular hemodynamics on O_2 extraction or acetazolamide challenge. During a mean follow-up of 43.7 months, 7 of 34 patients who did not receive surgery suffered a TIA, stroke, or intracranial hemorrhage. That is, the risk of asymptomatic patients becoming symptomatic was 3.2%.

◆ Medical Therapy for Moyamoya Phenomena

Platelet inhibitors and anticoagulation therapy are occasionally used in the treatment of moyamoya phenomena, but these treatments have not been shown to have a beneficial effect on the natural history. Antiplatelet therapy is most often used in patients with a mild form of the disease or in patients deemed poor surgical candidates. In a study of 651 patients with moyamoya disease who initially received medical therapy, 38% eventually received surgical therapy for symptom progression.[15,49] Antiplatelet agents are commonly used in patients whose ischemic symptoms are the result of embolic phenomena as well as in peri- or postoperative patients.[32,50,51] Calcium-channel blockers are often used in patients with migraines and intractable headaches, a relatively common manifestation of moyamoya phenomena.[50] Due to the risk of hemorrhage and the difficulty of maintaining therapeutic levels, anticoagulation therapy is not recommended except in select patients with frequent TIAs or multiple infarcts despite antiplatelet therapy (Class III recommendation).[35] Patients with epilepsy are often managed with anticonvulsant medications, but the best therapy for these patients remains to be determined.

◆ Natural History in Pediatric Patients with Treatment

Randomized clinical trials are the optimal means of assessing whether surgery or medical therapy is the best therapy, but such studies are difficult to perform when a condition is uncommon. It is also particularly difficult to judge outcome after surgery in patients with moyamoya disease because surgery is a form of palliative therapy in a disease associated with a poor natural history.[33] Despite the lack of randomized clinical trials, an overwhelming number of studies have demonstrated favorable outcomes after surgery in select pediatric patients with moyamoya phenomena.

Surgical therapies are often used to treat patients with radiographic disease progression; patients with hemodynamic insufficiency or failure on an oxygen extraction study, computed tomography perfusion, or acetazolamide challenge; patients with cognitive decline; or patients with clinical progression of disease. Indirect bypass procedures tend to be used in children because of the small size of their donor and recipient vessels, but both direct and combination procedures have been used successfully. In a study of 143 patients of whom 67% had a history of preoperative stroke, 7.7% of patients had perioperative strokes and only 3.2% had a stroke after at least 1 year of follow-up after undergoing pial synangiosis.[32] Of 46 patients with a minimum of 5 years of follow-up, 2 developed late onset strokes.

Three other large studies have demonstrated a low rate of perioperative stroke (4%) with a 96% or greater probability of remaining free of stroke over a 5-year follow-up.[16,20,32] In a recent meta-analysis of surgical therapy for moyamoya phenomena in children, 57 studies, which included 1,448 patients, were reviewed.[19] Most of the studies were of Japanese patients. Fewer than 10% were from Western institutions. The indications for surgery were reported in fewer than 15% of the studies and varied significantly across studies. Indirect procedures were performed in 73% of cases and combined with direct bypass in 23%. Overall rates of perioperative stroke and reversible ischemic events were 4.4% and 6.1%, respectively. In 87% of the patients, symptomatic cerebral ischemia was reduced or disappeared completely, although data on overall function and developmental status were lacking. There was no difference in the outcomes of patients undergoing the different surgical therapies, but good collateral formation was significantly more frequent in the direct/combined group than in the indirect group.

Although the rates of perioperative strokes in patients treated with bypass procedures appear low, ischemic phenomena have been reported in 4 to 31% of patients near the time of revascularization.[5,7,21,22,24,27,31,52] Children are at particular risk of ischemic events during the perioperative window because crying and hyperventilation can lower the $PaCO_2$, causing cerebral vasoconstriction. Techniques used to reduce hypocarbia, pain, hypotension, hypovolemia, and hyperthermia before, during, and after surgery are recommended.[32,53] A slight postoperative elevation in systemic blood pressure may be beneficial,[53] but patients with a direct bypass also may have an increased risk of developing cerebral hyperperfusion syndrome.

Current recommendations that appear to have a beneficial effect on the natural history of moyamoya phenomena in children include the use of revascularization to reduce the risk of stroke in select patients (Class I, Level B evidence).[35] Indications for surgical intervention include progression of ischemic symptoms or inadequate blood flow or cerebral perfusion reserve in an individual without a contraindication for surgery (Class I, Level B evidence).[35] During hospitalization, reducing pain and anxiety may reduce the incidence of hyperventilation-induced vasoconstriction and stroke (Class IIb, Level C evidence).[35] Peri- and postoperative management of systemic hypotension, hypovolemia, hyperthermia, and hypocarbia may reduce the incidence of stroke (Class IIb, Level C evidence).[35]

Despite the large number of publications demonstrating that surgical therapy may be performed safely in and provide benefits to pediatric patients with moyamoya phenomena, scant data assessing functional outcomes are available. Furthermore, the effects of surgery on the natural history of the disease remain unclear. A standardized approach for evaluation and treatment of patients is critical to determine the indications and appropriate timing of intervention.

◆ Natural History and Treatment of Moyamoya Syndrome

Unlike moyamoya disease, which is the idiopathic presentation of angiographic moyamoya changes, moyamoya syndrome is the development of these phenomena in the presence of a known pathological entity. Numerous conditions have been associated with moyamoya phenomena, and it is often difficult to assess whether the association is causal or causative. Diseases such as neurofibromatosis, Down syndrome, cranial irradiation, and sickle cell disease are most often associated with moyamoya phenomena. Based on discharge databases from the states of Washington and California, concomitant diagnoses include hypertension (31%), coronary artery disease (12%), diabetes mellitus (10%), peripheral vascular disease (3.0%), hyperlipidemia (1.3%), sickle cell disease (4.4%), Down syndrome (3.0%), and neurofibromatosis type 1 (2.3%).[54] Whether there is a difference in the natural history of patients with moyamoya disease and those with moyamoya phenomena remains unclear.

The only subgroup of patients with moyamoya syndrome that has received a fair amount of attention is those with sickle cell anemia. In the United States, ~100,000 patients have sickle cell anemia, and 1 in 10 children with sickle cell anemia will suffer a stroke before the age of 20 years.[35,55] Large randomized clinical trials support screening patients with sickle cell anemia with transcranial Doppler (TCD) ultrasonography. Patients with elevated TCD velocities (> 200 cm/second) or a history of previous stroke are started on a regimen of transfusions and have a 10-fold reduction in their stroke risk.[35,56–59] These patients, however, may have increased risks associated with chronic transfusion including iron overload, infection, and immune response, not to mention the high cost associated with therapy.[59]

As many as 43% of patients with sickle cell anemia and stroke may develop moyamoya phenomena associated with supraclinoid stenosis/occlusion.[55,60,61] These patients have a fivefold increased risk of stroke compared with patients with sickle cell anemia but without moyamoya collaterals.[55,60,61] Furthermore, children with severe stenotic lesions on cerebral magnetic resonance angiography were excluded from large trials assessing transfusion therapy.[57] A few small studies have demonstrated a beneficial role of surgical therapy in patients who develop ischemic phenomena despite transfusion therapy in the presence of sickle cell anemia and moyamoya syndrome.[62–64] Currently, the role of surgical therapy in the algorithm of patients with sickle cell anemia also with elevated velocity on TCD or inadequate cerebrovascular reserve remains unclear.

Current recommendations that likely have a beneficial effect on the outcome of both patients with sickle cell anemia and patients with sickle cell anemia and moyamoya collaterals include periodic transfusions. The transfusions reduce the percentage of sickle hemoglobin, thereby decreasing the risk of stroke in children 2 to 16 years old with abnormal velocity readings on TCD (Class I, Level A evidence).[35,57,58] Current guidelines from the American Heart Association note that children with sickle cell anemia and confirmed cerebral infarction should receive regular transfusions of red blood cells in conjunction with measures to prevent iron overload (Class I, Level B evidence).[35,57,58] In individuals with sickle cell anemia, the percentage of sickle hemoglobin should be reduced with transfusions before cerebral angiography is performed (Class I, Level C evidence).[35,57,58] In patients with sickle cell anemia who experience cerebral infarction, exchange transfusion designed to reduce sickle hemoglobin to less than 30% of total hemoglobin is appropriate (Class IIa, Level C evidence).[35,57,58] In children with sickle cell anemia and an intracerebral hemorrhage, it is reasonable to evaluate for a structural vascular lesion (Class IIa, Level B evidence).[35] In children with sickle cell anemia, it is reasonable to repeat a normal TCD annually and to repeat an abnormal study in 1 month (Class IIa, Level B evidence).[35,57,58] Borderline and mildly abnormal TCD studies may be repeated in 3 to 6 months. Hydroxyurea may be considered in children and young adults with sickle cell anemia and stroke who cannot continue on long-term transfusion (Class IIb, Level B Evidence).[35] Bone marrow transplantation may be considered for children with sickle cell anemia (Class IIb, Level C evidence).[35] Surgical revascularization procedures may be considered in children with sickle cell anemia who continue to have cerebrovascular dysfunction despite optimal medical management (Class IIb, Level C evidence).[35]

◆ Natural History in Adult Patients without Treatment

There is an overall paucity of information concerning the natural outcomes of adult patients with moyamoya phenomena who are left untreated. Compared with children, adults are more likely to present with hemorrhage, often with devastating consequences.[45,46] Approximately 60% of adult patients will experience hemorrhage, which is most likely in females and Hispanics.[1,2,12,13,15,37] Although the childhood form of moyamoya has been considered more likely to progress than the adult forms, the latter is not a stable process, as previously noted.[65] Over a 14-year period, Kuroda et al studied 120 adults with moyamoya phenomena, 15 of whom progressed. Overall, ~20% of adult patients have been noted to have disease progression, and the disease is more likely to progress in women than in men.[13,47]

Although the exact statistics are unclear, adult moyamoya phenomena have been associated with significant rates of morbidity and mortality and with poor outcomes. In a study by Hallemeier et al, patients receiving medical management for unilateral and bilateral moyamoya disease had 5-year stroke-free survival rates of only 35% and 18%, respectively.[7] The Kaplan-Meier risk for recurrent stroke after a first ischemic event (80%) was similar in a study by Kraemer et al.[9]

Although overall outcomes are quite poor, an assessment of hospital discharge outcomes in the United States is less discouraging. At discharge, 75% were classified as routine and 10% of patients required short-term hospital care or home health.[13] Fifty-three patients (2.32%) died in hospital. Hemorrhagic stroke, followed by ischemic stroke, was the most significant predictor of in-hospital death. However, analysis may be limited by the low rates of in-hospital death, and overall morbidity and mortality rates associated with moyamoya phenomena may be significantly higher because this study reflects only in-hospital morbidity and mortality.

Few studies have assessed functional and cognitive outcomes in adults, but we have found that two-thirds of untreated patients demonstrated neurocognitive dysfunction.[6] A large proportion of patients had pronounced cognitive dysfunction, including processing speed (29%), verbal memory (31%), verbal fluency (26%), and executive function (25%). Manual strength and dexterity were also affected in many patients. Furthermore, 28% of patients reported moderate-to-severe depression. The patterns of deficits suggest a mechanism of diffuse small vessel disease possibly caused by chronic hypoperfusion.

◆ Natural History of Unilateral Moyamoya Phenomena

Often, moyamoya phenomena may manifest as unilateral disease. It is unclear whether this unilateral manifestation is an earlier form of disease or a different disease entity. Regardless, progression to bilateral disease is relatively common. In three studies comprising 512 patients with moyamoya phenomena, 14% had unilateral disease. Of the cases with unilateral disease, 44% progressed to bilateral disease within a mean interval of 1.5 to 2.2 years.[47,48,66] Predictors of disease progression included abnormalities on the contralateral side of the anterior cerebral artery, middle cerebral artery, or internal carotid artery; cranial irradiation; Asian heritage; family history of moyamoya phenomena; previous cardiac abnormalities; and young age. Onset of disease before 7 years also predicted a faster progression of the disease. Consequently, these patients likely should be followed for both contralateral and overall disease progression.

◆ Natural History in Adult Patients with Treatment

Although no randomized clinical trials have compared the outcomes associated with observation, medical therapy, and surgical intervention for moyamoya disease, the reported outcomes in surgically treated patients are quite favorable. These patients are often symptomatic and experiencing disease progression or hemodynamic insufficiency. Therefore, their natural outcomes after surgical intervention are probably superior to those of observation alone. Some studies have demonstrated that most cases are treated surgically because of progression.[14,67] In the United States, rates of bypass increased over time along with overall rates of hospital admissions for patients with the diagnosis of moyamoya phenomena.[13]

It is often difficult to compare surgical series in adults because inclusion and selection criteria vary as has the severity of the disease. Surgical therapy includes direct bypass (superficial temporal artery-to-middle cerebral artery or superficial temporal artery-to-anterior cerebral artery), indirect procedures (encephaloduroarteriosynangiosis, encephalomyosynangiosis, encephalomyoarteriosynangiosis, encephaloarteriosynangiosis, durapexy, multiple cranial bur holes, and transplantation of omentum), or a combination of therapies. Thus far there is no evidence that indirect or direct bypass results in superior outcomes in adults.[68]

We reviewed our outcomes of 43 adult patients with moyamoya disease who underwent encephaloduroarteriosynangiosis (67 hemispheres total).[12] During a median follow-up of 41 months (range 4 to 126), 98% of the patients with available imaging developed collateral vessels and 82% had increased perfusion on single photon emission computed tomography. The 5-year infarction-free survival rate, including postoperative and follow-up infarctions, was 70%. The incidence of periprocedural hemisphere infarction (< 48 hours) was 3%. During follow-up, patients experienced 10 TIAs, 6 infarcts, and 1 intracranial hemorrhage. Although the hemisphere selected for surgery was based on patients' symptoms and the severity of their pathology, the 5-year infarction-free survival rate was 94% in operated hemispheres compared with 36% in nonoperated hemispheres ($p = 0.007$). After controlling for age and sex, operative hemispheres were 89% less likely to experience infarction than contralateral hemispheres (hazard ratio, 0.11; 95% confidence interval 0.02–0.56). Of the 43 patients, 38 (88%) had preserved or improved functional status as measured on the modified Rankin Scale.

One of the largest studies of revascularization procedures for moyamoya phenomena included 233 adult patients (389 procedures) and 96 pediatric patients (168 procedures); direct revascularization was used to treat 95.1% of the adults and 76.2% of the pediatric patients.[20] In 264 patients undergoing 450 procedures (mean follow-up 4.9 years), the surgical morbidity rate was 3.5% and the mortality rate was 0.7% per treated hemisphere. The cumulative 5-year risk of perioperative or subsequent stroke or death was 5.5%. Of the 171 patients presenting with a TIA, 91.8% were free of TIAs after 1 year or more. Overall, there was a significant improvement in the quality of life in the cohort as measured by the modified Rankin Scale.

Although some clinicians believe that revascularization surgery is less useful in patients presenting with hemorrhage, some studies have reported favorable outcomes in such circumstances. The best intervention remains unclear. In a series of patients with hemorrhagic moyamoya phenomena, 28.3% of patients who did not undergo surgery suffered further hemorrhage compared with 19.1% of those who received surgery.[69,70] Other studies have found similar decreased rates of hemorrhage in patients undergoing revascularization after hemorrhage.

◆ Conclusion

Although the natural history of patients with moyamoya phenomena is unclear, a significant number of patients continue to have disease progression. The overall outcome for both children and adults is often poor. Surgical revascularization is associated with a low rate of morbidity and mortality, and most patients experience favorable long-term outcomes. Further assessment of functional and cognitive outcomes of patients with moyamoya disease who are observed and of those who are medically and surgically treated is indicated. A standardized approach for the evaluation and treatment of these patients is needed to determine the indications and appropriate timing of intervention.

References

1. Nishimoto A. [Moyamoya disease(author's transl)]. Neurol Med Chir (Tokyo) 1979;19(3):221–228
2. Saeki N, Yamaura A, Hoshi S, Sunami K, Ishige N, Hosoi Y. [Hemorrhagic type of moyamoya disease]. No Shinkei Geka 1991;19(8):705–712
3. Andaluz N, Choutka O, Zuccarello M. Trends in the management of adult moyamoya disease: results of a nationwide survey. World Neurosurg 2010;73(4):361–364
4. Burke GM, Burke AM, Sherma AK, Hurley MC, Batjer HH, Bendok BR. Moyamoya disease: a summary. Neurosurg Focus 2009;26(4):E11
5. Chiu D, Shedden P, Bratina P, Grotta JC. Clinical features of moyamoya disease in the United States. Stroke 1998;29(7):1347–1351
6. Festa JR, Schwarz LR, Pliskin N, et al. Neurocognitive dysfunction in adult moyamoya disease. J Neurol 2010;257(5):806–815
7. Hallemeier CL, Rich KM, Grubb RL Jr, et al. Clinical features and outcome in North American adults with moyamoya phenomenon. Stroke 2006;37(6):1490–1496
8. Khan N, Schuknecht B, Boltshauser E, et al. Moyamoya disease and Moyamoya syndrome: experience in Europe; choice of revascularisation procedures. Acta Neurochir (Wien) 2003;145(12):1061–1071, discussion 1071
9. Kraemer M, Heienbrok W, Berlit P. Moyamoya disease in Europeans. Stroke 2008;39(12):3193–3200
10. Lee S, Lee S, Kim S, Pokorski R. Moyamoya disease: review of the literature and estimation of excess morbidity and mortality. J Insur Med 2009;41(3):207–212
11. Mesiwala AH, Sviri G, Fatemi N, Britz GW, Newell DW. Long-term outcome of superficial temporal artery-middle cerebral artery bypass for patients with moyamoya disease in the US. Neurosurg Focus 2008;24(2):E15
12. Starke RM, Komotar RJ, Hickman ZL, et al. Clinical features, surgical treatment, and long-term outcome in adult patients with moyamoya disease. Clinical article. J Neurosurg 2009;111(5):936–942
13. Starke RM, Crowley RW, Maltenfort M, et al. Moyamoya disorder in the United States. Neurosurgery 2012;71(1):93–99
14. Fukui M. Current state of study on moyamoya disease in Japan. Surg Neurol 1997;47(2):138–143
15. Fukui M. Guidelines for the diagnosis and treatment of spontaneous occlusion of the circle of Willis ('moyamoya' disease). Research Committee on Spontaneous Occlusion of the Circle of Willis (Moyamoya Disease) of the Ministry of Health and Welfare, Japan. Clin Neurol Neurosurg 1997;99(Suppl 2):S238–S240
16. Choi JU, Kim DS, Kim EY, Lee KC. Natural history of moyamoya disease: comparison of activity of daily living in surgery and non surgery groups. Clin Neurol Neurosurg 1997;99(Suppl 2):S11–S18
17. Kuroda S, Ishikawa T, Houkin K, Nanba R, Hokari M, Iwasaki Y. Incidence and clinical features of disease progression in adult moyamoya disease. Stroke 2005;36(10):2148–2153
18. Scott RM, Smith ER. Moyamoya disease and moyamoya syndrome. N Engl J Med 2009;360(12):1226–1237
19. Fung LW, Thompson D, Ganesan V. Revascularisation surgery for paediatric moyamoya: a review of the literature. Childs Nerv Syst 2005;21(5):358–364
20. Guzman R, Lee M, Achrol A, et al. Clinical outcome after 450 revascularization procedures for moyamoya disease. Clinical article. J Neurosurg 2009;111(5):927–935
21. Han DH, Nam DH, Oh CW. Moyamoya disease in adults: characteristics of clinical presentation and outcome after encephalo-duro-arterio-synangiosis. Clin Neurol Neurosurg 1997;99(Suppl 2):S151–S155
22. Houkin K, Ishikawa T, Yoshimoto T, Abe H. Direct and indirect revascularization for moyamoya disease surgical techniques and peri-operative complications. Clin Neurol Neurosurg 1997;99(Suppl 2):S142–S145
23. Houkin K, Kamiyama H, Abe H, Takahashi A, Kuroda S. Surgical therapy for adult moyamoya disease. Can surgical revascularization prevent the recurrence of intracerebral hemorrhage? Stroke 1996;27(8):1342–1346
24. Ishikawa T, Houkin K, Kamiyama H, Abe H. Effects of surgical revascularization on outcome of patients with pediatric moyamoya disease. Stroke 1997;28(6):1170–1173
25. Kim DS, Kye DK, Cho KS, Song JU, Kang JK. Combined direct and indirect reconstructive vascular surgery on the fronto-parieto-occipital region in moyamoya disease. Clin Neurol Neurosurg 1997;99(Suppl 2):S137–S141
26. Kim DS, Yoo DS, Huh PW, Kang SG, Cho KS, Kim MC. Combined direct anastomosis and encephaloduroarteriogaleosynangiosis using inverted superficial temporal artery-galeal flap and superficial temporal artery-galeal pedicle in adult moyamoya disease. Surg Neurol 2006;66(4):389–394, discussion 395
27. Matsushima T, Inoue T, Suzuki SO, Fujii K, Fukui M, Hasuo K. Surgical treatment of moyamoya disease in pediatric patients—comparison between the results of indirect and direct revascularization procedures. Neurosurgery 1992;31(3):401–405
28. Matsushima Y, Suzuki R, Yamaguchi T, Tabata H, Inaba Y. [Effects of indirect EC/IC bypass operations on adult moyamoya patients]. No Shinkei Geka 1986;14(13):1559–1566
29. Mizoi K, Kayama T, Yoshimoto T, Nagamine Y. Indirect revascularization for moyamoya disease: is there a

beneficial effect for adult patients? Surg Neurol 1996; 45(6):541–548, discussion 548–549

30. Morioka M, Hamada J, Todaka T, Yano S, Kai Y, Ushio Y. High-risk age for rebleeding in patients with hemorrhagic moyamoya disease: long-term follow-up study. Neurosurgery 2003;52(5):1049–1054, discussion 1054–1055

31. Nakashima H, Meguro T, Kawada S; Hirotsune N, Ohmoto T. Long-term results of surgically treated moyamoya disease. Clin Neurol Neurosurg 1997; 99(Suppl 2):S156–S161

32. Scott RM, Smith JL, Robertson RL et al. Long-term outcome in children with moyamoya syndrome after cranial revascularization by pial synangiosis. J Neurosurg 2004 February;100(2 Suppl Pediatrics): 142–9

33. Ueki K, Meyer FB, Mellinger JF. Moyamoya disease: the disorder and surgical treatment. Mayo Clin Proc 1994;69(8):749–757

34. Nagaraja D, Verma A, Taly AB, Kumar MV, Jayakumar PN. Cerebrovascular disease in children. Acta Neurol Scand 1994;90(4):251–255

35. Roach ES, Golomb MR, Adams R, et al; American Heart Association Stroke Council; Council on Cardiovascular Disease in the Young. Management of stroke in infants and children: a scientific statement from a Special Writing Group of the American Heart Association Stroke Council and the Council on Cardiovascular Disease in the Young. Stroke 2008;39(9): 2644–2691

36. Soriano SG, Sethna NF, Scott RM. Anesthetic management of children with moyamoya syndrome. Anesth Analg 1993;77(5):1066–1070

37. Baba T, Houkin K, Kuroda S. Novel epidemiological features of moyamoya disease. J Neurol Neurosurg Psychiatry 2008;79(8):900–904

38. Kuroda S, Houkin K. Moyamoya disease: current concepts and future perspectives. Lancet Neurol 2008; 7(11):1056–1066

39. Ezura M, Yoshimoto T, Fujiwara S, Takahashi A, Shirane R, Mizoi K. Clinical and angiographic follow-up of childhood-onset moyamoya disease. Childs Nerv Syst 1995;11(10):591–594

40. Kurokawa T, Tomita S, Ueda K, et al. Prognosis of occlusive disease of the circle of Willis (moyamoya disease) in children. Pediatr Neurol 1985;1(5):274–277

41. Maki Y, Enomoto T. Moyamoya disease. Childs Nerv Syst 1988;4(4):204–212

42. Lee JY, Phi JH, Wang KC, Cho BK, Shin MS, Kim SK. Neurocognitive profiles of children with moyamoya disease before and after surgical intervention. Cerebrovasc Dis 2011;31(3):230–237

43. Weinberg DG, Rahme RJ, Aoun SG, Batjer HH, Bendok BR. Moyamoya disease: functional and neurocognitive outcomes in the pediatric and adult populations. Neurosurg Focus 2011;30(6):E21

44. Yamada I, Matsushima Y, Suzuki S. Childhood moyamoya disease before and after encephalo-duro-arterio-synangiosis: an angiographic study. Neuroradiology 1992;34(4):318–322

45. Houkin K, Yoshimoto T, Kuroda S, Ishikawa T, Takahashi A, Abe H. Angiographic analysis of moyamoya disease— how does moyamoya disease progress? Neurol Med Chir (Tokyo) 1996;36(11):783–787, discussion 788

46. Ishii K, Isono M, Kobayashi H, Kamida T. Temporal profile of angiographical stages of moyamoya disease: when does moyamoya disease progress? Neurol Res 2003;25(4):405–410

47. Kuroda S, Hashimoto N, Yoshimoto T, Iwasaki Y; Research Committee on Moyamoya Disease in Japan. Radiological findings, clinical course, and outcome in asymptomatic moyamoya disease: results of multicenter survey in Japan. Stroke 2007;38(5):1430–1435

48. Kuriyama S, Kusaka Y, Fujimura M, et al. Prevalence and clinicoepidemiological features of moyamoya disease in Japan: findings from a nationwide epidemiological survey. Stroke 2008;39(1):42–47

49. Ikezaki K. Rational approach to treatment of moyamoya disease in childhood. J Child Neurol 2000; 15(5):350–356

50. Scott RM. Moyamoya syndrome: a surgically treatable cause of stroke in the pediatric patient. Clin Neurosurg 2000;47:378–384

51. Scott RM. Surgery for moyamoya syndrome? Yes. Arch Neurol 2001;58(1):128–129

52. Matsushima Y, Aoyagi M, Suzuki R, Tabata H, Ohno K. Perioperative complications of encephalo-duro-arterio-synangiosis: prevention and treatment. Surg Neurol 1991;36(5):343–353

53. Nomura S, Kashiwagi S, Uetsuka S, Uchida T, Kubota H, Ito H. Perioperative management protocols for children with moyamoya disease. Childs Nerv Syst 2001; 17(4–5):270–274

54. Uchino K, Johnston SC, Becker KJ, Tirschwell DL. Moyamoya disease in Washington State and California. Neurology 2005;65(6):956–958

55. Kirkham FJ, DeBaun MR. Stroke in children with sickle cell disease. Curr Treat Options Neurol 2004;6(5): 357–375

56. Adams R, McKie V, Nichols F, et al. The use of transcranial ultrasonography to predict stroke in sickle cell disease. N Engl J Med 1992;326(9):605–610

57. Adams RJ, Brambilla D; Optimizing Primary Stroke Prevention in Sickle Cell Anemia (STOP 2) Trial Investigators. Discontinuing prophylactic transfusions used to prevent stroke in sickle cell disease. N Engl J Med 2005;353(26):2769–2778

58. Adams RJ, McKie VC, Hsu L, et al. Prevention of a first stroke by transfusions in children with sickle cell anemia and abnormal results on transcranial Doppler ultrasonography. N Engl J Med 1998;339(1):5–11

59. Lee MT, Piomelli S, Granger S, et al; STOP Study Investigators. Stroke Prevention Trial in Sickle Cell Anemia (STOP): extended follow-up and final results. Blood 2006;108(3):847–852

60. Dobson SR, Holden KR, Nietert PJ, et al. Moyamoya syndrome in childhood sickle cell disease: a predictive factor for recurrent cerebrovascular events. Blood 2002;99(9):3144–3150

61. Roach ES. Etiology of stroke in children. Semin Pediatr Neurol 2000;7(4):244–260

62. Fryer RH, Anderson RC, Chiriboga CA, Feldstein NA. Sickle cell anemia with moyamoya disease: outcomes after EDAS procedure. Pediatr Neurol 2003;29(2): 124–130

63. Hankinson TC, Bohman LE, Heyer G, et al. Surgical treatment of moyamoya syndrome in patients with sickle cell anemia: outcome following encephaloduroarteriosynangiosis. J Neurosurg Pediatr 2008; 1(3):211–216

64. Smith ER, McClain CD, Heeney M, Scott RM. Pial synangiosis in patients with moyamoya syndrome and sickle cell anemia: perioperative management and surgical outcome. Neurosurg Focus 2009;26(4):E10

65. Suzuki J, Kodama N. Moyamoya disease—a review. Stroke 1983;14(1):104–109

66. Kelly ME, Bell-Stephens TE, Marks MP, Do HM, Steinberg GK. Progression of unilateral moyamoya disease: A clinical series. Cerebrovasc Dis 2006; 22(2–3):109–115

67. Vilela MD, Newell DW. Superficial temporal artery to middle cerebral artery bypass: past, present, and future. Neurosurg Focus 2008;24(2):E2

68. Starke RM, Komotar RJ, Connolly ES. Optimal surgical treatment for moyamoya disease in adults: direct versus indirect bypass. Neurosurg Focus 2009; 26(4):E8

69. Fujii K, Ikezaki K, Irikura K, Miyasaka Y, Fukui M. The efficacy of bypass surgery for the patients with hemorrhagic moyamoya disease. Clin Neurol Neurosurg 1997;99(Suppl 2):S194–S195

70. Yoshida Y, Yoshimoto T, Shirane R, Sakurai Y. Clinical course, surgical management, and long-term outcome of moyamoya patients with rebleeding after an episode of intracerebral hemorrhage: An extensive follow-Up study. Stroke 1999;30(11):2272–2276

3 The Natural History of Moyamoya Disease

4
Genetics of Moyamoya Angiopathy

Constantin Roder and Boris Krischek

◆ Introduction

The term *moyamoya* is used to describe different disease entities sharing distinctive findings (i.e., stenosis) and bypassing fragile collateral vessels of major intracranial arteries. Based on these pathological changes, diagnostic criteria define a bilateral appearance without known systemic diseases or exogenous disease–causing factors as definite moyamoya disease; a bilateral or unilateral appearance with a known systemic disease (such as Down syndrome or neurofibromatosis) or a history of possibly disease-causing events (such as radiation or infection of the brain) as moyamoya syndrome; and idiopathic unilateral appearance as probable moyamoya disease.[1] Differences in the clinical appearance of moyamoya disease reflect the type (familial versus sporadic), ethnic group (Asian versus Caucasian), age (juvenile versus adult), or manifestation (ischemic versus hemorrhagic cases).[2] Although several clinical differences within moyamoya disease are known, knowledge of the causes remains limited. Several reports on genetic factors causing the disease have been published.[2]

◆ Evidence for Genetic Contribution to Moyamoya Disease

The variable incidence of moyamoya disease across ethnic groups and known familial cases are the strongest evidence for a genetic contribution to the genesis of this disease.[2] Moyamoya disease is much more common in Asian countries (primarily Japan and Korea) than in Caucasian populations. Its incidence varies because of the rarity of the disease and because of technical progress in radiographic imaging. In Japan, the incidence is 0.3 to 1 per 100,000 population. In non-Asian countries, the incidence is a tenth of that in Japan.

An environmental or geographical influence on these rates seems unlikely, because the incidence of moyamoya disease in patients with an Asian heritage living in non-Asian countries is also higher than that of the local non-Asian population.[3] Among Asian-Americans in California, the incidence of 0.28/100,000 population is comparable to the incidence in Asia, a finding that supports the thesis of a genetic etiology of moyamoya disease. A familial history is present in 9 to 15% of all moyamoya disease cases. The mean age at onset of symptoms is 30 years in sporadic cases and 11.8 years in familial cases. Anticipation (i.e., symptoms of a genetic disorder become apparent at an earlier age as it is passed on to the next generation) can be found in affected families. The female-to-male ratio is 1.8:1 in sporadic cases and 5:1 in familial cases.[3]

Apart from the described regional differences and the familial occurrence of moyamoya disease, the association with other diseases with a known genetic background such as neurofibromatosis type 1 (NF-1) or Down syndrome, among others, also may provide clues about the genesis of this disease.[2] The prevalence of moyamoya disease in females (female-to-male ratio of 1.8:1) may be related to genetic factors, but hormonal factors could also be involved. Differences between Asian and Caucasian patients with moyamoya disease in terms of clinical presentation such as rates of subarachnoid hemorrhage, ischemic stroke, or age at onset of symptoms have been described. Genetic causes are likely to be involved in these differences, but this possibility remains conjectural because the available data are inconsistent and environmental, hormonal, and unknown factors cannot be ruled out.[4]

◆ Genetic Studies on Moyamoya Disease

Several genetic studies on moyamoya disease have been published (**Table 4.1**). However, the different techniques used in this research make comparing and understanding the findings challenging. To put the current knowledge on the genetics of moyamoya disease into perspective, this chapter briefly examines different study designs and discusses the available research data. The studies are classified by technique used. When a combination of techniques has been used, the discussion focuses on the most important finding.

Mode of Inheritance

The mode of inheritance can be determined by phenotyping affected families and by subsequent analysis of disease patterns throughout

generations. For example, Mineharu et al phenotyped 15 highly affected families with a total of 52 patients with moyamoya disease.[5] An autosomal dominant mode of inheritance with incomplete penetrance was found. This analysis also revealed an increased rate of maternal transmission compared with paternal transmission (3.44:1). The most common transmission was from mother to daughter (60%). These non-Mendelian patterns suggest that epigenetic factors such as genomic imprinting or the influence of sex-determining factors and/or genes are involved in the genesis of familial moyamoya disease.

Linkage Analysis

Linkage studies are used to identify cosegregation (the tendency for closely linked genes and genetic markers to be inherited together) of possible disease-causing genomic sequences in affected families by tracing known genomic markers in correlation to phenotype. If markers appear to be linked to affected patients, it is assumed that disease-causing genes are located nearby. The probability of separation between these markers and possible disease-causing genes, also known as crossing over during the prophase of meiosis, is very low. Analysis may be performed genome-wide or only within certain genomic regions depending on the chosen markers. However, linkage studies can only be performed with familial cases. Five linkage studies have been published.

In 1999, Ikeda et al analyzed 371 microsatellite markers across all 22 autosomes and found linkage to the marker D3S3050 on chromosome 3p24.2–p26.[6] Genes responsible for von Hippel-Lindau and Marfan syndrome are located in this genetic region. Consequently, the authors proposed that the region of chromosome 3p may encode a gene product that is fundamentally important for the formation and maintenance of vascular wall homeostasis and therefore may be involved in the genesis of inherited vascular disease.

Inoue et al performed linkage analysis with 15 microsatellite markers on chromosome 6 (human leukocyte antigen [HLA] genes).[7] The marker D6S441 was shared in affected family members in 16 of 19 families that were examined. Based on the occasional coincidence

Table 4.1 Genetic Studies on Moyamoya Angiopathy by Chromosome Location of Focus of Study

Reference	Chromosome Location	Study Type	Ethnicity of Patients	Number of Samples	Main Finding
Mineharu et al 2006[5]		Determination of inheritance pattern	Japanese	52 fMMD	Autosomal dominant with incomplete penetrance
Roder et al 2010[20]	1p13.3, 10q11.21	Association study	Caucasian	40 MMD	Disease association with *PSRC-1* (rs599839) and *CXCL12* (rs501120) polymorphisms
Ikeda et al 1999[6]	3p24.2–p26	Linkage analysis	Japanese	37 fMMD	Linkage to D3S3050
Roder et al 2010[22]	5q31–32, 19q31.1	Association study	Caucasian	40 MMD	Disease association with *PDG-FRB* (rs382861) and *TGFB1* (rs1800471) polymorphisms
Inoue et al 1997[16]	6p21.3	Association study	Japanese	71 MMD	Disease association with HLA-DQB1*0502, DRB1*0405, DQB1*0401 alleles
Inoue et al 2000[7]	6q25.2	Linkage analysis	Japanese	fMMD 20 affected sibling pairs	Linkage to D6S441
Han et al 2003[14]	6p21.3	Association study	Korean	28 MMD	Disease association with HLA-B35 allele
Hong et al 2009[15]	6p21.3	Association study	Korean	54 MMD, 16 fMMD	Disease association with HLA-DRB1*1302, DQB1*0609 alleles
Sakurai et al 2004[9]	8q23, 12p12	Linkage analysis	Japanese	fMMD 12 affected families	Linkage to D8S546, D12S1690
Guo et al 2009[25]	10q23.3	Genetic analysis of a hereditary multisystem disorder	Caucasian	5 MMD/HMD	Disease association with *ACTA2* (R258H/C) mutation
Shimojima et al 2009[26]	10q23.3	Association study	Japanese	46 MMD, 7 fMMD	No disease association with *ACTA2* mutation
Milewicz et al 2010[28]	10q23.3	Association study, genetic analysis of a hereditary multisystem disorder, other	Caucasian	5 MMD/HMD	Disease association with *ACTA2* (R179H) mutation, syndrome of multisystemic smooth muscle cell dysfunction

(Continued on page 38)

4 Genetics of Moyamoya Angiopathy

I Diagnosing Moyamoya Angiopathy: Definition, Classifications, Symptomatology

Reference	Chromosome Location	Study Type	Ethnicity of Patients	Number of Samples	Main Finding
Roder et al 2010[27]	10q23.3	Association study	Caucasian	40 MMD	One MMD patient with the *ACTA2* (R179H) mutation
Li et al 2010[19]	11q22.3	Association study	Han Chinese	177 MMD, 31 fMMD	Disease association with the 5A/6A genotype at −1171bp of *MMP3*
Yamauchi et al 2000[8]	17q25	Linkage analysis	Japanese	56 fMMD	Linkage to D17S939 and between D17S785–D17S836
Mineharu et al 2008[11]	17q25.3	Linkage analysis	Japanese	55 fMMD	Linkage to D17S704 and to D17S1806 and the telomere of 17q
Nanba et al 2005[17]	17q25	Association study	Japanese	4 fMMD	No association found in the analyzed genes (*DNAI2, AANAT, PSR, HCNGP, HN1, SGSH, SYNGR2, EVPL, TIMP2*)
Kang et al 2006[18]	17q25.3	Association study	Korean	50 MMD, 11 fMMD	Disease association with rs8179090 (*TIMP2, −418bp*) polymorphism
Liu et al 2009[21]	17q25.3	Linkage analysis, association study	Japanese, Korean, Chinese, Caucasian	179 MMD	Linkage to 17q25.3 and disease association of ss161110142 at −1480bp of the transcription site of *RAPTOR*
Kamada et al 2011[23]	17q25.3	Genome-wide association study	Japanese	72 MMD	Disease association with *RNF213* (p.R4859K) variant
Liu et al 2011[24]	17q25.3	Linkage analysis, association study, functional analysis	Japanese, Korean, Chinese, Caucasian	42 East Asian families, 207 East Asian MMD, 1 Caucasian family, 49 Caucasian MMD	Disease association with *RNF213* (p.R4810K) variant

Table 4.1 *(Continued)* Genetic Studies on Moyamoya Angiopathy by Chromosome Location of Focus of Study

Reference	Chromosome Location	Study Type	Ethnicity of Patients	Number of Samples	Main Finding
Hervé et al 2010[29]	X chromosome	Determination of inheritance pattern	Algerian	4 MMD/HMD	X-linked recessive pattern of inheritance
Miskinyte et al 2011[30]	Xq28	Determination of inheritance pattern, linkage analysis, genetic analysis of a hereditary multisystem disorder, functional analysis	Caucasian	10 MMD/HMD	*MTCP1/MTCP1NB* and *BRCC3* deletions, common phenotypic changes

Abbreviations: fMMD, familial moyamoya disease cases; MMD, sporadic moyamoya disease cases; MMD/HMD, syndromic moyamoya disease cases of families with hereditary multisystem disorders.

of moyamoya disease and NF-1, of which the causative gene has been assigned to chromosome 17q11.2, Yamauchi et al genotyped 22 microsatellite markers on chromosome 17 in 24 moyamoya disease families.[8] The marker D17S939 located within the 9-cM region between D17S785 and D17S836 on chromosome 17q25 showed strong linkage. The finding suggested the location of a disease-causing gene locus for familial moyamoya disease. However, the description of this genetic region did not support a direct involvement of the NF-1 gene in the genesis of moyamoya disease because of the physical distance between both loci.

In a genome-wide analysis of 12 families with moyamoya disease, Sakurai et al reported linkage to D8S546 (8q23) and suggestive linkage to D12S1690 (12p12).[9] As a possible candidate gene, the authors suggested transforming growth factor-β-inducible early growth response, located on 8q22.3. Previously, the expression of transforming growth factor β 1 (TGFB1) had been reported to increase in cultured smooth muscle cells of superficial temporal arteries and in the serum of patients with moyamoya disease.[10]

In 2008, Mineharu et al performed a genome-wide parametric linkage analysis with 15 extended Japanese families.[11] The results showed linkage to D17S704 located in a 3.5Mb region between D17S1806 and the telomere of 17q. Ninety-four genes have been described in this region, of which BAI1-associated protein 2 (BAIAP2), tissue-inhibitor metalloproteinase 2 (TIMP2), ras-related C3 botulinum toxin substrate 3 (RAC3), and RAB40B, a member of the ras oncogene family, have been chosen as putative candidate genes for further analysis. However, sequencing of the coding exons and adjacent intronic regions of these genes in probands of five of the families showed no new disease-associated variants.

Association Studies

Association studies are based on a case-control design and can be used for both sporadic and familial cases. The length of genomic sequences examined may vary from single base pairs (single nucleotide polymorphisms [SNPs]), to entire (candidate) genes, longer sequences, and up to genome-wide studies.

The HLA system contains essential elements for immunological functions because it encodes cell-surface antigen proteins for intercellular communication and recognition. Supported by the hypothesis of an involvement of immunological factors (e.g., an autoimmune disease or infection of the patient), serological[12,13] and genetic analyses[7,14-16] were undertaken to elucidate the role of HLA molecules in the genesis of moyamoya disease. HLA genotyping examines the association of allelic variants based on a case-control study design. It is noteworthy that all HLA genes are located on chromosome 6. Significant associations were described for HLA-DQB1*0502, HLA-DRB1*0405, HLA-DQB1*0401, HLA-B35, HLA-DRB1*1302, and HLA-DQB*0609.[14-16] However, none of these results were replicated in further studies. Given that the HLA system is heterogeneous, the possibility of association of certain variants with the disease must be weighed against the possibility of random coherency.

Nanba et al[17] performed sequence analyses of candidate genes in the 9-cM region between the markers D17S785 and D17S835 on chromosome 17q25, the region Yamauchi et al[8] described as linked to familial moyamoya disease. Nanba et al selected 9 of 65 known genes in this region for their analysis based on criteria such as plausible compatibility with the genesis of moyamoya disease or known specific expression patterns in the brain, among others.[17] Bioinformatics were also used for the analysis of ~2.100 expressed sequence tags with the goal of identifying candidate genes within 17q25. However, no disease-related mutations or new candidate genes were found.

Based on the results of linkage studies by Ikeda et al[6] (3p24.2–p26) and Yamauchi et al[8] (17q25), Kang et al analyzed the promoter regions, exon-intron junctions, and exons of TIMP4 (3p25) and TIMP2 (17q25) as candidate genes.[18] A polymorphism in the promoter region of TIMP2 (position −418bp, rs8179090) was described as significantly associated with familial moyamoya disease in the examined Korean cohort. However, these findings could not be replicated in other cohorts from different ethnic groups.[5,19,20]

In 2010, Liu et al published the results of a multicenter study with samples from Japan, Korea, China, and Europe.[21] After they extended their previous linkage analysis, the linkage signal was narrowed to a 2.1-Mb region on 17q25.3.[11] Within this region, the genes CARD14, RAPTOR, and AATK were

sequenced in four unrelated individuals. A new polymorphism (ss161110142) was found at position −1480 bp from the transcription site of the Raptor gene. Further analysis of this polymorphism in the different cohorts proved that the A allele was relatively common in Asian patients with moyamoya disease, but it was not found in the Caucasian samples. The authors concluded that the ss161110142 variant is a founder haplotype among East Asian patients with moyamoya disease. RAPTOR is known to be associated with vascular smooth muscle cell proliferation and intimal expansion mediated by interferon-γ as well as with HLA-mediated endothelial cell proliferation. Therefore, it might be a reasonable candidate gene to be involved in the etiology of moyamoya disease.

Based on the theory of abnormal synthesis of extracellular matrix components causing moyamoya disease, Li et al[19] analyzed five functional promoter polymorphisms in MMP2, MMP3, MMP9, and MMP13 as well as a potentially functional promoter polymorphism in TIMP2[18] in 208 patients. Significant association with the functional MMP3 promoter polymorphism at position −1171 was found in both familial and sporadic cases, underlining the possible role of an imbalance between MMPs and TIMPs in the genesis of moyamoya disease.

In 2010, Roder et al published the first genetic studies with exclusively Caucasian patients with moyamoya disease.[20,22] Their first study was based on the examination of SNPs in genes encoding for cytokines and growth factors with known histopathological changes in patients with moyamoya disease. They found a significant association for rs382861 in the promoter region of PDGFRB. There was also a significant association for rs1800471 and a trend for rs1800470, both located in the first exon of TGFB1. Among others, TGFB1 is known to be a potent angiogenic factor and responsible for the maintenance of the extracellular matrix. Allele combinations of rs1800470 and rs1800471, which were most common in patients with moyamoya disease in this study, are known to increase TGFB1 levels in vitro.[22]

The second study was based on the description of common histopathological changes, such as intimal thickening or smooth muscle cell migration, in the walls of vessels of patients with moyamoya disease and with atherosclerotic disease.[20] The authors analyzed SNPs in genes that had previously been described to be associated with atherosclerotic disease. Association of rs599839 and a trend toward significance for three other SNPs (rs8326, rs34208922, rs501120) was found. In patients with coronary heart disease, rs599839 is associated with levels of low-density lipoprotein. The SNP rs501120 is located upstream from *CXCL12*, which is known to be involved in stem cell homing and vasculogenesis in ischemic tissues. Therefore, it might be a reasonable gene to be involved in the genesis of moyamoya disease.

Kamada et al[23] published the first genome-wide association study on moyamoya disease, including the analysis of 785,720 SNPs. A strong association was found in the terminal region of 17q25, including seven SNPs at the *RNF213* locus, a gene encoding for a finger protein expressed in spleen and leukocytes. Mutational analysis of *RNF213* revealed a founder mutation (p.R4859K) and three further missense mutations, making it a strong candidate gene for being involved in the genesis of moyamoya disease.

Liu et al published a comprehensive paper on linkage analysis, exome analysis, association analysis of parts of 17q25.3, and functional analysis of *RNF213* knockdown zebrafish.[24] The authors suggested that *RNF213* was involved in the genesis of moyamoya disease because they found a strong association of the R4810K variant in Asian patients with moyamoya disease and irregular vessel formation in *RNF213* knockdown zebrafish. This variant was not identified in Caucasian samples.

Hereditary Multisystemic Diseases

Mutations of the vascular smooth muscle cell-specific isoform of α-actin (*ACTA2*) are known to be associated with familial thoracic aortic aneurysms and dissections. Guo et al[25] performed extended genotyping and phenotyping of affected families with thoracic aortic aneurysms and dissections. They found an increased frequency of patients with coronary heart disease, livedo reticularis, stroke, and moyamoya disease. Genetic analysis revealed variations, in particular involving *ACTA2* R258C/H, which was detected more frequently in patients with early onset stroke and moyamoya disease.

However, sequencing of *ACTA2* in a Japanese[26] and a European[27] cohort failed to replicate these findings. In a follow-up study, the same group[28] reported five syndromic patients with a de novo mutation of *ACTA2* (R179H) causing smooth muscle cell malfunction throughout the body. The pathological changes consisted of aortic and cerebrovascular disease (including changes similar to those seen in patients with moyamoya disease), fixed dilated pupils, hypotonic bladder, malrotation, hypoperistalsis of the gut, and pulmonary hypertension.

In 2010, Hervé et al first reported precise phenotyping of a family with a multisystemic disorder, including moyamoya syndrome.[29] In a follow-up study, two other families with these distinct multisystemic changes were found and all three families were analyzed. Phenotypic changes included moyamoya angiopathy, facial dysmorphism, hypergonadotropic hypogonadism, hypertension, premature graying of hair, short stature, dilated cardiomyopathy, premature coronary heart disease, and early bilateral cataracts.[30] Because the family tree analysis favored an X-linked pattern of inheritance, further genetic analysis of the X chromosome revealed an overlapping deletion of exon 1 of *MTCP1/MTCP1NB* and exons 1 to 3 of *BRCC3* in all three families. *MTCP1NB* and *BRCC3* knockdown zebrafish were examined. *MTCP1NB* knockdown did not result in changes of the vascular phenotype, but *BRCC3* knockdown led to defective angiogenesis. *BRCC3* is a ubiquitously expressed deubiquinating enzyme known to be part of DNA repair complexes. The authors suggested that this gene might play an important role in angiogenesis and vessel maintenance. However, the authors examined three additional families with familial moyamoya disease who exhibited no other systemic changes and were unable to identify these deletions.

◆ Conclusion

A genetic component involved in the genesis of moyamoya is likely. The quantity and comprehensiveness of genetic studies on the origin of moyamoya angiopathies have increased rapidly. However, the results are seldom replicable and seem to indicate a multifactorial cause for the disease. The most challenging part of genetic research on moyamoya angiopathy is the small number of patients available, reflecting the rarity of the disease. Comparisons of results and cooperation of international groups are needed to increase the statistical power of studies. Further research is needed to evaluate the role of moyamoya vasculopathy within syndromic patients compared with patients with definite moyamoya disease. As seen in the studies of patients with hereditary multisystemic disease, small numbers of patients, precisely phenotyped and analyzed, could be sufficient to identify further genes. Although such variations in genes have not yet been detected in patients with definite moyamoya disease, it may provide valuable insight into cascades that are responsible for the development of moyamoya-like changes.

References

1. Fukui M. Guidelines for the diagnosis and treatment of spontaneous occlusion of the circle of Willis ('moyamoya' disease). Research Committee on Spontaneous Occlusion of the Circle of Willis (Moyamoya Disease) of the Ministry of Health and Welfare, Japan. Clin Neurol Neurosurg 1997;99(Suppl 2):S238–S240

2. Roder C, Nayak NR, Khan N, Tatagiba M, Inoue I, Krischek B. Genetics of Moyamoya disease. J Hum Genet 2010;55(11):711–716

3. Kuroda S, Houkin K. Moyamoya disease: current concepts and future perspectives. Lancet Neurol 2008; 7(11):1056–1066

4. Krischek B, Kasuya H, Khan N, Tatagiba M, Roder C, Kraemer M. Genetic and clinical characteristics of Moyamoya disease in Europeans. Acta Neurochir (Wien) 2011;112:31–34

5. Mineharu Y, Takenaka K, Yamakawa H, et al. Inheritance pattern of familial moyamoya disease: autosomal dominant mode and genomic imprinting. J Neurol Neurosurg Psychiatry 2006;77(9):1025–1029

6. Ikeda H, Sasaki T, Yoshimoto T, Fukui M, Arinami T. Mapping of a familial moyamoya disease gene to chromosome 3p24.2–p26. Am J Hum Genet 1999; 64(2):533–537

7. Inoue TK, Ikezaki K, Sasazuki T, Matsushima T, Fukui M. Linkage analysis of moyamoya disease on chromosome 6. J Child Neurol 2000;15(3):179–182

8. Yamauchi T, Tada M, Houkin K, et al. Linkage of familial moyamoya disease (spontaneous occlusion of the circle of Willis) to chromosome 17q25. Stroke 2000;31(4):930–935

9. Sakurai K, Horiuchi Y, Ikeda H, et al. A novel susceptibility locus for moyamoya disease on chromosome 8q23. J Hum Genet 2004;49(5):278–281

10. Hojo M, Hoshimaru M, Miyamoto S, et al. Role of transforming growth factor-beta1 in the pathogenesis of moyamoya disease. J Neurosurg 1998;89(4):623–629

11. Mineharu Y, Liu W, Inoue K, et al. Autosomal dominant moyamoya disease maps to chromosome 17q25.3. Neurology 2008;70(24 Pt 2):2357–2363

12. Aoyagi M, Ogami K, Matsushima Y, Shikata M, Yamamoto M, Yamamoto K. Human leukocyte antigen in patients with moyamoya disease. Stroke 1995; 26(3):415–417

13. Kitahara T, Okumura K, Semba A, Yamaura A, Makino H. Genetic and immunologic analysis on moya-moya. J Neurol Neurosurg Psychiatry 1982;45(11):1048–1052

14. Han H, Pyo CW, Yoo DS, Huh PW, Cho KS, Kim DS. Associations of Moyamoya patients with HLA class I and class II alleles in the Korean population. J Korean Med Sci 2003;18(6):876–880

15. Hong SH, Wang KC, Kim SK, Cho BK, Park MH. Association of HLA-DR and -DQ Genes with Familial Moyamoya Disease in Koreans. J Korean Neurosurg Soc 2009;46(6):558–563

16. Inoue TK, Ikezaki K, Sasazuki T, Matsushima T, Fukui M. Analysis of class II genes of human leukocyte antigen in patients with moyamoya disease. Clin Neurol Neurosurg 1997;99(Suppl 2):S234–S237

17. Nanba R, Tada M, Kuroda S, Houkin K, Iwasaki Y. Sequence analysis and bioinformatics analysis of chromosome 17q25 in familial moyamoya disease. Childs Nerv Syst 2005;21(1):62–68

18. Kang HS, Kim SK, Cho BK, Kim YY, Hwang YS, Wang KC. Single nucleotide polymorphisms of tissue inhibitor of metalloproteinase genes in familial moyamoya disease. Neurosurgery 2006;58(6):1074–1080, discussion 1074–1080

19. Li H, Zhang ZS, Liu W, et al. Association of a functional polymorphism in the MMP-3 gene with Moyamoya Disease in the Chinese Han population. Cerebrovasc Dis 2010;30(6):618–625

20. Roder C, Peters V, Kasuya H, et al. Common genetic polymorphisms in moyamoya and atherosclerotic disease in Europeans. Childs Nerv Syst 2011;27(2):245–252

21. Liu W, Hashikata H, Inoue K, et al. A rare Asian founder polymorphism of Raptor may explain the high prevalence of Moyamoya disease among East Asians and its low prevalence among Caucasians. Environ Health Prev Med 2010;15(2):94–104

22. Roder C, Peters V, Kasuya H, et al. Polymorphisms in TGFB1 and PDGFRB are associated with Moyamoya disease in European patients. Acta Neurochir (Wien) 2010;152(12):2153–2160

23. Kamada F, Aoki Y, Narisawa A, et al. A genome-wide association study identifies RNF213 as the first Moyamoya disease gene. J Hum Genet 2011;56(1):34–40

24. Liu W, Morito D, Takashima S, et al. Identification of RNF213 as a susceptibility gene for moyamoya disease and its possible role in vascular development. PLoS ONE 2011;6(7):e22542

25. Guo DC, Papke CL, Tran-Fadulu V, et al. Mutations in smooth muscle alpha-actin (ACTA2) cause coronary artery disease, stroke, and Moyamoya disease, along with thoracic aortic disease. Am J Hum Genet 2009;84(5):617–627

26. Shimojima K, Yamamoto T. ACTA2 is not a major disease-causing gene for moyamoya disease. J Hum Genet 2009;54(11):687–688

27. Roder C, Peters V, Kasuya H, et al. Analysis of ACTA2 in European Moyamoya disease patients. Eur J Paediatr Neurol 2011;15(2):117–122

28. Milewicz DM, Østergaard JR, Ala-Kokko LM, et al. De novo ACTA2 mutation causes a novel syndrome of multisystemic smooth muscle dysfunction. Am J Med Genet A 2010;152A(10):2437–2443

29. Hervé D, Touraine P, Verloes A, et al. A hereditary moyamoya syndrome with multisystemic manifestations. Neurology 2010;75(3):259–264

30. Miskinyte S, Butler MG, Hervé D, et al. Loss of BRCC3 deubiquitinating enzyme leads to abnormal angiogenesis and is associated with syndromic moyamoya. Am J Hum Genet 2011;88(6):718–728

5

Clinical Assessment of Cerebral Perfusion in Moyamoya Disease

James R. Sagar and Colin P. Derdeyn

◆ Introduction

Hemodynamic impairment likely plays a major role in the risk for stroke in patients with moyamoya disease.[1-4] Chronic hypoperfusion leading to metabolic downregulation and clinical cognitive decline has been suggested as another potential mechanism of neurological injury in these patients.[5] Surgical revascularization is a mainstay of treatment for these patients, and the rationale is based on improving perfusion. Preoperative hemodynamic assessment is typically used to justify invasive treatment. This chapter describes and evaluates current modalities for the assessment of cerebral perfusion.

◆ Cerebral Perfusion Pressure

When an artery becomes narrowed or completely occluded, the mean arterial pressure (MAP) in the distal circulation may fall. This response is a function of both the degree of stenosis and the adequacy of collateral sources of blood flow.[6] However, cerebral arterial occlusion does not consistently predict a reduction in MAP, even when the occlusions are distal to the circle of Willis.[7] When sources of collateral flow are inadequate, MAP decreases, leading to a reduction in cerebral perfusion pressure (CPP).

When CPP falls, the cerebrovasculature can respond with two compensatory mechanisms serving to maintain the normal delivery of oxygen and nutrients (**Fig. 5.1**). The first is autoregulation: reflex changes in vascular resistance in response to changing arterial blood pressure that maintain cerebral blood flow (CBF) over a wide range of CPP values. The site of this regulation is resistance arterioles that can dilate to reduce vascular resistance and to maintain CBF at near normal levels.[8,9]

The second compensatory mechanism is an increased oxygen extraction fraction (OEF).[10,11] When the CBF and thus the delivery of oxygen falls, the amount of available oxygen extracted from the blood can increase to maintain normal oxygen metabolism (cerebral metabolic rate of oxygen [$CMRO_2$]). OEF can increase from a baseline of 30% to up to 80%.

In the autoregulatory range (region between points A and B in **Fig. 5.1**), CBF falls at a slight[12,13] but constant rate, and normal $CMRO_2$ is maintained by slight increases in OEF.[14] Once autoregulatory capacity is exceeded (point B), CBF falls sharply, inducing a sharp increase in OEF. This situation has been called "misery perfusion.[15] Vascular mean transit time (MTT) is defined as the ratio of cerebral blood volume (CBV) to CBF. An increase in MTT may be used to detect autoregulatory arteriole dilation. It is critical to note that these compensatory responses were largely defined in animal studies involving acute and global reductions in MAP or CPP. The extent to which they are valid in humans with chronic regional reductions in CPP is unclear.

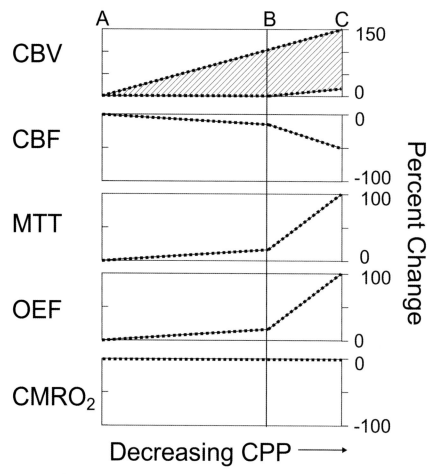

Fig. 5.1 Schematic of hemodynamic changes in response to reduced cerebral perfusion pressure (CPP; left to right at bottom) in the oligemic range. A to B is the autoregulatory range. Cerebral blood volume (CBV) either increases or remains stable, depending on the modality used for measurement. Cerebral blood flow (CBF) falls slightly. Mean transit time (MTT) and oxygen extraction fraction (OEF) increase slightly, and cerebral metabolic rate of oxygen ($CMRO_2$) is maintained. Once autoregulatory capacity is exceeded, further reductions in pressure lead to a passive reduction in flow (B to C). Cerebral blood volume increases further. Mean transit time and OEF increase dramatically, and $CMRO_2$ is maintained. Further reductions in pressure will exceed the ability of OEF to compensate, and true ischemia will result.

◆ Cerebral Metabolic Downregulation and Cognitive Impairment

Chronic cerebral oligemia has been linked to cognitive impairment in patients with carotid occlusion. These patients typically manifest decreased measures of global cerebral functioning on neuropsychological testing, such as attention, processing speed, and learning, that cannot be attributed to focal infarction.[5] It has been theorized that chronic oligemia may result in cerebral metabolic downregulation (decreased $CMRO_2$) as an adaptive mechanism to reduce the need for CBF. The cognitive impairment is then a manifestation of decreased cerebral metabolism. Whether this phenomenon exists and is reversible remains to be established.

◆ Clinical Assessment of Cerebral Perfusion

Certain patterns of collateral blood flow have been correlated with hemodynamic impairment, but the ability of these findings to identify individual patients with hemodynamic compromise has been poor.[7,16] The primary issue is that anatomic imaging, such as angiography, is limited to demonstrating the pathways of blood flow but not the amount of blood delivered.

It is also difficult to correlate clinical condition with hemodynamic impairment. Symptoms such as limb shaking or orthostatic transient ischemic attacks are strongly associated with hemodynamic impairment (high specificity); however, most patients with hemodynamic impairment do not have these symptoms (low sensitivity).[17] On magnetic resonance imaging (MRI), a linear pattern of white matter infarctions of the centrum semiovale or corona radiata ipsilateral to the occluded carotid artery is highly specific, but not sensitive, for hemodynamic impairment in that cerebral hemisphere (**Fig. 5.2**).[18,19] This pattern of infarction is common in patients with moyamoya disease, suggesting a hemodynamic mechanism.

Single measurements of CBF alone do not adequately assess cerebral hemodynamic status. First, normal values may be found when perfusion pressure is reduced, but CBF is maintained by autoregulatory vasodilation.

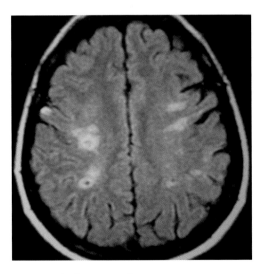

Fig. 5.2 Fluid-attenuated inversion recovery image of a 35-year-old woman with moyamoya disease demonstrating bilateral infarctions in the centrum semiovale white matter. A small infarction of the right motor cortex is also present, corresponding to a minor stroke affecting her left hand.

Second, CBF may be low when perfusion pressure is normal. This situation can occur when the metabolic demands of the tissue are low. Reduced blood flow related to reduced metabolic demand may not cause confusion when low regional CBF is measured in areas of frank tissue infarction; however, blood flow can also be reduced in normal, noninfarcted tissue due to the destruction of afferent or efferent fibers by a remote lesion.[20] As a consequence of these issues, three basic strategies of hemodynamic assessment have been developed: paired blood flow measurements, CBV measurement, and direct measurement of the OEF.[21] These are indirect methods, and the presence of hemodynamic impairment is inferred when a test is abnormal.[22]

Paired Blood Flow Measurements

The first strategy relies on paired blood flow measurements: an initial measurement obtained at rest and a second measurement obtained after a cerebral vasodilatory stimulus. These studies are commonly referred to as tests of cerebrovascular reactivity or reserve. Hypercapnia, acetazolamide, and physiologic tasks such as hand movement have been used as vasodilatory stimuli. Normally, each results in a robust increase in CBF. If the CBF response is muted or absent, preexisting autoregulatory cerebral vasodilation related to reduced CPP is inferred.

Quantitative or qualitative (relative) measurements of CBF can be made using a variety of methods, including inhalation or intravenous injection of ^{133}Xe, with single photon emission computed tomography (SPECT), stable xenon computed tomography (CT), positron emission tomography (PET), computed tomography perfusion with iodinated contrast, and MRI. Changes in the velocity of blood in the middle cerebral artery trunk or internal carotid artery can also be measured with transcranial Doppler ultrasonography and MRI. Changes in blood oxygen level–dependent MRI signals also may be measured.[23] Inhalation or injection of xenon blood flow tracers may cause arterial dilation and error in hemodynamic measurements, especially when used with acetazolamide.[24] Furthermore, blood velocity in the middle cerebral artery cannot be measured in many patients with advanced moyamoya disease because of the absence or stenosis of these vessels.

The blood flow responses to these vasodilatory stimuli have been categorized into grades of hemodynamic impairment: Stage 1, reduced augmentation (relative to the contralateral hemisphere or normal controls); Stage 2, absent augmentation (same value as baseline); and Stage 3, paradoxical reduction in regional blood flow compared with baseline measurement. The latter phenomenon has been labeled cerebrovascular steal.

Cerebral Blood Volume Measurement

The second strategy measures either regional CBV alone or in combination with measurements of CBF in the resting brain to detect reduced perfusion pressure. As discussed earlier, the CBV/CBF ratio (or, inversely, the CBF/CBV ratio) is mathematically equivalent to the vascular MTT. Measurement of MTT may be more sensitive than CBV alone for the identification of autoregulatory vasodilation; however, it may be less specific. The CBV/CBF ratio may increase in low-flow conditions with normal perfusion pressure, such as hypocapnia. Quantitative regional measurements of CBV and CBF can be made with PET or SPECT. MRI and computed tomography (CT) techniques

for the quantitative measurement of CBV have been developed. Patients are identified as abnormal with these techniques based on comparison of absolute quantitative values or hemispheric ratios of quantitative values to the range observed in normal control subjects. One issue that remains unresolved is to what extent autoregulatory vasodilation of arterioles gives rise to measurable increases in the CBV. Experimental data have produced conflicting results.[25–27] Although increases in CBV almost certainly indicate autoregulatory vasodilation, the significance of normal CBV in patients with increased OEF—a frequent finding—is unclear.[28] Thus, the sensitivity and specificity of CBV measurements for detecting reduced CPP are unknown. The use of dynamic susceptibility-based MRI methods of measurement for CBF and CBV in the setting of moyamoya disease may be problematic due to the delay and dispersion of the contrast bolus.[29]

Direct Measurement of Oxygen Extraction Fraction

The third strategy relies on direct measurements of OEF to identify patients with increased oxygen extraction (**Fig. 5.3**). At present, regional measurements of OEF can

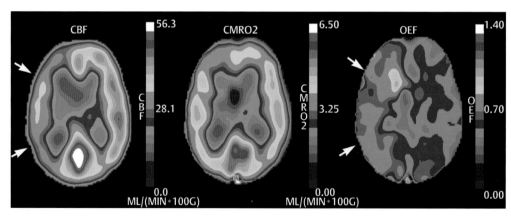

Fig. 5.3 Compensatory increase in oxygen extraction fraction (OEF) as identified by positron emission tomography. These images are from a neurologically normal patient with a unilateral carotid occlusion due to atherosclerosis. Cerebral blood flow (CBF) is reduced on the left image (*arrows*). Although oxygen metabolism (CMRO$_2$, middle image) is normal and symmetric, it reflects a compensatory increase in OEF (right image, *arrows*). *Source:* Derdeyn CP, Videen TO, Simmons NR, et al. Count-based PET method for predicting ischemic stroke in patients with symptomatic carotid arterial occlusion. Radiology 1999;212:499–506. (Used with permission from The Radiological Society of North America.)

be made only with PET using ^{15}O-labeled radiotracers. MRI measurements using pulse sequences sensitive to deoxyhemoglobin (which is increased in regions with increased oxygen extraction) are being developed to provide similar information.[30]

Magnetic Resonance Imaging and Computed Tomography Methods of Hemodynamic Assessment

The widespread availability of CT and MRI over PET facilities has created increasing interest in using these modalities to evaluate cerebral blood supply. Several studies have utilized acetazolamide and paired blood flow measurements with CT or MRI SPECT to increase the contrast between regions of varying perfusion by dilating the cerebral vasculature. Unfortunately, SPECT is not a purely quantitative measurement: The blood flow map it provides is a statistical comparison to a normalized control.[31] Further drawbacks to SPECT include tracer kinetics that often require a 2-day study and the lack of anatomic-spatial resolution, the presence of which is the main advantage of MRI and CT.[32]

CBV measurements using CT perfusion sequences have several advantages, including the availability of CT and the use of contrast rather than a radioactive tracer. Perfusion sequences use continuous image acquisition to track the first pass of a contrast bolus through the cerebral vasculature. These data can then be used to create maps of CBV, CBF, and MTT.[31] This method also provides accurate anatomical data to correlate to perfusion measurements.

Diffusion susceptibility contrast-weighted and arterial spin-labeled MRI sequences are the latest methods for hemodynamic assessment. Similar to CT perfusion imaging, diffusion susceptibility contrast MRI tracks the dispersion of the first pass of a contrast bolus. The resulting image gives a map of relative cerebral perfusion. Arterial spin-labeled MRI has the added benefit of not requiring contrast medium to be administered. Instead, water molecules in the carotid bloodstream are labeled magnetically, and continuous imaging tracks the bolus of labeled water through the brain. CBF maps are then calculated as in the other modalities.

Although CT and MRI perfusion methods have great utility in many clinical disease states, the complex collateral network of the moyamoya vasculature presents significant obstacles. As stated, blood flow through collateral channels can delay the dispersion of contrast and preclude accurate measurement of perfusion with CT and diffusion susceptibility contrast MRI. Furthermore, arterial spin-labeled imaging may be inaccurate if MTT is so prolonged that a portion of an arterial spin-labeled water bolus has lost its magnetic labeling by the time it reaches the parenchyma (**Fig. 5.4**). Finally, many patients have comorbid conditions that preclude the use of iodinated or gadolinium-based contrast media.[29,31]

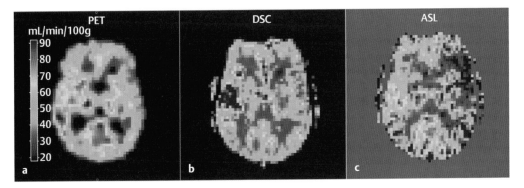

Fig. 5.4a–c A 79-year-old woman with moyamoya disease and an infarction of the left middle cerebral artery. (**a**) Positron emission tomography perfusion map using H_2O^{15}-labeled water. (**b**) Diffusion susceptibility contrast magnetic resonance imaging (MRI). (**c**) Arterial spin-labeled (ASL) MRI. Note that arterial spin-labeled MRI may overestimate perfusion deficits if arterial transit time is prolonged because magnetic labeling may be lost during slower flow through collateral channels.

Correlation among Methods of Hemodynamic Assessment

The correlation among methods that compare impaired vasodilatory capacity and increased OEF in patients with cerebrovascular disease has been inconsistent.[22] To what extent maximal autoregulatory vasodilation persists when OEF is elevated remains unclear, particularly in humans with chronic reductions in perfusion pressure. Patients have been observed with increased OEF who did not have increased CBV or MTT.[28] Whether this latter finding represents a variable vasodilatory capacity or some form of long-term compensatory response remains to be determined. Therefore, both the independence of the mechanisms of autoregulatory vasodilation and oxygen extraction and the changes occurring over time may be sources of difficulty in comparing the outcomes across methods. The clinical validity of CT- and MRI-based assessments in moyamoya disease is still under investigation. No studies have evaluated patients with these methods and compared the data to PET measurements of CBV or MTT.

◆ Conclusion

Several methods are available to assess the hemodynamic status of patients with moyamoya phenomena. These methods include tests of vasodilatory capacity and measurements of vasodilation and oxygen extraction. In the future, research will likely focus on the ability of these tests to identify patients at risk for future stroke or cognitive impairment. This research has great potential to improve patient selection for revascularization procedures and to improve patient outcomes.

References

1. Zipfel GJ, Sagar J, Miller JP, et al. Cerebral hemodynamics as a predictor of stroke in adult patients with moyamoya disease: a prospective observational study. Neurosurg Focus 2009;26(4):E6
2. Ikezaki K, Matsushima T, Kuwabara Y, Suzuki SO, Nomura T, Fukui M. Cerebral circulation and oxygen metabolism in childhood moyamoya disease: a perioperative positron emission tomography study. J Neurosurg 1994;81(6):843–850
3. Yamashita T, Kashiwagi S, Nakashima K, et al. Modulation of cerebral hemodynamics by surgical revascularization in patients with moyamoya disease. Acta Neurol Scand Suppl 1996;166:82–84
4. Kuroda S, Houkin K, Kamiyama H, Abe H, Mitsumori K. Regional cerebral hemodynamics in childhood moyamoya disease. Childs Nerv Syst 1995;11(10):584–590
5. Chmayssani M, Festa JR, Marshall RS. Chronic ischemia and neurocognition. Neuroimaging Clin N Am 2007;17(3):313–324, viii viii
6. Powers WJ, Press GA, Grubb RL Jr, Gado M, Raichle ME. The effect of hemodynamically significant carotid artery disease on the hemodynamic status of the cerebral circulation. Ann Intern Med 1987;106(1):27–34
7. Derdeyn CP, Shaibani A, Moran CJ, Cross DT III, Grubb RL Jr, Powers WJ. Lack of correlation between pattern of collateralization and misery perfusion in patients with carotid occlusion. Stroke 1999;30(5):1025–1032
8. Rapela CE, Green HD. Autoregulation Of Canine Cerebral Blood Flow. Circ Res 1964 August;15:Suppl-12
9. MacKenzie ET, Farrar JK, Fitch W, Graham DI, Gregory PC, Harper AM. Effects of hemorrhagic hypotension on the cerebral circulation. I. Cerebral blood flow and pial arteriolar caliber. Stroke 1979;10(6):711–718
10. Lennox WG, Gibbs FA, Gibbs EL. Relationship of unconsciousness to cerebral blood flow and to anoxemia. Arch Neurol Psychiatry 1934;34(5):1001–1013
11. Kety SS, King BD, Horvath SM, Jeffers WS, Hafkenschiel JH. The effects of an acute reduction in blood pressure by means of differential spinal sympathetic block on the cerebral circulation of hypertensive patients. J Clin Invest 1950;29(4):402–407
12. Kontos HA, Wei EP, Navari RM, Levasseur JE, Rosenblum WI, Patterson JL Jr. Responses of cerebral arteries and arterioles to acute hypotension and hypertension. Am J Physiol 1978;234(4):H371–H383
13. Dirnagl U, Pulsinelli W. Autoregulation of cerebral blood flow in experimental focal brain ischemia. J Cereb Blood Flow Metab 1990;10(3):327–336
14. Schumann P, Touzani O, Young AR, Morello R, Baron JC, MacKenzie ET. Evaluation of the ratio of cerebral blood flow to cerebral blood volume as an index of local cerebral perfusion pressure. Brain 1998;121(Pt 7):1369–1379
15. Baron JC, Bousser MG, Rey A, Guillard A, Comar D, Castaigne P. Reversal of focal "misery-perfusion syndrome" by extra-intracranial arterial bypass in hemodynamic cerebral ischemia. A case study with 15O positron emission tomography. Stroke 1981;12(4):454–459
16. van Everdingen KJ, Visser GH, Klijn CJ, Kappelle LJ, van der Grond J. Role of collateral flow on cerebral hemodynamics in patients with unilateral internal carotid artery occlusion. Ann Neurol 1998;44(2):167–176
17. Levine RL, Lagreze HL, Dobkin JA, et al. Cerebral vasocapacitance and TIAs. Neurology 1989;39(1):25–29
18. Waterston JA, Brown MM, Butler P, Swash M. Small deep cerebral infarcts associated with occlusive internal carotid artery disease. A hemodynamic phenomenon? Arch Neurol 1990;47(9):953–957
19. Derdeyn CP, Khosla A, Videen TO, et al. Severe hemodynamic impairment and border zone—region infarction. Radiology 2001;220(1):195–201
20. Feeney DM, Baron JC. Diaschisis. Stroke 1986;17(5):817–830
21. Powers WJ. Cerebral hemodynamics in ischemic cerebrovascular disease. Ann Neurol 1991;29(3):231–240
22. Derdeyn CP, Grubb RL Jr, Powers WJ. Cerebral hemodynamic impairment: methods of measurement and association with stroke risk. Neurology 1999;53(2):251–259

23. Mikulis DJ, Krolczyk G, Desal H, et al. Preoperative and postoperative mapping of cerebrovascular reactivity in moyamoya disease by using blood oxygen level-dependent magnetic resonance imaging. J Neurosurg 2005;103(2):347–355

24. Hartmann A, Dettmers C, Schuier FJ, Wassmann HD, Schumacher HW. Effect of stable xenon on regional cerebral blood flow and the electroencephalogram in normal volunteers. Stroke 1991;22(2):182–189

25. Tomita M. Significance of cerebral blood volume. In: Tomita M, Sawada T, Naritomi H, Heiss W-D, editors. Cerebral hyperemia and ischemia: From the standpoint of cerebral blood volume. Amsterdam: Elsevier Science Publishers; 1988.

26. Ferrari M, Wilson DA, Hanley DF, Traystman RJ. Effects of graded hypotension on cerebral blood flow, blood volume, and mean transit time in dogs. Am J Physiol 1992;262(6 Pt 2):H1908–H1914

27. Zaharchuk G, Mandeville JB, Bogdanov AA Jr, Weissleder R, Rosen BR, Marota JJ. Cerebrovascular dynamics of autoregulation and hypoperfusion. An MRI study of CBF and changes in total and microvascular cerebral blood volume during hemorrhagic hypotension. Stroke 1999;30(10):2197–2204, discussion 2204–2205

28. Derdeyn CP, Videen TO, Yundt KD, et al. Variability of cerebral blood volume and oxygen extraction: stages of cerebral haemodynamic impairment revisited. Brain 2002;125(Pt 3):595–607

29. Calamante F, Ganesan V, Kirkham FJ, et al. MR perfusion imaging in Moyamoya Syndrome: potential implications for clinical evaluation of occlusive cerebrovascular disease. Stroke 2001;32(12):2810–2816

30. An H, Lin W. Cerebral oxygen extraction fraction and cerebral venous blood volume measurements using MRI: effects of magnetic field variation. Magn Reson Med 2002;47(5):958–966

31. Lee M, Zaharchuk G, Guzman R, Achrol A, Bell-Stephens T, Steinberg GK. Quantitative hemodynamic studies in moyamoya disease: a review. Neurosurg Focus 2009;26(4):E5

32. Kang KH, Kim HS, Kim SY. Quantitative cerebrovascular reserve measured by acetazolamide-challenged dynamic CT perfusion in ischemic adult Moyamoya disease: initial experience with angiographic correlation. AJNR Am J Neuroradiol 2008;29(8):1487–1493

6

Worldwide Epidemiology of Moyamoya Disease

Norberto Andaluz and Mario Zuccarello

◆ Introduction

Spontaneous occlusion of the circle of Willis, also known as moyamoya disease, is a rare cerebrovascular disorder of unknown etiology with a progressive clinical course. The Japanese term "moyamoya" means puffy, hazy, obscure, or vague, and best describes the abnormal vascular network at the base of the brain as typically depicted on cerebral angiography. First reported in 1961 in Japan,[1,2] where it is most prevalent, patterns of distribution of age at onset show two peaks. A higher peak of incidence at 5 years of age and a lower peak at 30 to 49 years of age are used to classify moyamoya disease into two types: the juvenile and adult types, respectively. The pathophysiology of the juvenile type is cerebral ischemia from the progressive steno-occlusive changes that occur at the circle of Willis, and that of the adult type is cerebral hemorrhage as the result of breakdown of collateral vessels formed at a younger age. A total of 10 to 15% of cases of moyamoya disease are familial.[3,4]

◆ Worldwide Epidemiology of Moyamoya Disease

The incidence of moyamoya disease is high in countries in eastern Asia, such as Japan and Korea.[5] In Japan, a nationwide survey conducted in 1994 estimated the total number of patients treated for moyamoya disease at 3,900, with prevalence and incidence rates of 3.16/100,000 and 0.35/100,000, respectively.[6] The female-to-male ratio was 1.8:1, and 10% of patients had a family history of the disease. A more recent survey from 2003 shows a dramatic increase in the number of patients treated for moyamoya disease in Japan. An estimated 7,700 cases represented an almost 100% increase relative to the 3,900 patients reported in 1994. The female-to-male ratio remained at 1.8:1, and 12.1% of patients had a positive family history of moyamoya disease. The prevalence was estimated at 6.03/100,000, and the incidence of newly diagnosed cases was 0.54/100,000.[7] Furthermore, an analysis of the regional all-inclusive epidemiological data performed in 2008 in Hokkaido, a major island of Japan with a population of 5.63 million at the time of the study, reported the prevalence and incidence at 10.5/100,000 and 0.94/100,000, respectively—both of which largely exceeded the results of previous surveys. The female-to-male ratio was 2.18:1. Age at onset occurred in two peaks: the highest was observed between 45 and 49 years old, and the second occurred between 5 and 9 years old. A family history was observed in 15.4% of patients.[8]

Although these epidemiological findings show significant differences compared with previous studies, several explanations for these discrepancies were theorized. First, the survey methods were different from previous reports. The previous studies were based on data obtained from surveys in large hospitals, whereas the Hokkaido study included all patients diagnosed with moyamoya disease in the region. Second, the widespread use of magnetic resonance imaging in more recent years is likely to have improved the diagnosis of asymptomatic patients. Finally, a gradual change of epidemiological features was proposed. Although the reasons are unclear, the incidence of pediatric moyamoya disease seems to have started to decrease.[5] Nevertheless, moyamoya disease remains the most common pediatric cerebrovascular disorder in Japan, with a prevalence of 3/100,000 children.[6–9]

To date, only Japan and the Republic of Korea have conducted large-scale, nationwide surveys of moyamoya disease.[6–8,10] The Korean cooperative study from 2000 reported 334 patients with definite moyamoya disease diagnosed before 1995. In this study, epidemiological and clinical features essentially resembled those of the Japanese population.[10,11] In contrast, the clinical features of moyamoya disease in China differ somewhat from those in other Asian countries.[12] Although the age distribution among Chinese patients is similar to that of Japanese and Korean patients, the Chinese exhibited a male preponderance over females (1.16:1), and the incidence of moyamoya disease in adults is higher than that of children (3.5:1). A more recent survey identified 202 patients with moyamoya disease in the Nanjing provincial capital of China.[13] Results showed an equal incidence in male and female patients, and a higher incidence in adults than in children. The overall prevalence in that study, estimated at 3.92/100,000, was lower than the 6.03/100,000 found in Japan, but it was similar to that reported in Taiwan.[14]

This ethnicity pattern suggests that a genetic predisposition may be involved. A notable phenomenon observed in this study was a higher percentage of hemorrhage than ischemia; hemorrhage was more common in males aged 35 to 45 years than in females in this age range. The percentage of asymptomatic patients in this study was low, although the authors recognized that economic limitations preclude the widespread use of magnetic resonance imaging and digital subtraction angiography in this large population. Finally, the familial

occurrence of moyamoya disease was only 1.48%.[13] These findings further support the theory that genetic factors may play a role in the differences in the incidence of moyamoya disease.

Originally considered to affect predominantly persons of Asian heritage, moyamoya disease has now been observed throughout the world in people of many ethnic backgrounds, including American and European populations. A survey of the literature published between 1972 and 1989 found 1,053 cases reported outside Japan, including 625 cases in Asia, 201 in Europe, 176 in North and South America, 52 in Africa, and 9 in Oceania.[15] Unfortunately, this study included not only cases of moyamoya disease, but also those of "moyamoya phenomenon," and a true estimate of moyamoya disease could not be established.

Moyamoya disease is extremely uncommon in non-Asian populations. Limited data about Caucasian patients also suggest noticeable differences in terms of clinical presentation and course of the disease. A survey of high-volume neurovascular centers across the United States recently found that 72% of respondents evaluated fewer than 10 adults during the 12 months preceding the survey, and that only two centers (6%) evaluated more than 30 patients during the same period.[16] Another survey in the states of Washington and California reported an annual incidence of 0.086/100,000.[17] In this survey, ethnicity-specific incidences were highest among individuals of Asian-American heritage (0.28/100,000), followed by African Americans (0.13/100,000), Caucasians (0.06/100,000), and Hispanics (0.03/100,000). These findings seem to indicate that ethnic differences in the incidence of moyamoya disease appear to remain unchanged after immigration to the United States.

Several differences between moyamoya disease in the United States and eastern Asian countries have been noted. Cases in the United States show the following features: (1) a preponderance of ischemic over hemorrhagic stroke in adults, with only 20.5% of adults presenting with hemorrhagic stroke; (2) the absence of a peak in incidence in childhood years; (3) a more pronounced female predominance than in Asian countries, representing a 2.7:1 female-to-male ratio; and (4) a remarkably high rate of recurrent stroke in the first few

Table 6.1 Main Differences in Worldwide Distribution of Moyamoya Disease

	Japanese Patients	Chinese Patients	Western Patients
Prevalence	6–10/100,000	4/100,000	0.1/100,000
Female:male ratio	1.8:1	1:1.6	2.7:1
Bimodal age presentation	Yes	No	No
Frequency	More common in children than adults	More common in adults than children	More common in adults than children
Presentation in children	Ischemic stroke	Infrequent, ischemic stroke	Rare, ischemic stroke
Presentation in adults	Hemorrhagic stroke	High chance of hemorrhagic stroke	High chance of ischemic stroke; high chance of recurrence
Familial cases	10–15%	1.5%	6%

years after presentation. In medically treated symptomatic hemispheres, the 5-year risk of recurrent ipsilateral stroke was 65% after the initial presentation and 27% after angiographic diagnosis.[18–20]

The epidemiological setting in Europe, where the estimated incidence is reported to represent 10% that of Japan, has proven to be similar to that in the United States. In 2008, a detailed analysis of demographic and clinical data of white Europeans with moyamoya disease presented the following highlights: (1) older age at onset, with a median age of 34 years; (2) absence of an age distribution peak in childhood; (3) rarity of hemorrhagic stroke, with an incidence of 5%; (4) high risk of recurrence of ischemic stroke after the onset of symptoms, with a 61.9% recurrence at 1 year; and (5) a high risk of perioperative stroke, estimated at 27.3%.[21–23] **Table 6.1** summarizes the main differences in worldwide distribution of moyamoya disease.

Although the cause and pathogenesis of moyamoya disease are poorly understood, it is evident, based on the ethnic and familial penetration of the disease, that genetic factors play a major role. The familial incidence of affected first-degree relatives in Japan is 10 to 15% and that in the United States has been reported at 6%.[4–8,24,25] Associations with loci in chromosomes 3, 6, 8, and 17 as well as specific human leukocyte antigen haplotypes have been described.[26–31] The coincidence of mutations in the vascular smooth muscle cell–specific isoform of α-actin (ACTA-2) with thoracic aortic aneurysms and dissections and moyamoya disease was reported in patients of northern European descent with a positive family history of the two conditions.[32]

Epidemiological analyses have shown distinctive features of familial moyamoya disease: (1) a female-to male ratio of 5:1, as opposed to 1.6:1 in sporadic cases; (2) a younger mean age at onset, 11.8 in familial versus 30 years in sporadic cases; and (3) a strong association with anticipation in familial moyamoya disease.[5] In a report of eight parent-offspring pairs, all were mother-offspring pairs. The parents presented with symptoms of moyamoya disease between 22 and 36 years of age, whereas their offspring presented with symptoms between 5 and 11 years of age.[5] However, despite evidence strongly suggesting a genetic basis of moyamoya disease, significant questions remain.[3] Identical twins with only one affected sibling suffering from moyamoya disease have been reported.[33] This fact may support the concept that environmental factors may precipitate the development of the disease in genetically susceptible patients.

◆ Conclusion

Moyamoya disease is a rare condition with a proteiform presentation that affects all individuals, regardless of age, ethnicity, and gender. However, clear epidemiological differences have been identified among different populations, as summarized previously. At present, it is unclear whether Asians and Caucasians develop an identical form of moyamoya disease. Further research is required to better understand the pathophysiology and the multiple forms of presentation of this disease in hosts with differing genetic and environmental characteristics.

References

1. Takeuchi K, Shimizu K. Hypoplasia of the bilateral internal carotid arteries. Brain Nerve 1957;9:37–43
2. Suzuki J, Takaku A. Cerebrovascular "moyamoya" disease. Disease showing abnormal net-like vessels in base of brain. Arch Neurol 1969;20(3):288–299
3. Smith ER, Scott RM. Moyamoya: epidemiology, presentation, and diagnosis. Neurosurg Clin N Am 2010; 21(3):543–551
4. Takahashi JC, Miyamoto S. Moyamoya disease: recent progress and outlook. Neurol Med Chir (Tokyo) 2010; 50(9):824–832
5. Kuroda S, Houkin K. Moyamoya disease: current concepts and future perspectives. Lancet Neurol 2008; 7(11):1056–1066
6. Wakai K, Tamakoshi A, Ikezaki K, et al. Epidemiological features of moyamoya disease in Japan: findings from a nationwide survey. Clin Neurol Neurosurg 1997;99(Suppl 2):S1–S5
7. Kuriyama S, Kusaka Y, Fujimura M, et al. Prevalence and clinicoepidemiological features of moyamoya disease in Japan: findings from a nationwide epidemiological survey. Stroke 2008;39(1):42–47
8. Baba T, Houkin K, Kuroda S. Novel epidemiological features of moyamoya disease. J Neurol Neurosurg Psychiatry 2008;79(8):900–904
9. Nagaraja D, Verma A, Taly AB, Kumar MV, Jayakumar PN. Cerebrovascular disease in children. Acta Neurol Scand 1994;90(4):251–255
10. Han DH, Kwon OK, Byun BJ, et al; Korean Society for Cerebrovascular Disease. A co-operative study: clinical characteristics of 334 Korean patients with moyamoya disease treated at neurosurgical institutes (1976–1994). Acta Neurochir (Wien) 2000;142(11): 1263–1273, discussion 1273–1274
11. Ikezaki K, Han DH, Kawano T, Kinukawa N, Fukui M. A clinical comparison of definite moyamoya disease between South Korea and Japan. Stroke 1997; 28(12):2513–2517
12. Matsushima Y, Qian L, Aoyagi M. Comparison of moyamoya disease in Japan and moyamoya disease (or syndrome) in the People's Republic of China. Clin Neurol Neurosurg 1997;99(Suppl 2):S19–S22
13. Miao W, Zhao PL, Zhang YS, et al. Epidemiological and clinical features of Moyamoya disease in Nanjing, China. Clin Neurol Neurosurg 2010;112(3):199–203
14. Hung CC, Tu YK, Su CF, Lin LS, Shih CJ. Epidemiological study of moyamoya disease in Taiwan. Clin Neurol Neurosurg 1997;99(Suppl 2):S23–S25
15. Goto Y, Yonekawa Y. Worldwide distribution of moyamoya disease. Neurol Med Chir (Tokyo) 1992; 32(12):883–886
16. Andaluz N, Choutka O, Zuccarello M. Trends in the management of adult moyamoya disease in the United States: results of a nationwide survey. World Neurosurg 2010;73(4):361–364
17. Uchino K, Johnston SC, Becker KJ, Tirschwell DL. Moyamoya disease in Washington State and California. Neurology 2005;65(6):956–958
18. Chiu D, Shedden P, Bratina P, Grotta JC. Clinical features of moyamoya disease in the United States. Stroke 1998;29(7):1347–1351
19. Hallemeier CL, Rich KM, Grubb RL Jr, et al. Clinical features and outcome in North American adults with moyamoya phenomenon. Stroke 2006;37(6): 1490–1496
20. Numaguchi Y, Gonzalez CF, Davis PC, et al. Moyamoya disease in the United States. Clin Neurol Neurosurg 1997;99(Suppl 2):S26–S30
21. Kraemer M, Heienbrok W, Berlit P. Moyamoya disease in Europeans. Stroke 2008;39(12):3193–3200
22. Khan N, Yonekawa Y. Moyamoya angiopathy in Europe. Acta Neurochir Suppl (Wien) 2005;94:149–152
23. Yonekawa Y, Ogata N, Kaku Y, Taub E, Imhof HG. Moyamoya disease in Europe, past and present status. Clin Neurol Neurosurg 1997;99(Suppl 2):S58–S60
24. Scott RM, Smith JL, Robertson RL et al. Long-term outcome in children with moyamoya syndrome after cranial revascularization by pial synangiosis. J Neurosurg 2004 February;100(2 Suppl Pediatrics):142–9
25. Fukui M, Kono S, Sueishi K, Ikezaki K. Moyamoya disease. Neuropathology 2000;20(Suppl):S61–S64
26. Ikeda H, Sasaki T, Yoshimoto T, Fukui M, Arinami T. Mapping of a familial moyamoya disease gene to chromosome 3p24.2–p26. Am J Hum Genet 1999; 64(2):533–537
27. Nanba R, Tada M, Kuroda S, Houkin K, Iwasaki Y. Sequence analysis and bioinformatics analysis of chromosome 17q25 in familial moyamoya disease. Childs Nerv Syst 2005;21(1):62–68
28. Inoue TK, Ikezaki K, Sasazuki T, Matsushima T, Fukui M. Linkage analysis of moyamoya disease on chromosome 6. J Child Neurol 2000;15(3):179–182
29. Inoue TK, Ikezaki K, Sasazuki T, Matsushima T, Fukui M. Analysis of class II genes of human leukocyte antigen in patients with moyamoya disease. Clin Neurol Neurosurg 1997;99(Suppl 2):S234–S237
30. Han H, Pyo CW, Yoo DS, Huh PW, Cho KS, Kim DS. Associations of Moyamoya patients with HLA class I and class II alleles in the Korean population. J Korean Med Sci 2003;18(6):876–880
31. Sakurai K, Horiuchi Y, Ikeda H, et al. A novel susceptibility locus for moyamoya disease on chromosome 8q23. J Hum Genet 2004;49(5):278–281
32. Roder C, Peters V, Kasuya H, et al. Analysis of ACTA2 in European Moyamoya disease patients. Eur J Paediatr Neurol 2011;15(2):117–122
33. Tanghetti B, Capra R, Giunta F, Marini G, Orlandini A. Moyamoya syndrome in only one of two identical twins. Case report. J Neurosurg 1983;59(6): 1092–1094

7

Implications of Cortical Microvasculature in Adult Moyamoya Disease

Marcus Czabanka and Peter Vajkoczy

◆ Introduction

Moyamoya angiopathy refers to bilateral steno-occlusive lesions of the basal cerebral arteries leading to chronic cerebrovascular hemodynamic impairment and subsequent ischemia.[1,2] Patients also may become symptomatic with intracranial hemorrhage.[1] Just as contradictory as the clinical manifestations of the disease is the predominating pathophysiology. The metaphor "moyamoya" describes the typical cloudy appearance of the angiographic picture, which is caused by the presence of small moyamoya vessels that arise from the base of the brain and are known as potential compensation routes.[1,3] Moyamoya disease combines two pathophysiologies: progressive vascular occlusive disease leading to cerebral ischemia paralleled by a disease-specific proarteriogenic mechanism that causes diverse intracranial-to-intracranial as well as extracranial-to-intracranial collaterals.[1,4]

Surgical revascularization represents the most efficient therapy for patients with moyamoya and neurological symptoms.[1,5] During surgery, one of the most impressive observations is the reddish appearance of the brain of patients with moyamoya disease. This observation led Takeuchi et al to investigate this phenomenon and to analyze cortical vasculature.[6] They postulated an increased number of leptomeningeal anastomoses and dilated pial arteries in patients with moyamoya disease, which in turn lead to the highly vascularized "reddish" appearance of the cortex (**Fig. 7.1**).[6]

◆ Cerebral Blood Flow, Perfusion Patterns, and Clinical Presentation

In moyamoya disease, the reddish appearance of the cerebral cortex, a result of an increased number of cortical vessels, questions the role of cortical vascularization as a potential compensation route for the decreased cerebral blood flow associated with the disease. Indeed, assessment of cerebral blood flow is one of the common diagnostic tests used in patients with moyamoya disease.

Besides digital subtraction angiography, cerebral perfusion is a key parameter that can help guide treatment decisions, the most important aspect of which is cerebrovascular reserve capacity (CVRC).[7,8] Surgical revascularization is a promising strategy to restore CVRC in patients with cerebrovascular disease.[7] Different techniques are available to assess CVRC. The most important techniques are xenon computed tomography (CT) and positron emission tomography (PET). Xenon CT has been the workhorse for measuring and quantifying regional cerebral blood flow in patients with moyamoya disease. Reduced CVRC, as assessed

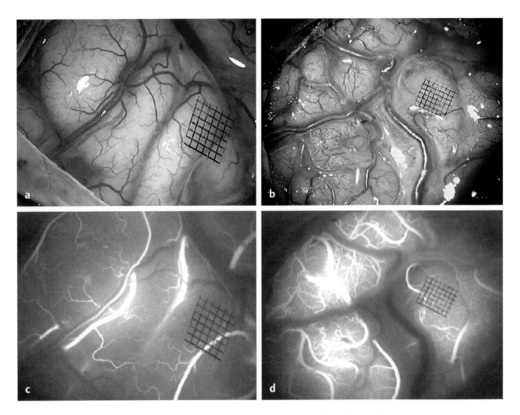

Fig. 7.1a–d (**a**) Intraoperative image of cortical surface (territory of middle cerebral artery) during revascularization surgery (directly after the dura mater was opened) in a patient suffering from atherosclerotic cerebrovascular disease associated with significant hemodynamic compromise. The millimeter grid was placed intraoperatively for postoperative analysis. Cortical microvascularization does not show increased cortical vascular density, and the color of the cortex is normal. (**b**) Intraoperative image of cortical surface (vascular territory of middle cerebral artery) during revascularization surgery (directly after the dura mater was opened) in a patient with moyamoya disease. The millimeter grid was placed for postoperative analysis. Note the reddish appearance of the cortical surface related to increased cortical vascularization in comparison to Fig. 7.1a. (**c**) Intraoperative indocyanine green (ICG) videoangiography corresponding to the operative view shown in Fig. 7.1a showing visualization of cortical vascularization during the arterial phase in the same patient as shown in Fig. 7.1a. As shown, cortical vascularization in the middle cerebral artery territory is not increased despite significant hemodynamic compromise. (**d**) Intraoperative ICG videoangiography corresponding to the operative view shown in Fig. 7.1b showing visualization of cortical vascularization in the vascular territory of the middle cerebral artery during the arterial phase in the same patient as shown in Fig. 7.1b. Note the increased fluorescence signal, which reflects an increase in cortical microvessels compared with Fig. 7.1c.

by xenon CT, is a predictor of stroke in patients with occlusive cerebrovascular disease.[9] PET studies identifying misery perfusion (i.e., reduced CVRC and increased oxygen extraction fraction from the blood) correlate with an increased risk of stroke after carotid occlusion.[9] Nevertheless, other techniques such as Doppler ultrasonography and magnetic resonance imaging–based techniques contribute to the assessment of CVRC in patients with moyamoya disease.

Recent insights into the pathophysiology of moyamoya disease show that CVRC is not the single deciding parameter for predicting clinical symptoms. We found no difference in CVRC between 13 symptomatic and asymptomatic patients with moyamoya disease.[10] When xenon CT was used to analyze CVRC according to specific cerebral hemisphere, CVRC below -5% represented an independent factor for identifying a hemisphere affected by moyamoya disease as symptomatic or asymptomatic.[11] However, receiver operating characteristic analysis showed that its predictive value for clinical symptoms is comparable or even slightly inferior to that of magnetic resonance imaging or digital subtraction angiography.[11] Therefore, the clinical decision to treat patients with moyamoya disease may not be based on cerebral perfusion characteristics such as CVRC alone.

The reduction of CVRC in moyamoya disease and its influence on the clinical course of the disease are complex pathophysiological phenomena governed by the reduction of cerebral blood flow in response to the typical steno-occlusive lesions and a variety of different compensation mechanisms that are not fully understood.[12] For example, the angiographic picture of the disease does not provide functional information about the reduction of cerebral blood flow.[9] In turn, the maximum reduction of CVRC may occur in a vascular territory that does not show the most prominent occlusion on digital subtraction angiography.[11] Consequently, functional perfusion patterns must not correlate with angiographic findings and they do not reliably allow estimation of clinical symptoms.[11] The individual availability and effectiveness of different cerebral compensation mechanisms in moyamoya disease might be responsible for this complex relationship. The role of cortical vascularization is unknown partly because cortical vascularization is seldom visualized in clinical diagnostic images in detail. Therefore, cortical vascularization might represent a clinically relevant, but so far unknown compensation route in moyamoya disease.

◆ Analysis of Cortical Microvasculature using Indocyanine Green Fluorescence

In 1984, Takeuchi et al showed that cortical vascularization is significantly altered in moyamoya disease[6] when they found an increased number and diameter of cortical vessels in patients with moyamoya disease.[6] With the introduction of intraoperative indocyanine green (ICG) videoangiography, visualization and investigation of cortical vascularization have become possible.[13] During surgery, the ICG dye is injected intravenously and later can be detected by a microscope incorporating a fluorescence detection camera. Using a computer-based analysis system used for experimental microvascular analysis, morphological and functional vascular parameters can be detected.[4]

For analysis of cortical vascularization using ICG videoangiography, arterial and venous macrovascularization as well as cortical microvascularization can be characterized according to functional aspects of ICG angiography. The early filling arteries (A1) and their direct branches (A2) and the last draining veins (V1) and their direct branches (V2) are referred to as cortical macrovascularization.[4] All vessels appearing between A2 and V2 vessels are regarded as cortical microvascularization (**Fig. 7.2**).[4]

Microvascularization was quantified postoperatively using a computer-assisted analysis system (CAPIMAGE, Zeintl Software Engineering, Heidelberg, Germany).[4] Microvascular density (MD) is calculated by measuring the ratio between the length of all microvessels in a predefined region of interest (cm/cm^2). Furthermore, microvascular diameter (D) is analyzed, and microvascular surface (MVS) per analyzed region of interest is calculated based on following formula: $MVS = \pi * D/2 * MD$.[4]

◆ Microhemodynamic Analysis of Cortical Microvascularization

Microhemodynamic analysis using ICG videoangiography can be performed using a computer-based analysis software (IC-CALC 1.1 software, Pulsion Medical Systems, Munich, Germany). This software allows specific and time-dependent functional analysis of the intensity of fluorescence in regions of interest that can be defined by the user.[4] Cortical microhemodynamic fluorescence intensity was evaluated in three distinct compartments in a time-dependent manner: the arterial compartment (A2 vessels), capillary compartment (brain parenchyma), and venous compartment (V2 vessels).[4] By comparing time points of peak fluorescence intensity in the arterial (A2 vessel) and venous (V2 vessel) compartments, the transit time for the fluorescent dye to pass through the microvasculature can be assessed (**Fig. 7.2**).[4] This time was defined as the microvascular

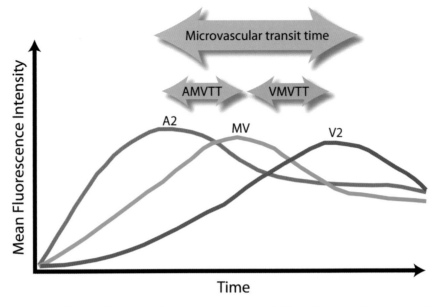

Fig. 7.2 Schematic illustration of analysis protocol and definitions. The graph demonstrates the fluorescence curves for regions of interest placed in the arterial compartment (*A2* vessels), the microvascular compartments (MV), and the venous compartment (*V2* vessels). Time difference between maximum fluorescence intensity in the arterial and venous compartment reflects microvascular transit time. The time difference between maximum fluorescence intensity in the arterial and microvascular segment represents arterial microvascular transit time (AMVTT). The time difference between maximum fluorescence intensity in the microvascular and venous segment represents venous microvascular transit time (VMVTT).

transit time (see **Fig. 7.2**).[4] Furthermore, the time difference of the peak fluorescence intensity between the arterial (A2 vessel) and capillary compartment was analyzed. This time was defined as arterial microvascular transit time. According to this procedure, venous microvascular transit time was defined as the time difference between the capillary and venous (V2 vessel) compartment.

◆ Cortical Microvasculature Compensates for Reduced Cerebral Blood Flow

Cortical microvasculature is an important regulator of cerebral perfusion. More than half of the total cerebrovascular resistance is located in the extraparenchymal vessel segments.[14] In moyamoya disease, the vascular density of cortical microvasculature is significantly higher compared with that of hemodynamically healthy patients.[4] Increased microvascular density is accompanied by an increased diameter and microvascular surface area.[4] Although these observations may be pure responses to chronic hemodynamic cerebrovascular impairment, patients suffering from atherosclerotic occlusive cerebrovascular disease with hemodynamic compromise comparable to that observed in moyamoya disease do not demonstrate comparable microvascular characteristics (see **Fig. 7.1**).[4] Therefore, increased cortical microvascular density, diameter, and microvascular surface area represent moyamoya-specific phenomena that may be associated with proarteriogenic mechanisms observed in this disease.

Although these anatomic observations demonstrate morphological criteria, the function of these vessels is also different. Microvascular transit time was significantly increased in the arterial microvascular compartment of patients with moyamoya disease compared with patients suffering from atherosclerosis.[4] That is, the fluorescent dye traveled at a slower rate through the arterial microvascular segment in

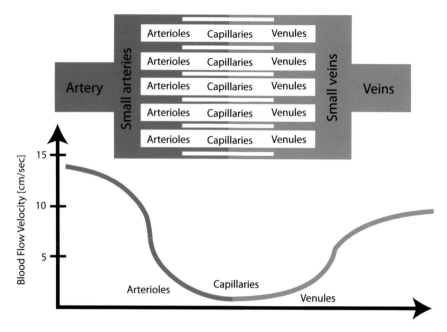

Fig. 7.3 Schematic illustration of the physiology among vascular segments, resistance, and corresponding velocity of blood flow. As vascular density and vascular surface area increase, a declining vascular resistance leads to a reduction in the velocity of blood flow in the corresponding vascular segment. Arterioles represent the resistance-controlling vascular segments.

patients with moyamoya disease. According to physiological concepts, this finding translates into significantly reduced microvascular blood flow velocity and consequently into reduced vascular resistance in the arterial microvascular segment in patients with moyamoya disease (**Fig. 7.3**). Arterioles represent the resistance-controlling vascular segment. Therefore, this observation might represent a potential mechanism in moyamoya disease leading to reduced microvascular resistance to maintain cortical blood flow in the presence of proximal steno-occlusion in the large basal arteries.[4]

◆ Clinical Role of Cortical Microvasculature as a Compensation Mechanism for Reduced Cerebral Blood Flow

The clinical relevance of cortical microvasculature and its effects on compensatory cerebral blood flow remain elusive. Currently, we can only rely on the data obtained from 13 patients with moyamoya disease who underwent detailed analysis of their cortical microvasculature. When cortical microvascular density was analyzed in terms of clinical symptoms, asymptomatic patients demonstrated higher cortical microvascular density and significantly increased arterial microvascular transit time than symptomatic patients.[10] This observation does not represent a causal relationship, but it provides preliminary evidence that cortical microvascular density might represent a potential clinically relevant mechanism for compensating for reduced cerebral blood flow. Obviously, patients with moyamoya disease characterized by a strong arteriogenic potential for altered cortical vascularization (i.e., increased cortical microvascular density) demonstrate improved cerebrovascular hemodynamics and fewer clinical symptoms.[10] Furthermore, there is a positive correlation between cortical microvascular density (as measured by intraoperative ICG videoangiography) and hemodynamic compromise (i.e., CVRC) assessed via xenon-enhanced CT.[10] This correlation between hemodynamic impairment and cortical microvascular density underlines the potential compensatory role of cerebral microvascularization in moyamoya disease. Further studies detailing this relationship are needed to characterize the clinical significance of cortical microvascular compensatory mechanisms in patients with moyamoya disease.

◆ Conclusion

Patients with moyamoya disease are characterized by significantly altered cortical vascularization, which might contribute to the compensation process for reduced cerebral blood flow by reducing the vascular resistance of cortical arteries.

References

1. Kuroda S, Houkin K. Moyamoya disease: current concepts and future perspectives. Lancet Neurol 2008; 7(11):1056–1066
2. Suzuki J, Takaku A. Cerebrovascular "moyamoya" disease. Disease showing abnormal net-like vessels in base of brain. Arch Neurol 1969;20(3):288–299
3. Yamauchi H, Kudoh T, Sugimoto K, Takahashi M, Kishibe Y, Okazawa H. Pattern of collaterals, type of infarcts, and haemodynamic impairment in carotid artery occlusion. J Neurol Neurosurg Psychiatry 2004; 75(12):1697–1701
4. Czabanka M, Peña-Tapia P, Schubert GA, Woitzik J, Vajkoczy P, Schmiedek P. Characterization of cortical microvascularization in adult moyamoya disease. Stroke 2008;39(6):1703–1709
5. Burke GM, Burke AM, Sherma AK, Hurley MC, Batjer HH, Bendok BR. Moyamoya disease: a summary. Neurosurg Focus 2009;26(4):E11
6. Takeuchi S, Ishii R, Tsuchida T, Tanaka R, Kobayashi K, Ito J. Cerebral hemodynamics in patients with moyamoya disease. A study of the epicerebral microcirculation by fluorescein angiography. Surg Neurol 1984; 21(4):333–340
7. Schmiedek P, Piepgras A, Leinsinger G, Kirsch CM, Einhäupl K. Improvement of cerebrovascular reserve capacity by EC-IC arterial bypass surgery in patients with ICA occlusion and hemodynamic cerebral ischemia. J Neurosurg 1994;81(2):236–244
8. Yonas H, Smith HA, Durham SR, Pentheny SL, Johnson DW. Increased stroke risk predicted by compromised cerebral blood flow reactivity. J Neurosurg 1993; 79(4):483–489
9. Lee M, Zaharchuk G, Guzman R, Achrol A, Bell-Stephens T, Steinberg GK. Quantitative hemodynamic studies in moyamoya disease: a review. Neurosurg Focus 2009;26(4):E5
10. Czabanka M, Peña-Tapia P, Schubert GA, et al. Clinical implications of cortical microvasculature in adult Moyamoya disease. J Cereb Blood Flow Metab 2009; 29(8):1383–1387
11. Czabanka M, Peña-Tapia P, Schubert GA, et al. Proposal for a new grading of Moyamoya disease in adult patients. Cerebrovasc Dis 2011;32(1):41–50
12. Vajkoczy P. Moyamoya disease: collateralization is everything. Cerebrovasc Dis 2009;28(3):258
13. Woitzik J, Peña-Tapia PG, Schneider UC, Vajkoczy P, Thomé C. Cortical perfusion measurement by indocyanine-green videoangiography in patients undergoing hemicraniectomy for malignant stroke. Stroke 2006;37(6):1549–1551
14. Baumbach GL, Heistad DD. Regional, segmental, and temporal heterogeneity of cerebral vascular autoregulation. Ann Biomed Eng 1985;13(3-4):303–310

8

Neuropsychological Considerations in the Assessment of Children and Adults with Moyamoya Disease

Jeannine V. Morrone-Strupinsky and George P. Prigatano

◆ Introduction

Moyamoya disease is a rare condition that results in occlusion of the cerebrovasculature, particularly of the internal carotid arteries.[1] Vessels distal to the blockage then expand, particularly in the deep watershed territory of the white matter. On angiography, the disease creates the appearance of a "puff of smoke." The finding is typically bilateral, although one hemisphere can show greater severity of disease than the other.[2] The initial symptoms can result from ischemia (i.e., stroke, transient ischemic attack, seizure) or from the expansion of vessels distal to the blockage (i.e., hemorrhage, headache).[2] Ischemia typically occurs in regions of the brain supplied by the internal carotid arteries and the middle cerebral arteries (MCAs) (i.e., frontal, parietal, and portions of the temporal lobes). After a stroke, lesions are most commonly found in the frontal lobes in both children and adults.[3] The peak for the onset of symptoms is bimodal: during early childhood (approximately age 5) and middle adulthood (mid-40s).[2] Rates of hemorrhage are much higher in adults (20%) than in children.[2] The ratio of females-to-males with moyamoya disease is 1-to-1 during young childhood, but changes to 3-to-1 starting in the second decade of life.[4] Genetic factors can contribute to moyamoya disease, but the disease also can develop secondary to other conditions, such as sickle cell disease.[5] This chapter focuses on primary moyamoya disease, although some group studies reviewed included participants with moyamoya disease related to both types of origins.

◆ Neurocognitive Changes in Adults with Moyamoya Disease

Because moyamoya disease is a rare condition, there are few group studies, particularly those assessing functional outcomes. Even fewer studies include a neuropsychological component. Most of the literature consists of case studies. Moreover, few studies have examined the natural course of moyamoya disease in the absence of surgery. In the event of stroke, it is difficult to isolate the effects of moyamoya disease, per se, on cognitive functioning. Based on a PubMed search covering the years 1980 to 2010, we found 14 papers using the search terms *moyamoya* and *cognition*, 26 papers using the search terms *moyamoya* and *cognitive*, and 23 papers using the search terms *moyamoya* and *neuropsychological*.

◆ Case Reports

Case reports illustrate that moyamoya disease can have deleterious effects on both cognition and mood. Schwarz et al[5] presented a 25-year-old woman with moyamoya disease and depression who had sustained an ischemic stroke at the age of 15 years. She had cognitive sequelae and continued to experience chronic headaches. Magnetic resonance imaging (MRI) of the brain showed microangiopathic changes and an old infarct involving the head of the caudate. Regions of hyperintense signal were present in the periventricular area and scattered through the deep white matter (significantly advanced for age). Based on a neuropsychological assessment, her intellectual functioning was below average, as was her performance in most other areas. She had noteworthy deficits in executive functioning (i.e., verbal abstraction, inhibition, and problem solving).

Lubman et al[6] presented a young man with a 2-year history of paranoid schizophrenia, who subsequently was incidentally diagnosed with moyamoya disease. Neuropsychological evaluation revealed significant executive dysfunction (high-level attention, reasoning, problem solving, and difficulty organizing information during an encoding task). These findings were considered to reflect the interaction of the two conditions.

More unusual neurological sequelae have been reported in other case studies. Rabbani et al[7] presented a young woman with bilateral moyamoya disease who developed enhancing lesions in the anterior midbody, splenium (left worse than right), and rostrum and posterior midbody of the corpus callosum. She demonstrated signs of callosal disconnection (i.e., unilateral tactile anomia and ideomotor apraxia), intermanual conflict, and alien limb features. Anjaneyulu and Bhaskar[8] reported a case of cortical blindness as a rare presentation of moyamoya disease. Hayashi et al[9] presented a 52-year-old woman who sustained a right frontal lobe infarction, and cerebral angiography revealed moyamoya vessels. The woman exhibited geographical mislocation, person misidentification, and fantastic confabulation, which persisted for 1.5 months and gradually resolved. Neuropsychological examination revealed memory impairment and frontal lobe dysfunction.

Moore et al[10] studied neurorehabilitation outcomes of four patients with moyamoya disease who had sustained strokes. Their scores on the Functional Independence Measure were assessed at admission and during the week of discharge. The scores were also estimated for premorbid function. The functional area scores

on the Functional Independence Measure include self-care, sphincter control, mobility, locomotion, communication, and social cognition. All patients showed improved functional independence after their rehabilitation stay. Variability in presentation and outcome is expected due to differential type, location, and extent of the cerebrovascular accident.

Patients with moyamoya disease are typically younger than the average stroke patient; hence, their life expectancy with disability is much longer than that of the average stroke patient.[10] Their significant loss of earning potential supports the economic value of neuropsychologically guided rehabilitation to help patients return to productive activity.[11,12]

◆ Group Studies

Natural Course of Moyamoya Disease

Two group studies of patients with moyamoya disease who have not undergone surgery have been discussed in the English literature. Karzmark et al[13] studied 36 patients who underwent preoperative neuropsychological assessment. To be classified as having mild impairment, at least half of a subject's test scores had to be between 1 and 2 standard deviations below the mean. To be classified as having moderate to severe impairment, at least half of a subject's test scores had to be at least 2 standard deviations below the mean. The authors found cognitive impairment in 11 (31%) patients and moderate to severe impairment in 4 (11%) patients. The highest rates of impairment were observed on the FAS (a measure of verbal fluency), Animal Naming, Trail Making Test (TMT)-Part B, Boston Naming Test, and the Grooved Pegboard. The lowest rates of impairment were observed on memory measures, the Tactile Finger Recognition Test, Delis-Kaplan Executive Function System Design Fluency, and Wechsler Adult Intelligence Scale (WAIS)-III Vocabulary. On the Beck Depression Inventory-II, the mean score was within normal limits. Of the 36 patients tested, 7 subjects obtained scores in the clinical range for depression (5 mild, 2 moderate); 1 did not complete the questionnaire.

The study by Karzmark et al[13] suggests that executive functioning was most vulnerable to the effects of moyamoya disease. Almost half of the patients in their study showed impairment on tests of executive functioning (TMT-B and verbal fluency), whereas memory was fairly well preserved. That only 11% of the patients had a Full Scale Intelligence Quotient (FSIQ) of < 80 supports the notion that in adulthood, the effects of the disorder are usually milder than with early onset based on this measure (which is limited; see the following discussion). The authors concluded that relative strength in memory suggested that the medial temporal region of the brain and associated structures tend to be spared by moyamoya disease, perhaps reflecting the geographic distribution of the underlying vascular pathology. In this study, however, neuropsychological data were not correlated with imaging findings, and the number of patients who may have had preexisting strokes is unknown.

Festa et al[1] evaluated 29 patients with moyamoya disease before surgery. Most of the patients (83%) had a history of stroke, but the incidence of impairment did not differ between patients who had had strokes (84%) and those who had not (75%). Two-thirds of the patients showed cognitive dysfunction. Pronounced dysfunction was observed on tests of processing speed (29%), verbal memory (31%), verbal fluency (26%), and executive function (25%). Manual strength and dexterity also were affected. Twenty-eight percent of patients reported moderate to severe depression. The authors concluded that moyamoya disease produces a "subcortical-frontal pattern" of impairment, which is consistent with the findings of Karzmark et al.[13]

Calviere et al[14] studied 10 adults before surgery. The seven patients who had sustained ischemic strokes were evaluated at least 3 months after stroke. Three patients were diagnosed with moyamoya disease due to severe headache; one of these patients developed a cortical subarachnoid hemorrhage. The patients completed a neuropsychological battery that focused on executive functions but also assessed processing speed, naming, visuospatial perception and construction, and verbal/visual memory. Patients were considered to have executive dysfunction if they were impaired on three or more tests in that domain (classified as mildly impaired or severely impaired). The 10 patients also underwent perfusion-weighted MRI. Six patients met the criteria for executive dysfunction, and regional cerebrovascular reserve (rCVR) of the frontal lobes was lower in patients with executive dysfunction. Five patients with executive dysfunction showed reduced frontal rCVR, whereas frontal rCVR was positive in the patients with no executive dysfunction. Cognitive functioning was unimpaired in other domains.

◆ Postoperative Outcome Studies in Patients with Moyamoya Disease

Case Reports

Jefferson et al[15] used neuropsychological testing and perfusion MRI to demonstrate a temporal relationship between the vascular effects of the superficial temporal artery-to-MCA bypass procedure and an improvement in neurocognitive status. They presented a 48-year-old attorney who sustained a right hemisphere infarction related to moyamoya disease. She underwent a neuropsychological evaluation 3 months before bypass surgery and 5 weeks after surgery (1 year after her stroke). On her preoperative evaluation, consistent with her premorbid history, the patient demonstrated strong language and verbal reasoning abilities, including intact naming, verbal fluency, abstract verbal reasoning, and expressive word knowledge. Consistent with a right hemispheric stroke, her visuospatial perception, organizational skills, and constructional skills were impaired. Her visuospatial memory was significantly impaired, and her verbal memory was mildly impaired. On postoperative assessment, her visuospatial analysis/constructional skills improved to the normal range, and her visuospatial memory improved considerably. Her verbal learning/recall skills also improved. In tandem with the improvement in her cognitive performance, her postoperative cerebral blood flow (CBF) values on perfusion MRI increased to normal levels in both hemispheres.

Restoration of perfusion after surgery, however, is associated with potential risks. Ogasawara et al[16] suggested that "rapid restoration of normal perfusion pressure after vascular reconstruction may result in regional hyperperfusion secondary to impaired autoregulation that occurs in the context of chronic ischemia." They presented a 48-year-old Japanese man who developed an infarct in the right temporo-occipital region and was diagnosed with moyamoya disease. One month later, he underwent a superficial temporal artery-to-MCA anastomosis. Four days after surgery, the patient experienced severe headache and agitated delirium. Diffusion-weighted MRI obtained 6 hours after the onset of these symptoms revealed hyperintensity in the right temporal lobe. Follow-up perfusion computed tomography showed increased CBF and cerebral blood volume in the right temporal lobe; indeed, CBF in the right temporal lobe was double that in the left temporal lobe. T2-weighted MRI and perfusion computed tomography performed 15 days after the patient became symptomatic confirmed resolution of the hyperintensity and hyperperfusion in the right temporal lobe. MRI obtained 3 months after surgery showed brain atrophy only in the right temporal lobe.

On admission, this patient underwent a preoperative neuropsychological evaluation. The neuropsychological battery was readministered 3 and 6 months after surgery. Preoperative evaluation of intelligence and memory (using the WAIS-revised [WAIS-R] and Wechsler Memory Scale [WMS]) showed that the patient's performance IQ was impaired (PIQ = 68), but his verbal IQ was intact (VIQ = 97). His memory was spared (MQ = 110). His attention was average (digit span = 8; 5 digits forward, 3 digits backward). Three months after surgery, testing demonstrated a decline in his attention (digit span of 5 on the WAIS-R and 3 on the WMS), and no areas of improvement. Six months after surgery, his attention was still impaired (digit span of 5 on the WAIS-R and 3 on the WMS). His processing speed was slow across assessments (WAIS-R Symbol Search = 4, 3, 4). The patient's quality of life, including his ability to work, was adversely affected by his cognitive impairment.

Group Studies

Starke et al[17] used the modified Rankin Scale (mRS) to evaluate the functional status of 43 patients with moyamoya disease after surgical treatment. The mRS emphasizes motor impairment, and function is rated on a 0 to 6 scale from intact functioning to death. The scale is not specific to cognitive issues. As the authors stated, "it does not measure higher cortical function and postoperative cognitive decline," (p. 941). After undergoing an indirect bypass, most patients had improved or preserved functional status. After 67 surgical procedures, 17 patients (25%) had significant disability (mRS > 2) at discharge and 13 patients (18%) had significant disability at long-term follow-up. From the time of admission to follow-up, the functional independence of four patients (9%) declined based on the mRS related to progression of their moyamoya disease. Of the 43 patients, 38 (88%) improved or showed no change in their functional independence.

Modified Rankin Scale scores were obtained at baseline, after surgery, and at long-term follow-up (median follow-up 41 months).[17] At baseline, 80% of patients had a score of at least 2 on the mRS (45%, 2; 25%, 3; and 10%, 4). After surgery, 55% of patients had a score of at least 2 on the mRS (30%, 2; 18%, 3; and 7%, 4). At long-term follow-up, 39% had a score of at least 2 on the mRS (excluding two deaths, one unrelated to progression of the moyamoya disease; 24%, 2; 10%, 3; 3%, 4; and 2%, 5). Clearly, postoperative neuropsychological evaluation could help in the assessment of outcomes of patients with moyamoya disease because the mRS score provides only a rough estimate of overall functional outcome.

Hallemeier et al[18] followed 34 patients with moyamoya disease for a median of 5.1 years. Twenty-two patients had sustained an ischemic or hemorrhagic stroke. During follow-up, 14 patients were treated with surgical revascularization, 6 of whom underwent the procedure on both hemispheres. Of the 19 patients for whom functional outcome was assessed at last follow-up, there were no differences in scores on the mRS, Barthel Scale, or Stroke Specific Quality of Life (SS-QOL) Scale between those who had undergone surgery and those who had not or between those who had presented with ischemia and those who had presented with hemorrhage. However, patients with bilateral symptomatic involvement had a worse functional outcome than those with unilateral involvement. Patients with unilateral involvement were more likely to have an mRS score of 0 or 1 than those with bilateral involvement (48%; $p = 0.04$). The Barthel Scale assesses basic activities of daily living and does not address higher-level cognition. Likewise, the SS-QOL scale does not adequately assess higher-level cognition.

Guzman et al[4] studied outcomes after revascularization procedures in 264 patients (for a minimum of 6 months), which included both children and adults. Follow-up was conducted 1 week, 6 months, 36 months, and 10 years after surgery. When pre- and postoperative status was compared, 71.2% of patients reported a significant improvement in quality of life as measured using the mRS ($p < 0.0001$). Neuropsychological findings were not reported, although a significant proportion of patients reported increased energy level and an improved ability to concentrate.

◆ Neuropsychological Studies of Moyamoya Disease in Adults

Given the relative rarity of moyamoya disease in adults, the neuropsychological literature is limited. However, a wide variety and degree of neuropsychological deficits have been reported in this patient group, depending on the location and extent of the disease. These patients have complicated medical histories, and the role of multiple factors in producing their neuropsychological test findings remains unclear. These adults need to be studied carefully before and after surgery with clear documentation of comorbid neurological and related medical conditions that might influence neuropsychological test findings.

◆ Neurocognitive Changes in Children with Moyamoya Disease

The literature on the neuropsychological consequences of moyamoya disease in children is also limited. This paucity partially reflects the low incidence of the disease in infants and children. In Japan, the incidence is estimated at ~3 cases per 100,000; the rates are even lower in other populations.[2] In contrast, there are ~180 cases of traumatic brain injury per 100,000 children.[19]

Hogan et al[20] summarized the literature on how measures of intelligence are affected by stroke in childhood. A major conclusion from their review was that the well-established finding of a lower WAIS verbal IQ after a left hemisphere stroke (versus performance IQ) and lower performance IQ following onset of right hemisphere stroke (versus verbal IQ) in adults has not been found in children. Furthermore, children with a stroke who have average IQ scores on the WAIS may still have notable cognitive and behavioral problems that negatively affect their school performance. The findings are similar in children who have sustained a traumatic brain injury.[21] The conclusion from this review is that a wide variety of neuropsychological measures, in addition to standard IQ tests, is needed to assess neuropsychological correlates of moyamoya disease before and after surgery in children.

Case Studies

Bowen et al[22] have emphasized that the neuropsychological assessment of children with moyamoya disease must include measures beyond standard IQ scores. They reported on two children who underwent extensive neuropsychological testing. Interestingly, performance on the Tactual Performance Test (of the Halstead-Reitan Neuropsychological Test Battery) was thought specifically to identify important neurocognitive impairments not detected by standard IQ scores. Although the authors suggest that patients' performance on this test may specifically reveal important visuospatial and visuomotor deficits, other studies on this test with adults argue that it may simply be a very sensitive overall marker of severity and presence of brain dysfunction.[23] Bowen et al[22] also noted that speed of finger tapping with the nondominant left hand remained impaired in one child with a relatively good neurocognitive status. Whether finger tapping measures subtle motor performance per se or reflects the integrity of the right hemisphere remains unclear.

Ganesan et al[24] studied monovular female twins who were diagnosed with moyamoya disease. At the ages of 7 and 8 years, their verbal IQs were significantly higher than their performance IQs as were their executive dysfunction. Twin A was worse off cognitively than her sister, likely reflecting focal cerebral infarctions.

Klasen et al[25] examined a 12-year-old boy with acute transient psychosis coincident with physical exertion. His evaluation revealed moyamoya disease and an occluded left MCA. After his psychosis resolved, he underwent a neuropsychological examination, which revealed low average spelling, borderline impaired recall of a word list, and impaired visual scanning speed and set-shifting. Apparently, he had made a full recovery by 1 year after the psychotic event.

Group Studies

Hogan et al[20] assessed intellectual decline in children with moyamoya syndrome. There were four groups in this study: (1) children with moyamoya syndrome who sustained a stroke, (2) children with moyamoya syndrome and sickle cell anemia who sustained a stroke, (3) children with sickle cell anemia but no evidence of stroke, and (4) normally developing children. The children were studied at two time points to determine whether functioning declined and whether the groups differed. The authors concluded that some evidence suggests a decline in IQ in patients diagnosed with moyamoya syndrome and stroke, but whether chronic bilateral hypoperfusion also contributed to the symptom picture is unknown. They further noted that their results ". . .suggest that the presence of moyamoya vasculopathy may have a deleterious effect on the capacity to develop intellectual functions consistent with increasing chronological age" (pg. 828). Whether this relationship is unique to moyamoya disease or to any major brain disorder in childhood remains to be seen.

Ishii et al[26] reported IQ scores in 20 children with moyamoya disease, from ages 5 to 16 years. Children were studied before and after surgery. The FSIQ score of these children was quite variable, ranging from as low as 66 to as high as 125. Mean scores were in the low range of average. They noted that preoperative FSIQ scores correlated with mean CBF, but they reported no correlation coefficient. After surgery, children again showed variable outcomes, but the greatest improvements were observed on the performance IQ measure of the WAIS.

Matsushima et al[27] studied 65 pediatric moyamoya disease patients before and after surgery. Again, preoperative WAIS IQ scores (presumably FSIQ scores) were highly variable, ranging from severe restriction of intellectual development to children with superior intelligence. Postoperatively, a few children showed improvement, but the authors concluded there was no significant difference across all of the IQ measures when studied. The authors suggested, however, that without surgery the functioning of children may well deteriorate over time.

Kim et al[28] studied 410 consecutive pediatric patients with moyamoya disease who underwent bilateral encephaloduroarteriosynangiosis augmented by bifrontal encephalogaleoperiosteal synangiosis. Preoperatively, IQ was assessed in 276 patients (FSIQ < 90 [$n = 67$, 24%] and FSIQ IQ $\geq$ 90 [$n = 209$, 76%]), and neurocognitive function (unspecified) was assessed in 258 patients (19 [7%] were deemed "normal," and 239 [93%] were deemed "abnormal"). Postoperatively, FSIQ was assessed in 106 patients (mean time after surgery 44 months, range 2–176 months; 71 [67%] patients had a FSIQ $\geq$ 90 and 35 patients [33%] had a FSIQ < 90). Clinical outcome was dichotomized into favorable (excellent and good outcomes) and unfavorable (fair and poor outcomes) based on degree and frequency of neurological deficits. Eighty-one percent of the patients had favorable outcomes. FSIQ < 90 was identified as one predictor of unfavorable surgical outcome (odds ratio, 4.09; 95% confidence interval, 2.06–8.11; $p < 0.001$), but abnormal performance on the "cerebral function test" was not predictive (odds ratio, 1.46; 95% confidence interval, 0.32–6.59; $p = 0.62$).

Although they did not specifically include a measure of neuropsychological functioning, Darwish and Besser[29] studied the long-term outcomes of 16 children with moyamoya disease in Australia. Like other investigators, they noted that long-term functional outcome was related to the child's preoperative functional status. Outcomes were unrelated to the type of surgical procedure or age at presentation. All of these children had suffered strokes or transient ischemic attacks, and several had a seizure disorder. It remains unclear if the surgical treatment of moyamoya disease improves the neuropsychological status of children who have not developed stroke or a seizure disorder.

As is true with adult studies, a wide range and degree of intellectual impairment have been associated with moyamoya disease in children. Although sparse, the literature has argued for the importance of expanding the neuropsychological examination beyond IQ measures to include a wide variety of tests that may be sensitive to underlying brain dysfunction. In the limited reports available, tests sensitive to overall severity of brain injury and the presence of brain injury (the Tactual Performance Test) have shown some promising results, at least in two cases. Interestingly, speed of finger tapping in the nondominant hand may provide useful information about right hemisphere dysfunction that is not obvious using other measures of intelligence.

◆ Implications for Future Assessment of Neuropsychological Functioning in Children and Adults with Moyamoya Disease

The literature on both adults and children suggests that a wide range and degree of neuropsychological deficits can be associated with moyamoya disease. Patients with hypoperfusion (which predominantly affects the frontal lobes given the vascular territories affected by moyamoya disease) may perform differently than patients who have hypoperfusion and ischemic or hemorrhagic strokes, which can occur anywhere in the brain.

Within the confines of the patient's clinical condition, a neuropsychological examination should be performed before and after surgery to be of maximum help. **Table 8.1** lists 10 dimensions of a clinical neuropsychological examination.[30] The tests administered to sample these dimensions may vary widely, depending on the clinical experience (and biases) of different neuropsychological examiners.

In our setting, we find it practical to use a two-tiered approach that incorporates standardized neuropsychological tests, which are useful in our typical examination procedures (**Table 8.2**). The first tier is a "short" battery of neuropsychological tests that can be administered to school-aged children through the later years of life. We use the BNI Screen for Higher

Table 8.1 Ten Dimensions of a Clinical Neuropsychological Examination

1. Speech and language functions
2. Perceptual skills (auditory, visual, and tactual)
3. Attention and concentration skills
4. Learning capacity
5. Memory
6. Intellectual level and executive function
7. Speed of new learning
8. Speed and coordination of simple motor responses
9. Emotional and motivational characteristics
10. Self-awareness of level of functioning and judgments regarding psychosocial implications

Source: Reproduced with permission from Prigatano and Pliskin.[30]

Cerebral Functions, Adult and Children's versions. This screen samples speech and language functions, orientation to time and place, attention and concentration skills, visuospatial and visual problem-solving skills, memory, affect expression and perception, and awareness (or prediction of performance) on a verbal memory task. We then sample simple motor speed using the Halstead Finger Tapping Test supplemented with measures of cognitive processing speed using the TMT-Part A and the Digit Symbol Coding subtest from the WAIS, Adult and Children's versions. Executive functions are sampled by using the TMT-Part B, which particularly assesses ability to shift cognitive set in a flexible manner without making errors. This basic battery is used for both children and adults as a screening assessment when patients can only be examined for 20 to 30 minutes

A longer battery of neuropsychological tests can be used to sample a full range of abilities subsumed under the term "intelligence" utilizing the WAIS scales. We also incorporate tests of verbal fluency using the Controlled Oral Word Association subtest of the Multilingual Aphasia Examination or subtests from A Developmental Neuropsychological Assessment-II. We also recommend using demanding tests of verbal learning and memory, which can help assess an individual's capacity to learn and retain information in the presence of a distraction. In our

Table 8.2 Suggested Test Battery to Assess Cognitive Functioning in Patients with Moyamoya Disease*

Group	Cognitive Domain		Short Battery	Long Battery
Children (< age 16)	General screening		BNI Screen for Children	BNI Screen for Children
	Intelligence		—	WPPSI-III/WISC-IV
	Motor speed		Halstead Finger Tapping Test	Halstead Finger Tapping Test
	Processing speed		TMT-A, WISC-IV Digit Symbol-Coding	TMT-A, WPPSI-III/WISC-IV Digit Symbol-Coding
	Learning and memory (verbal and visuospatial)		—	CVLT-C, Rey Complex Figure Test
	Executive functioning	Attention/working memory	—	WISC-IV Digit Span/ NEPSY Visual Attention
		Verbal fluency	—	COWAT
		Set-shifting	TMT-B	TMT-B
		Concept formation	—	WCST
	Mood		—	BASC-2, Children's Depression Inventory
Adults (≥ age 16)	General screening		BNI Screen for Higher Cerebral Functions	BNI Screen for Higher Cerebral Functions
	Estimate of verbal and visuospatial intelligence		—	WAIS-IV Vocabulary and Block Design subtests, or full index for each
	Motor speed		Halstead Finger Tapping Test	Halstead Finger Tapping Test
	Processing speed		TMT-A, WAIS-IV Digit Symbol-Coding	TMT-A, WAIS-IV Digit Symbol-Coding
	Learning and memory (verbal and visuospatial)		—	RAVLT, BVMT-R
	Executive functioning	Attention/working memory	—	WAIS-IV Digit Span
		Verbal fluency	—	COWAT
		Set-shifting	TMT-B	TMT-B
		Concept formation	—	WCST
		Planning/ organization	—	Rey Complex Figure copy, Tower of London
	Mood and quality of life		—	BDI-2, SS-QOL

Abbreviations: BASC-2, Behavioral Assessment System for Children-2; BDI, Beck Depression Inventory; BVMT-R, Brief Visuospatial Memory Test–Revised; COWAT, Controlled Oral Word Association Test; CVLT-C, California Verbal Learning Test–Children's Version; NEPSY, A Developmental Neuropsychological Assessment; RAVLT, Rey Auditory Verbal Learning Test; SS-QOL, Stroke Specific Quality of Life; TMT, Trail Making Test; WAIS, Wechsler Adult Intelligence Scale; WCST, Wisconsin Card Sorting Test; WISC, Wechsler Intelligence Scale for Children; WPPSI, Wechsler Preschool and Primary Scale of Intelligence.

*A detailed description of the tests listed in this table and the functions they purportedly measure can be found in Lezak.[31]

clinical setting, we use the Rey Auditory Verbal Learning Test and the Brief Visuospatial Memory Test-Revised for these purposes. Tests of concept formation and planning are limited. Nevertheless, we sometimes find it useful to administer the Wisconsin Card Sorting Test, the Tower of London, and the Rey Complex Figure Test.

It also may be useful to sample a child's mood state by having parents complete the Behavioral Assessment System for Children-2. Adult patients can complete the Beck Depression Inventory-2 and the SS-QOL.

There is, however, no consensus on the actual tests that should be administered to this patient group. We do not include the Tactual Performance Test in our list of proposed measures because it is time consuming. Sometimes, however, this test can be extremely helpful and should be seriously considered, particularly when clinical research projects are conducted in this population.

◆ Conclusion

The literature characterizing the cognitive profiles of both children and adults with moyamoya disease before and after surgery is growing. The methods used in the cognitive assessment of these patients are becoming increasingly sophisticated, moving beyond IQ measures, brief screening measures, or self-report inventories, which are inadequate for measuring the cognitive outcomes of adults. Collaboration among neurologists, neurosurgeons, and neuropsychologists should prove fruitful for predicting treatment outcomes and for thoughtfully guiding patients during postoperative rehabilitation.

References

1. Festa JR, Schwarz LR, Pliskin N, et al. Neurocognitive dysfunction in adult moyamoya disease. J Neurol 2010;257(5):806–815
2. Scott RM, Smith ER. Moyamoya disease and moyamoya syndrome. N Engl J Med 2009;360(12):1226–1237
3. Cho HJ, Jung YH, Kim YD, Nam HS, Kim DS, Heo JH. The different infarct patterns between adulthood-onset and childhood-onset moyamoya disease. J Neurol Neurosurg Psychiatry 2011;82(1):38–40
4. Guzman R, Lee M, Achrol A, et al. Clinical outcome after 450 revascularization procedures for moyamoya disease. Clinical article. J Neurosurg 2009;111(5):927–935
5. Schwarz LR, Thurstin AH, Levine LA. A single case report of Moyamoya disease presenting in a psychiatric setting. Appl Neuropsychol 2010;17(1):73–77
6. Lubman DI, Pantelis C, Desmond P, Proffitt TM, Velakoulis D. Moyamoya disease in a patient with schizophrenia. J Int Neuropsychol Soc 2003;9(5):806–810
7. Rabbani O, Bowen LE, Watson RT, Valenstein E, Okun MS. Alien limb syndrome and moya-moya disease. Mov Disord 2004;19(11):1317–1320
8. Anjaneyulu A, Bhaskar G. Cortical blindness: a rare presentation of moya moya disease. Neurol India 1993; 41(2):118–119
9. Hayashi R, Watanabe R, Mimura M, Kato M, Katsumata Y. [A case of moyamoya disease presenting with geographic mislocation, person misidentification and fantastic confabulation]. No To Shinkei 2000;52(12):1091–1096
10. Moore DP, Lee MY, Macciocchi SN. Neurorehabilitation outcome in moyamoya disease. Arch Phys Med Rehabil 1997;78(6):672–675
11. Prigatano GP. Principles of Neuropsychological Rehabilitation. New York: Oxford University Press; 1999
12. Prigatano GP, Fordyce DJ, Zeiner HK, et al. Neuropsychological Rehabilitation After Brain Injury. Baltimore: Johns Hopkins University; 1986
13. Karzmark P, Zeifert PD, Tan S, Dorfman LJ, Bell-Stephens TE, Steinberg GK. Effect of moyamoya disease on neuropsychological functioning in adults. Neurosurgery 2008;62(5):1048–1051, discussion 1051–1052
14. Calviere L, Catalaa I, Marlats F, et al. Correlation between cognitive impairment and cerebral hemodynamic disturbances on perfusion magnetic resonance imaging in European adults with moyamoya disease. Clinical article. J Neurosurg 2010;113(4):753–759
15. Jefferson AL, Glosser G, Detre JA, Sinson G, Liebeskind DS. Neuropsychological and perfusion MR imaging correlates of revascularization in a case of moyamoya syndrome. AJNR Am J Neuroradiol 2006;27(1): 98–100
16. Ogasawara K, Komoribayashi N, Kobayashi M, et al. Neural damage caused by cerebral hyperperfusion after arterial bypass surgery in a patient with moyamoya disease: case report. Neurosurgery 2005;56(6):E1380, discussion E1380
17. Starke RM, Komotar RJ, Hickman ZL, et al. Clinical features, surgical treatment, and long-term outcome in adult patients with moyamoya disease. Clinical article. J Neurosurg 2009;111(5):936–942
18. Hallemeier CL, Rich KM, Grubb RL Jr, et al. Clinical features and outcome in North American adults with moyamoya phenomenon. Stroke 2006;37(6):1490–1496
19. Kraus JF, McArthur DL. Epidemiology of brain injury. In: Evans RW, editor. Neurology and Trauma. Philadelphia: WB Saunders Company; 1996. p. 3–17.
20. Hogan AM, Kirkham FJ, Isaacs EB, Wade AM, Vargha-Khadem F. Intellectual decline in children with moyamoya and sickle cell anaemia. Dev Med Child Neurol 2005;47(12):824–829
21. Hawley CA, Ward AB, Magnay AR, Mychalkiw W. Return to school after brain injury. Arch Dis Child 2004;89(2):136–142
22. Bowen M, Marks MP, Steinberg GK. Neuropsychological recovery from childhood moyamoya disease. Brain Dev 1998;20(2):119–123
23. Reitan RM. Investigation of the validity of Halstead's measures of biological intelligence. AMA Arch Neurol Psychiatry 1955;73(1):28–35
24. Ganesan V, Isaacs E, Kirkham FJ. Variable presentation of cerebrovascular disease in monovular twins. Dev Med Child Neurol 1997;39(9):628–631
25. Klasen H, Britton J, Newman M. Moyamoya disease in a 12-year-old Caucasian boy presenting with acute

transient psychosis. Eur Child Adolesc Psychiatry 1999; 8(2):149–153

26. Ishii R, Takeuchi S, Ibayashi K, Tanaka R. Intelligence in children with moyamoya disease: evaluation after surgical treatments with special reference to changes in cerebral blood flow. Stroke 1984;15(5):873–877

27. Matsushima Y, Aoyagi M, Koumo Y, et al. Effects of encephalo-duro-arterio-synangiosis on childhood moyamoya patients—swift disappearance of ischemic attacks and maintenance of mental capacity. Neurol Med Chir (Tokyo) 1991;31(11):708–714

28. Kim SK, Cho BK, Phi JH, et al. Pediatric moyamoya disease: An analysis of 410 consecutive cases. Ann Neurol 2010;68(1):92–101

29. Darwish B, Besser M. Long term outcome in children with Moyamoya disease: experience with 16 patients. J Clin Neurosci 2005;12(8):873–877

30. Prigatano GP, Pliskin N. Clinical Neuropsychology and Costs Outcome Research: A Beginning. New York: Psychology Press; 2003

31. Lezak MD. Neuropsychological assessment. 4th ed. New York: Oxford University Press; 2004

II

Treatment Options: Medical, Endovascular, Perioperative, and Surgical Management

9

Medical Management of Childhood Moyamoya

Joanne Ng and Vijeya Ganesan

◆ Introduction

Currently, no medical treatments can halt or reverse the arteriopathic process in moyamoya disease. This chapter focuses on medical strategies for the secondary prevention of stroke and the management of headache and hypertension in childhood moyamoya disease. It also discusses clinical outcomes.

Secondary Prevention of Arterial Ischemic Stroke in Childhood Moyamoya Disease

Although a randomized controlled trial is lacking, surgical revascularization to prevent recurrent arterial ischemic stroke in children with moyamoya disease is supported by a strong body of clinical evidence. In contrast, although antiplatelet agents are administered to children with moyamoya disease, in whom the primary presentations are related to cerebral ischemia, there has been relatively little evaluation of their efficacy or safety.

The rationale for using aspirin is to prevent the formation of microthrombus at sites of arterial stenosis. Aspirin inhibits the enzyme cyclooxygenase and prevents the production of thromboxane A2, which is a platelet agonist. Increasing evidence suggests that aspirin might have additional antithrombotic effects that are independent of cyclooxygenase.[1,2] There are even fewer data about the safety and efficacy profile of other antiplatelet agents such as clopidogrel, dipyridamole, ticlopidine, and glycoprotein IIb/IIIa antagonists when used in children.

Conventional wisdom advises against the use of antiplatelet agents in adults because hemorrhagic complications associated with moyamoya disease are predominant in this age group. However, this belief is based on the natural history of Japanese patients. Adult patients in other countries have ischemic manifestations of moyamoya disease more frequently than hemorrhagic symptoms. Anticoagulation therapy is usually avoided at all ages because of concerns about an increased risk of cerebral hemorrhage.

Our clinical practice is to begin aspirin therapy at diagnosis in children with nonhemorrhagic presentations of moyamoya disease and to continue the treatment until the age of 18 years, even in patients who undergo surgical revascularization.

Moyamoya in Sickle Cell Disease

As many as 43% of people who develop arterial ischemic stroke in the context of sickle cell disease demonstrate moyamoya arteriopathy; this manifestation is associated with a recurrence in more than 60% of patients, despite chronic blood transfusions.[3] Children with sickle cell disease and moyamoya disease have significant cognitive impairment compared with those with sickle cell disease alone. The impairment is not solely related to cerebral infarction; chronic hypoperfusion is also likely to contribute.[4] Several studies have reported revascularization of patients with sickle cell disease associated with moyamoya disease with positive results.[5-7] The American Heart Association Guidelines now recommend that surgical revascularization procedures be considered "as a last resort" in children with sickle cell disease who continue to have cerebrovascular dysfunction despite optimal medical management.[8]

We view surgical revascularization as an adjunct to established medical therapies to prevent a recurrence of arterial ischemic stroke in patients with sickle cell disease rather than as a replacement. Thus, we advocate continuing blood transfusion and considering additional medical therapies, such as hydroxyurea, as in patients with sickle cell disease with arterial ischemic stroke who do not have the moyamoya morphology of arteriopathy.

There is a real issue about the diagnosis of moyamoya disease in this group of patients and the radiological cut-off between the proximal occlusive arteriopathy of sickle cell disease and the ominous moyamoya pattern. In particular, future studies should include more detailed radiological analyses to identify consistent features that separate these groups and to inform prognosis.

Headache

A quarter to half of patients with moyamoya disease experience headache,[9,10] which is increasingly recognized as a significant symptom requiring medical management. The headaches reported suggest a vascular origin with migrainous features, a relationship with transient ischemic attacks (TIAs), hyperventilation, and resolution with revascularization. However, cluster and tension-type headaches have also been reported.[11,12] The interpretation of headache and its correlation with cerebral perfusion remains perplexing. Headaches arise at

any stage—as a presenting symptom or during the disease course. Headaches may be unmodified or recur after surgery, or they may develop de novo after surgery.

Headache as a presenting symptom of moyamoya disease is reported in 6.3% of Japanese patients.[9] However, its incidence may be underreported because patients categorized with asymptomatic moyamoya disease also complain of headache without other ischemic symptoms.[11] The largest series reviewing headache associated with moyamoya disease in children who have undergone surgical revascularization found that 44 of 204 children (22%) had preoperative headache, 28 of the 44 (64%) continued to have headache a year after surgery, and 10 of 160 (6.3%) without preoperative headache developed headache after surgery. Significantly, assessment of cerebral blood flow did not predict the course of headache.[12] The pathophysiology of headache in moyamoya disease remains poorly understood. It is presumed to be related to chronic hypoperfusion,[13] which could lower the threshold for migraines to develop.[14]

The series reported by Seol et al[10] suggests that headache could also reflect successful revascularization with the development of new leptomeningeal collateral vessels stimulating dural nociceptor structures. With this hypothesis in mind, Shirane and Fujimura treated 13 patients with moyamoya disease, significant headache, and hemodynamic compromise with direct revascularization (rather than indirect procedures).[15] After surgery, the headaches of 11 patients improved markedly. The authors suggested that direct revascularization improves headache by rapidly improving cerebral blood flow and ameliorates the demand related to the development of pial synagiosis. No studies have compared the effect of direct revascularization to indirect revascularization procedures specifically on headache symptoms.

The headaches associated with moyamoya disease can be incapacitating and refractory to simple analgesia and migraine treatments. Migraine prophylactic agents associated with lowering blood pressure (e.g., propranolol, clonidine, flunarizine) and triptans with vasoconstrictory effects are relatively contraindicated.

Calcium-channel blockers with vasodilatory action have also been used to treat patients with persistent TIAs and intractable headaches.[16] Intravenous verapamil has been reported to improve neurologic deficit in a single case.[17] Oxygen was administered in 10 children with moyamoya disease to examine the effects on the rebuild-up phenomenon on electroencephalography and on the development of TIAs. In four children with partial pressure of oxygen in the blood > 150 mm Hg, symptoms of TIA and headache were prevented.[18] The findings suggest that oxygen may have a role in aborting headache. In our center, anticonvulsant medications are used for migraine prophylaxis. In particular, topiramate and sodium valproate have been used with encouraging results.[19]

Hypertension

Hypertension is increasingly recognized in moyamoya disease with or without renovascular disease. Renovascular disease has been identified in 5 to 10% of patients with moyamoya disease, of whom most have been normotensive.[20,21] The management of hypertension is complex with the goals of counterbalancing adequate cerebral perfusion, the risk of end-organ damage, and specific neurological sequelae associated with hypertension itself.

Renovascular hypertension can be sufficiently severe that acute treatment with renal angioplasty or surgery can be necessary. If elective renovascular intervention is considered, there may be a role for undertaking cerebral revascularization because blood pressure tends to decrease in children without renovascular disease who have undergone revascularization.[22] Presumably, this tendency reflects that the cerebral circulation is no longer as reliant on systemic blood pressure.

Many children have a "pressure passive" cerebral circulation and rely on systemic blood pressure to maintain adequate cerebral blood flow.[19] Thus, it may be necessary to accept higher levels of blood pressure than typical in a child without moyamoya disease. The specific acceptable level in individual patients is often hard to define, but many patients are symptomatic at what might be considered "normal" blood pressure and thus declare their own limits. Rigorous management of blood pressure around the time of revascularization is critical to minimize the risk of perioperative arterial ischemic stroke.

◆ Outcome

In Japan and eastern Asia, the natural history of moyamoya disease is one of a high rate of recurrent ischemic and hemorrhagic stroke and cognitive impairment associated with high rates of death and disability.[23,24] The natural history of secondary cases is controversial, although at least a proportion of such patients will also have a progressive course.[25] As cases are now recognized in all ethnicities, whether the natural history of moyamoya disease is more benign in some ethnic groups than in others has been debated.[26] The increasing identification of asymptomatic cases in Japan[11,27] suggests the full spectrum of the disease is yet to be established and that patients with a benign course are likely to be underreported in the literature. However, the presence of moyamoya disease has been found to predict a high rate of recurrence in large series of childhood arterial ischemic stroke outside eastern Asia[28,29] as well as in people with sickle cell disease. Thus, the overall rate of morbidity is likely to be significant.[3]

At present, there are no clinical, angiographic, or radiological predictors of the natural history in individual cases. The 5-year cumulative risk for any recurrent ipsilateral stroke among medically treated hemispheres with impaired hemodynamic reserve (increased oxygen extraction fraction on positron emission tomography) is estimated to be 65%. If stratified for patients with bilateral disease only, the stroke risk increases to 82% over 5 years.[30] A nationwide survey in Japan focused on asymptomatic patients with moyamoya disease and found that the risk of stroke in medically treated hemispheres was 3.2%/year.[11] Clinically silent reinfarction has also been reported in patients with sickle cell disease[31] and moyamoya disease, in whom it may be associated with cognitive morbidity.[4,32] The data suggest that even asymptomatic patients should be reimaged after an interval, particularly if they have preexisting disease.[28]

◆ **Conclusion**

The medical management of moyamoya disease is limited to unproven but widely used strategies to prevent the recurrence of arterial ischemic stroke. There are evidence-based treatments for those with sickle cell disease–related disease. Symptomatic medical management of headache and hypertension are challenging and require a clear understanding of the pathophysiology and potential unwanted effects of intervention. At present, there are no clinical, angiographic, or radiological predictors of the natural history of moyamoya disease in individual cases. There are likely to be differences in Japanese and other patient groups, but overall the associated morbidity appears to be significant across all ethnic groups.

References

1. Monagle P, Chan A, Massicotte P, Chalmers E, Michelson AD. Antithrombotic therapy in children: the Seventh ACCP Conference on Antithrombotic and Thrombolytic Therapy. Chest 2004;126(3, Suppl)645S–687S

2. Gurbel PA, Bliden KP, DiChiara J, et al. Evaluation of dose-related effects of aspirin on platelet function: results from the Aspirin-Induced Platelet Effect (ASPECT) study. Circulation 2007;115(25):3156–3164

3. Dobson SR, Holden KR, Nietert PJ, et al. Moyamoya syndrome in childhood sickle cell disease: a predictive factor for recurrent cerebrovascular events. Blood 2002;99(9):3144–3150

4. Hogan AM, Kirkham FJ, Isaacs EB, Wade AM, Vargha-Khadem F. Intellectual decline in children with moyamoya and sickle cell anaemia. Dev Med Child Neurol 2005;47(12):824–829

5. Fryer RH, Anderson RC, Chiriboga CA, Feldstein NA. Sickle cell anemia with moyamoya disease: outcomes after EDAS procedure. Pediatr Neurol 2003;29(2):124–130

6. Hankinson TC, Bohman LE, Heyer G, et al. Surgical treatment of moyamoya syndrome in patients with sickle cell anemia: outcome following encephaloduroarteriosynangiosis. J Neurosurg Pediatr 2008;1(3):211–216

7. Smith ER, McClain CD, Heeney M, Scott RM. Pial synangiosis in patients with moyamoya syndrome and sickle cell anemia: perioperative management and surgical outcome. Neurosurg Focus 2009;26(4):E10

8. Roach ES, Golomb MR, Adams R, et al; American Heart Association Stroke Council; Council on Cardiovascular Disease in the Young. Management of stroke in infants and children: a scientific statement from a Special Writing Group of the American Heart Association Stroke Council and the Council on Cardiovascular Disease in the Young. Stroke 2008;39(9):2644–2691

9. Smith ER, Scott RM. Moyamoya: epidemiology, presentation, and diagnosis. Neurosurg Clin N Am 2010;21(3):543–551

10. Seol HJ, Wang KC, Kim SK, Hwang YS, Kim KJ, Cho BK. Headache in pediatric moyamoya disease: review of 204 consecutive cases. J Neurosurg 2005;103(5, Suppl)439–442

11. Kuroda S, Hashimoto N, Yoshimoto T, Iwasaki Y; Research Committee on Moyamoya Disease in Japan. Radiological findings, clinical course, and outcome in asymptomatic moyamoya disease: results of multicenter survey in Japan. Stroke 2007;38(5):1430–1435

12. Sewell RA, Johnson DJ, Fellows DW. Cluster headache associated with moyamoya. J Headache Pain 2009;10(1):65–67

13. Grindal AB, Toole JF. Headache and transient ischemic attacks. Stroke 1974;5(5):603–606

14. Olesen J, Friberg L, Olsen TS, et al. Ischaemia-induced (symptomatic) migraine attacks may be more frequent than migraine-induced ischaemic insults. Brain 1993;116(Pt 1):187–202

15. Shirane R, Fujimara M. Headaches in moyamoya disease. In: Cho B-K, Tominaga T, editors. Moyamoya Disease Update 2010.Tokyo: Springer; 2010:110–113.

16. Hosain SA, Hughes JT, Forem SL, Wisoff J, Fish I. Use of a calcium channel blocker (nicardipine HCl) in the treatment of childhood moyamoya disease. J Child Neurol 1994;9(4):378–380

17. McLean MJ, Gebarski SS, van der Spek AF, Goldstein GW. Response of moyamoya disease to verapamil. Lancet 1985;1(8421):163–164

18. Fujiwara J, Nakahara S, Enomoto T, Nakata Y, Takita H. The effectiveness of O2 administration for transient ischemic attacks in moyamoya disease in children. Childs Nerv Syst 1996;12(2):69–75

19. Ganesan V. Moyamoya: to cut or not to cut is not the only question. A paediatric neurologist's perspective. Dev Med Child Neurol 2010;52(1):10–13

20. Togao O, Mihara F, Yoshiura T, et al. Prevalence of stenoocclusive lesions in the renal and abdominal arteries in moyamoya disease. AJR Am J Roentgenol 2004;183(1):119–122

21. Yamada I, Himeno Y, Matsushima Y, Shibuya H. Renal artery lesions in patients with moyamoya disease: angiographic findings. Stroke 2000;31(3):733–737

22. Willems CE, Salisbury DM, Lumley JS, Dillon MJ. Brain revascularisation in hypertension. Arch Dis Child 1985;60(12):1177–1179

23. Kurokawa T, Tomita S, Ueda K, et al. Prognosis of occlusive disease of the circle of Willis (moyamoya disease) in children. Pediatr Neurol 1985;1(5):274–277

24. Imaizumi T, Hayashi K, Saito K, Osawa M, Fukuyama Y. Long-term outcomes of pediatric moyamoya disease monitored to adulthood. Pediatr Neurol 1998;18(4):321–325

25. Cramer SC, Robertson RL, Dooling EC, Scott RM. Moyamoya and Down syndrome. Clinical and radiological features. Stroke 1996;27(11):2131–2135

26. Chiu D, Shedden P, Bratina P, Grotta JC. Clinical features of moyamoya disease in the United States. Stroke 1998;29(7):1347–1351

27. Ikeda K, Iwasaki Y, Kashihara H, et al. Adult moyamoya disease in the asymptomatic Japanese population. J Clin Neurosci 2006;13(3):334–338

28. Ganesan V, Prengler M, Wade A, Kirkham FJ. Clinical and radiological recurrence after childhood arterial ischemic stroke. Circulation 2006;114(20):2170–2177

29. Fullerton HJ, Wu YW, Sidney S, Johnston SC. Risk of recurrent childhood arterial ischemic stroke in a

population-based cohort: the importance of cerebro-vascular imaging. Pediatrics 2007;119(3):495–501

30. Hallemeier CL, Rich KM, Grubb RL Jr, et al. Clinical features and outcome in North American adults with moyamoya phenomenon. Stroke 2006;37(6):1490–1496

31. Pegelow CH, Colangelo L, Steinberg M, et al. Natural history of blood pressure in sickle cell disease: risks for stroke and death associated with relative hypertension in sickle cell anemia. Am J Med 1997;102(2):171–177

32. Thompson RJ Jr, Armstrong FD, Link CL, Pegelow CH, Moser F, Wang WC. A prospective study of the relationship over time of behavior problems, intellectual functioning, and family functioning in children with sickle cell disease: a report from the Cooperative Study of Sickle Cell Disease. J Pediatr Psychol 2003;28(1):59–65

10

Pediatric Moyamoya

Edward R. Smith

◆ Introduction

Moyamoya is a progressive arteriopathy of the cerebral vasculature, initially described in 1957 in Japan as "hypoplasia of the internal carotid arteries" and named as a distinct disease in 1969.[1,2] The term is Japanese, meaning "puff of smoke." It is derived from the angiographic appearance of a network of characteristic small collateral vessels found in the most common form of the disorder in the region of the basal ganglia and skull base (**Fig. 10.1**). Development of these collaterals parallels the ongoing stenosis of the major branches of the anterior circulation, a process divided into six distinct stages by Suzuki and Takaku.[2] In rare cases, the arteriopathy and concomitant collateral development can also involve the posterior branches of the circle of Willis.

Much of the literature on moyamoya, including the name itself and how to define the condition, is controversial. Some groups have proposed "spontaneous occlusion of the circle of Willis" as an alternative to moyamoya (the term currently recognized by the International Classification of Diseases).[3] The definition of moyamoya is often unclear, with abundant examples of "moyamoya," "moyamoya disease," and "moyamoya syndrome" all being used interchangeably. Each is distinct, with moyamoya being the most general term and commonly defined as the characteristic radiographic findings on angiography, independent of any clinical qualifiers. Moyamoya *disease* is the bilateral presence of the arteriopathy, in the absence of any other associated systemic disorder. In contrast, all unilateral cases are defined as moyamoya syndrome, as are any bilateral cases that are found in conjunction with the presence of well-recognized systemic disorders (see the following).[4]

◆ Etiology

The underlying cause of the arteriopathy characterized as moyamoya remains unclear. It is likely that the radiographic findings seen on angiography are the common result of many different primary causes. This hypothesis is supported by the wide range of clinical presentations of affected patients, a population that includes individuals with genetic disorders, those with exposure to environmental insults, and others with no apparent predisposing factors. This heterogeneity is important because it suggests that subpopulations of patients may exist, with distinct natural histories and differing capacities to respond to therapy.[4]

Initial studies of moyamoya focused on pathology in the internal carotid arteries. Microscopic examination revealed hyperplasia of smooth muscle cells in the media of the wall

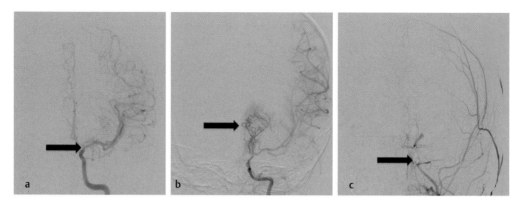

Fig. 10.1a–c Representative anteroposterior projection angiograms with injections of the internal carotid artery (ICA) show the progressive stages of moyamoya. (**a**) Suzuki stage I-II with ICA narrowing (*arrow*) but before extensive collateral vessels have developed. (**b**) Suzuki stage III-IV with significant ICA narrowing and characteristic "puff-of-smoke" appearance (*arrow*). (**c**) Suzuki stage V-VI with obliteration of ICA flow (*arrow*; common carotid artery injection). This occlusion of the ICA results in concomitant disappearance of the "puff-of-smoke" collaterals, because they are supplied by the ICA.

with associated thrombosis—a marked contrast to the atherosclerotic and inflammatory changes seen in patients with hyperlipidemia (**Fig. 10.2**).[5–7] The pathognomonic collateral vessels are derived from dilated preexisting channels and de novo angiogenesis.[8,9] The fragility of these collaterals, coupled with shear stresses from altered flow patterns in cerebral circulation, have been implicated in the formation of aneurysms, rupture resulting in hemorrhage, and thrombosis causing stroke.[10,11]

The presence of these dynamic processes of vessel development, extracellular matrix remodeling, and shifting patterns of ischemia have prompted study of related molecules, including cell-adhesion proteins, angiogenic peptides, and proteinases. Elevated levels of basic fibroblast growth factor, transforming growth factor β-1, metalloproteinases, intracellular adhesion molecules, and hypoxia-inducing factor-1 α have all been reported in moyamoya patients.[9,12–18]

These proteomic findings corroborate several ongoing genetic studies that implicate abnormalities in upstream regulatory elements in these pathways. TIMP2 (tissue inhibitor of metalloproteinase-2; a metalloproteinase inhibitor); ACTA2 (actin, α2, smooth muscle, aorta; a smooth muscle peptide); and mutations on chromosome 17 (near the neurofibromatosis-1 gene) have all been identified in

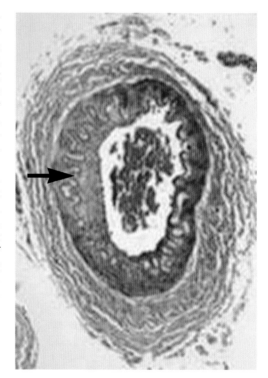

Fig. 10.2 Cross-sectional image of moyamoya vessel (middle cerebral artery) demonstrates progressive luminal occlusion from a combination of media hyperplasia (*arrow*) and thrombosis (Eosin, 100×).

select patients with moyamoya.[9,19–25] Unfortunately, there are no unifying patterns. A wide range of other mutated genes on multiple chromosomes has been correlated with the presence of moyamoya.[26–30]

It remains unclear whether the presence of moyamoya heralds a systemic predisposition to vascular disease (as is seen in Alagille syndrome and patients with cardiac anomalies or renal artery stenosis) or if moyamoya is an isolated disorder of the central nervous system (as with patients with moyamoya disease or those who have been treated with cranial radiation). In addition to the obvious implications regarding genetic causes, the risk of systemic vascular disease could affect the clinical management of patients.

The underlying cause of the arteriopathy described as moyamoya remains elusive. As discussed, it seems likely that many different factors—both genetic and environmental—contribute to the disorder. Series of familial cases need to be balanced against reports of identical twins with only one affected sibling when attempting to ascribe genetic causes to moyamoya.[31,32] Ultimately, the radiographic and clinical condition of moyamoya may result from environmental triggers initiating the arteriopathy in genetically susceptible individuals.

relatives.[5,31] This likelihood is increased in those of Asian ancestry, although multiple cases within families of many ethnicities have been reported. Interestingly, there have been reports of identical twins in which only one sibling has moyamoya. Such cases support a role for environmental influences in the development of this disorder.[31,32]

In addition to age, gender, and ethnic variations in the diagnosis of moyamoya, there are also known associations of specific conditions with the arteriopathy (**Table 10.1**). Moyamoya has been found in children with congenital malformations, genetic syndromes, and after exposure to the environmental stressor of cranial radiation.[24,31,42–47] The wide range of these associations, coupled with unknown rates of incidence and prevalence within each group, has sparked debate over the potential role of screening for moyamoya and the very definition of the condition itself. For example, children with sickle cell disease are one of the potentially largest affected groups. Ten percent of such children will have a stroke before they are 20 years old, and many of these children—perhaps up to 40%—demonstrate "moyamoya-like" changes on imaging.[48] These statistics have prompted substantive discussions among radiologists, hematologists, and neurosurgeons on the role of imaging in this population.

◆ Epidemiology

The original description of moyamoya was written in Japan. The condition remains strongly associated with individuals of east Asian heritage, affecting 3/100,000 children in Japan.[33–35] Moyamoya has since been found around the world, albeit with a far lower prevalence than in Japan (3/1,000,000 in Europe and ~1/1,000,000 in the United States).[36–39] The condition seems to affect females about twice as often as males. The age of presentation clusters in two major groups: 5-year-old children and adults in their 40s.[31,33,35,40,41] There are ethnic differences in those diagnosed with moyamoya. Compared with whites, those of Asian ancestry are diagnosed nearly five times more frequently, African Americans more than twice as often, while Hispanic children have half the rate.[37]

For individuals with moyamoya, there is a 6 to 10% chance of finding affected first-degree

Table 10.1 Moyamoya Syndrome: Associated Conditions

Sickle cell disease
Neurofibromatosis type I
Previous cranial therapeutic radiation
Down syndrome
Primary dwarfism
Congenital cardiac anomaly
Renal artery stenosis
Giant cervicofacial hemangiomas/PHACE/S syndrome (posterior fossa abnormalities, hemangioma, arterial lesions, cardiac abnormalities/aortic coarctation, and abnormalities of the eye)
Hyperthyroidism
Alagille syndrome

◆ Clinical Presentation

Two primary physiologic events occur in moyamoya. The major branches of the internal carotid arteries narrow, producing ischemia, and the brain attempts to compensate for this reduced flow through the development of collateral circulation. The presenting findings of moyamoya can usually be ascribed to one of these two events. In children, the most common symptoms are related to ischemia, transient ischemic attacks (TIAs), and stroke.[31] Compensatory mechanisms, such as the dilation and genesis of collateral vessels with concomitant changes in blood flow, have been implicated in the onset of headache (possibly through meningeal pain receptors triggered by engorged collaterals), aneurysm development, intracranial hemorrhage, and more typical symptoms such as choreiform movements (thought to be secondary to collaterals in the basal ganglia) and seizures.[4,31,49]

Typical presentations include the appearance of new neurologic deficits without apparent cause, intermittent "spells" suggestive of TIA (often in settings associated with reduced cerebral blood flow, such as dehydration- or hyperventilation-induced vasoconstriction, especially with crying) or gradual cognitive decline (particularly in children with preexisting cognitive limitations; for example, patients with Down syndrome).[44,50] Hemorrhage is extremely rare in children with moyamoya. It is present in fewer than 3% of cases (in contrast to a sevenfold increase in this rate in adults).[31,40,51] Outside the clinical manifestations of stroke, there is often no evidence of moyamoya on clinical examination, with the unusual exception of an enlarged optic disk associated with retinal vascular malformations—the so-called "morning glory disk."[52]

For children who develop an unexpected stroke, immediate evaluation protocols are outlined in the recent American Heart Association guidelines.[53] However, the level of concern for findings suggestive of ischemic events may be blunted when children have coexisting conditions that can mask symptoms (such as the cognitive delays associated with Down syndrome). Or, preexisting conditions may serve as facile explanations for stroke and thus lull clinicians into complacency (such as ascribing stroke to cardiac disease in children with cardiac anomalies or citing encephalopathy instead of TIAs as the source of intermittent deficits in brain tumor patients). In the United States, it is likely that moyamoya is underdiagnosed because its clinical manifestations are poorly recognized.

◆ Diagnostic Evaluation

If patients have neurologic symptoms suggestive of ischemia, they should be evaluated promptly. A delay in diagnosis can delay treatment and increase the risk of permanent disability from stroke. Initial studies often include computed tomography (CT) or magnetic resonance imaging (MRI). Although CT may demonstrate completed strokes (especially in the basal ganglia or watershed territories) or hemorrhage, it often appears normal, especially in the setting of TIA.[31] CT angiography can help identify narrowing of the branches of the internal carotid artery, especially when MRI or catheter angiography is not readily available.

MRI (with magnetic resonance angiography [MRA]) is a mainstay in the diagnosis and follow-up of moyamoya.[54–56] Acute and chronic infarction can be identified in great detail (with diffusion-weighted and fluid-attenuated inversion recovery images, respectively), along with changes in caliber of the affected vessels (with T2-weighted sequences and MRA).[57] The presence of the "ivy sign," a bright signal in the sulci of affected areas, indicates sluggish blood flow.[58] Magnetic resonance perfusion studies can further quantify blood flow.

Catheter-based digital subtraction angiography is a critical tool for both diagnosis of and therapeutic planning for moyamoya. A complete six-vessel study (both internal and external carotid arteries and both vertebral arteries) should be performed when possible. This study allows a definitive diagnosis, identification of associated vascular anomalies (such as aneurysms or arteriovenous malformations), and preoperative visualization of collateral vessels so that they can be preserved during surgery. Angiography can be performed safely in children. When possible, however, angiography should be performed by experienced radiologists to maximize the accuracy of diagnosis and to minimize the risk of complications (reported as < 1% at pediatric referral centers).[59] Disease severity is frequently classified into one of six progressive stages, as originally defined by Suzuki (**Fig. 10.1**).[2]

Many other studies have been used in the diagnostic evaluation of moyamoya, including electroencephalography (EEG), which often shows a "rebuild-up" phenomenon after hyperventilation, transcranial Doppler ultrasonography (used in sickle cell patients), and xenon-enhanced CT.[4,60] Perhaps one of the most commonly used studies is single-photon emission CT with an acetazolamide challenge—that is, a functional challenge of cerebral blood flow.[4,61]

One area of controversy centers on screening at-risk populations for the presence of moyamoya. Current American Heart Association guidelines do not support widespread screening and state that imaging should be reserved for individuals with specific symptoms that suggest the presence of moyamoya.[53] In contrast, several high-volume pediatric centers offer MRI or MRA to first-degree relatives in families with two or more affected members, to individuals with sickle cell disease that demonstrate elevated velocities on transcranial Doppler ultrasonography (> 175 cm/sec) refractory to exchange transfusion, and to patients with neurofibromatosis-1 if they have not previously undergone imaging.[44,62–64] This practice is supported by data demonstrating that a lower Suzuki stage is associated with a decreased stroke burden, both clinically and radiographically, when screening is performed in select populations.[65]

◆ Natural History

The temporal course of moyamoya is difficult to predict. Clinically, some children can remain asymptomatic for years while others have multiple, severe strokes within weeks. Some data indicate that younger children (especially infants) often have a more malignant presentation with short intervals between events. Overall, the disease worsens in almost all individuals. More than two-thirds of patients diagnosed with moyamoya will have clear symptomatic progression within 5 years and will have poor outcomes without treatment.[2,66–69]

Based on these data, many institutions in the United States and Japan have adopted an aggressive approach to treatment.[70] Neurological status at treatment is the most important predictor of long-term outcome.[31] The inconsistent results of attempted medical therapy do not match the marked success of surgical treatment, which reduces symptomatic progression from > 66% to < 3%, based on a multicenter meta-analysis.[71]

◆ Treatment

The treatment of moyamoya is predicated on restoring blood flow to the affected hemisphere. There are no known methods of arresting the underlying arteriopathy. There are three major therapeutic modalities: medical, surgical, and, more recently, endovascular. All three treatments share the goal of reducing the risk of ischemic and hemorrhagic injury by improving cerebral perfusion.

Medical Therapy

Medical therapy has three major components: prevention of thrombosis, maintenance of intravascular volume, and mitigation of nonischemic symptoms (such as headache and seizure). At many moyamoya centers, antithrombotic agents are used to prevent microthrombi at sites of arterial stenosis.[31] Aspirin is used most commonly, and its dosage is based on weight (usually 81 mg daily in children). Some clinicians prefer the use of low-molecular-weight heparin.[72,73]

Maintenance of intravascular volume often does not require administration of medication, but it does involve careful monitoring of fluid balance in children. The primary focus is more on avoiding of dehydration than on supplementing overall intake. Care must be taken in children at risk of fluid loss from illness (e.g., from diarrhea, vomiting), exercise, or activity in hot weather.[4] Mitigation of nonischemic symptoms usually involves treatment of seizures with antiepileptic medication in affected patients and management of headache with analgesics. Calcium-channel blockers can be very effective in ameliorating headache. However, they also can increase the risk of stroke through their propensity to induce hypotension.[74]

It is important to note that few data suggest that medical therapy alone is adequate for the long-term treatment of moyamoya. In studies attempting to manage moyamoya without surgery, almost 40% of patients failed during the period of observation.[3,75] This finding is in marked contrast to surgical treatment, which benefits 87% of treated patients.[71]

Surgical Therapy

Operative indications. Operative indications for moyamoya vary across institutions. Many advocate early surgery in patients with moyamoya, even if patients are asymptomatic, based on data that indicate that neurological status at time of surgery is the most important predictor of long-term outcome.[31] In patients with recent stroke, surgery is often deferred for ~6 weeks to allow swelling to decrease and to allow recovery in anticipation of the physiologic stress of surgery.

Surgical techniques. Surgery for moyamoya is predicated on the finding that the branches of the external carotid artery are not affected in the disorder. Thus, these branches can be used as a source of blood supply to the ischemic brain. The two major approaches commonly used are direct and indirect. Some surgeons opt to combine the two strategies in single procedures. Direct approaches employ a branch of the external carotid artery (usually the superficial temporal artery) as a graft and anastomose it to a cortical artery (usually a branch of the middle cerebral artery [MCA]). Indirect approaches such as pial synangiosis place vascularized tissue (e.g., the dura, muscle, or an artery with a cuff of adventitia) in contact with the brain to stimulate the growth of a new vascular network (**Fig. 10.3**).[4] Both types of approaches have been

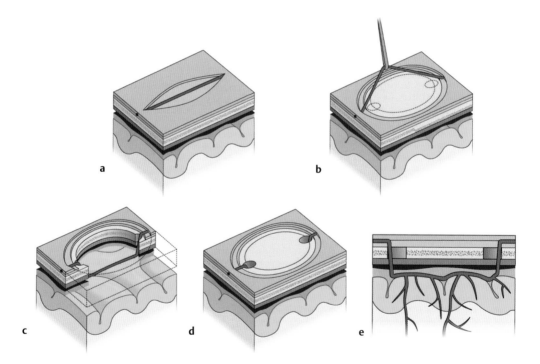

Fig. 10.3a–e Schematic representation of pial synangiosis, a method of indirect revascularization. (**a**) Dissection of the superficial temporal artery. (**b**) The vessel is mobilized (but left intact) to allow exposure of the bone for a craniotomy. (**c**) The bone is removed and the vessel is sutured to the pia after wide dissection of the arachnoid, after which (**d**) the bone is replaced to allow entry and egress of the vessel. (**e**) Image showing a cross-section with a stylized view of new collateral vessels growing from the graft to the brain. (Used with permission from Boston Children's Hospital.)

used with great success in children and have markedly reduced the risk of stroke when performed at experienced centers.[71]

Considerable debate exists over the selection of an individual operative approach. In the United States, most centers initially revascularize the territory of the MCA. At some Asian hospitals, anterior cerebral artery revascularization is included as part of the initial surgery.[76] Direct procedures such as an superficial temporal artery-to-MCA bypass immediately restore blood flow at the time of surgery. In contrast, indirect procedures require weeks or months to establish collateral vessels. However, the bypass can be difficult to perform in young children and may increase the risk of reperfusion hemorrhage, making indirect procedures more appealing. There are numerous indirect revascularization procedures, including encephaloduroarteriosynangiosis, encephalomyoarteriosynangiosis, pial synangiosis, and the drilling of bur holes without vessel synangiosis.[31,77–82]

When performed at experienced centers on carefully selected patients, all surgical treatments offer excellent outcomes compared with the expected natural history of moyamoya.[71] Long-term follow-up of patients treated with surgical revascularization (pial synangiosis) revealed that 67% had strokes preoperatively, but the rate was only 4.3% after surgery in patients with 5 years of follow-up.[31] This finding mirrors data from other centers, including a meta-analysis of more than 1,100 treated individuals, supporting the premise that surgical treatment of moyamoya confers durable, marked reductions in stroke.[4,71] Overall, indirect techniques are used in ~75% of all pediatric moyamoya cases; the remainder are direct or combined approaches.[71] This same meta-analysis showed little difference in outcomes between the two approaches (although placement of bur holes alone was the least successful) when performed at experienced centers. This finding suggests that surgeon and institutional experience may be more important in determining outcomes than any specific surgical technique.[4,31,71]

One of the greatest concerns regarding surgery is the risk of perioperative stroke, reported to occur in 4 to 10% of operations.[4] Meticulous surgical technique, adequate perioperative hydration, skilled anesthetic monitoring, and effective pain management all help reduce complication rates. Intraoperative coordinated care with anesthesia and the EEG team is critical. Selective use of anesthetic agents such as propofol to reduce cerebral metabolism during periods of EEG slowing, coupled with tight blood pressure control, may reduce the risk of stroke.[83] Institutions have adopted and published standardized protocols for the management of patients with moyamoya to maximize safe delivery of care to these complex children (**Fig. 10.4**).

---

1 day before surgery:

Continue aspirin therapy (usually 81 mg once a day orally if < 70 kg, 325 mg once a day orally if 70 kg or more).
Admit patient to hospital for overnight intravenous hydration (isotonic fluids 1.25-1.5 x maintenance).

At induction of anesthesia:

Institute electroencephalographic monitoring.
Maintain noromotension during induction; also normothermia (especially with smaller children), normocarbia (avoid hyperventilation to minimize cerebral vasoconstriction, $pCO_2 > 35$ mm Hg), and normal pH.
Placement of additional intravenous lines, arterial line, Foley catheter, and pulse oximeter.

During surgery:

Maintain normotension, normocarbia, normal pH, adequate oxygenation, normothermia, and adequate hydration.
Electroencephalographic slowing may respond to incremental blood pressure increases or other maneuvers to improve cerebral blood flow.

Postoperatively:

Avoid hyperventilation (relevant with crying in children); pain control is important.
Maintain aspirin therapy on postoperative Day 1.
Maintain intravenous hydration at 1.2-1.5 x maintenance until child is fully recovered and drinking well (usually 48-72 hours).

Fig. 10.4 Representative standardized protocol for the perioperative management of patients with moyamoya (modified from previous publications). From Smith et al.[48] (Used with permission from AANS.)

Centers differ in their philosophy of treating bilateral disease with single or staged craniotomies. In favor of doing both sides in one sitting is the hypothesis that the induction and awakening from anesthesia are greater risks to blood pressure shifts than the overall length of the surgery. Experience from Boston Children's Hospital suggests that performing both sides under a single anesthesia is safe. More than 200 cases have been performed with no increase in the stroke rate.

Endovascular Therapy

An evolving field is the application of endovascular techniques to the treatment of both primary moyamoya disease as well as its associated complications. Recent attempts to open stenosed vessels with endovascular tools such as stents have been associated with mixed results.[84,85] With current technology, it appears that sustained patency of vessels is not possible, likely reflecting the progressive nature of moyamoya involving long stretches of multiple vessels. More intriguing is the possibility of using endovascular treatments to manage acute ischemic events with direct application of angioplasty and intra-arterial vasodilators of thrombolytic agents.[86] The application of endovascular techniques to treat technically challenging moyamoya-associated vascular lesions such as aneurysms and arteriovenous malformations could improve the outcomes of patients afflicted with these disorders.[45,87]

◆ Follow-up and Outcome

After moyamoya is diagnosed, patients are often followed by neurosurgeons or neurologists for life because the primary arteriopathy is not arrested, even with surgery, and the risk of stroke is lifelong. Surgery, however, markedly reduces this risk. The probability of remaining stroke-free over the subsequent 5 years is 96%.[4,31,67] Patients are often maintained on aspirin therapy for life because microthrombi can still form in collateral vessels. Furthermore, its antithrombotic effect is helpful in maintaining patency of any surgical grafts. MRI or MRA is usually obtained 3 to 6 months after surgery as a baseline study, with annual studies for at least 5 years thereafter. Many centers obtain an angiogram at 1 year after surgery to assess the degree of surgical collateralization. Activity is liberalized over 6 to 12 weeks following surgery. Long-term patients have been able to engage in full lives, with normal exercise, active professional careers, and the ability to have children of their own.[31]

Unilateral Disease

A challenging area is the follow-up of moyamoya patients with unilateral disease. It is unclear which patients will develop bilateral moyamoya and which will remain stable. Data suggest that about a third will need surgery within 5 years. Risk factors for progression include young age and the presence of arteriographic anomalies on the initially unaffected side.[65,88] If these children have any of the associated risk factors for progression, it is prudent to follow them more closely, often by additional MRI or MRA studies during the first few years.

Management of Acute Neurologic Symptoms in the Patient with Moyamoya

The acute treatment of potential TIA or stroke in patients with moyamoya varies across centers. Initial steps often include administration of fluids (at 1–1.5 times maintenance), supplemental oxygen, and an additional dose of aspirin if the presence of hemorrhage has been excluded radiographically. Diagnostic evaluation includes electrolytes, glucose levels, and consideration of a MRI to exclude stroke. If seizure is suspected, EEG may be useful, along with administration of antiepileptic medication. It can be useful to admit children to the hospital overnight for observation and continued intravenous fluids. To date, use of thrombolytic therapy in these cases remains of unproven benefit, although it is worthy of further study.

◆ Conclusion

Moyamoya remains a complex condition to diagnose and treat. Its presence should be suspected whenever a child presents with symptoms of cerebral ischemia, especially in at-risk groups. Diagnosis should consist of MRI or MRA and digital subtraction angiography when possible. Management should be instituted as quickly as feasible. Timely referral to experienced centers is critical to optimize the outcomes of children with moyamoya. Surgical revascularization constitutes the mainstay of treatment and is associated with excellent long-term outcomes. Ongoing clinical and translational research efforts promise improvements in the understanding and treatment of this disorder in the near future.

References

1. Shimizu K, Takeuchi K. Hypoplasia of the bilateral internal carotid arteries. (in Japanese) No To Shinkei 1957;9:37–43
2. Suzuki J, Takaku A. Cerebrovascular "moyamoya" disease. Disease showing abnormal net-like vessels in base of brain. Arch Neurol 1969;20(3):288–299
3. Fukui M. Guidelines for the diagnosis and treatment of spontaneous occlusion of the circle of Willis ('moyamoya' disease). Research Committee on Spontaneous Occlusion of the Circle of Willis (Moyamoya Disease) of the Ministry of Health and Welfare, Japan. Clin Neurol Neurosurg 1997;99(Suppl 2):S238–S240
4. Scott RM, Smith ER. Moyamoya disease and moyamoya syndrome. N Engl J Med 2009;360(12):1226–1237
5. Fukui M, Kono S, Sueishi K, Ikezaki K. Moyamoya disease. Neuropathology 2000;20(Suppl):S61–S64
6. Takagi Y, Kikuta K, Nozaki K, Hashimoto N. Histological features of middle cerebral arteries from patients treated for Moyamoya disease. Neurol Med Chir (Tokyo) 2007;47(1):1–4
7. Takagi Y, Kikuta K, Sadamasa N, Nozaki K, Hashimoto N. Proliferative activity through extracellular signal-regulated kinase of smooth muscle cells in vascular walls of cerebral arteriovenous malformations. Neurosurgery 2006;58(4):740–748, discussion 740–748
8. Kono S, Oka K, Sueishi K. Histopathologic and morphometric studies of leptomeningeal vessels in moyamoya disease. Stroke 1990;21(7):1044–1050
9. Lim M, Cheshier S, Steinberg GK. New vessel formation in the central nervous system during tumor growth, vascular malformations, and Moyamoya. Curr Neurovasc Res 2006;3(3):237–245
10. Yamashita M, Tanaka K, Matsuo T, Yokoyama K, Fujii T, Sakamoto H. Cerebral dissecting aneurysms in patients with moyamoya disease. Report of two cases. J Neurosurg 1983;58(1):120–125
11. Oka K, Yamashita M, Sadoshima S, Tanaka K. Cerebral haemorrhage in Moyamoya disease at autopsy. Virchows Arch A Pathol Anat Histol 1981;392(3):247–261
12. Takagi Y, Kikuta K, Nozaki K, et al. Expression of hypoxia-inducing factor-1 alpha and endoglin in intimal hyperplasia of the middle cerebral artery of patients with Moyamoya disease. Neurosurgery 2007;60(2):338–345, discussion 345
13. Malek AM, Connors S, Robertson RL, Folkman J, Scott RM. Elevation of cerebrospinal fluid levels of basic fibroblast growth factor in moyamoya and central nervous system disorders. Pediatr Neurosis 1997;27(4):182–189
14. Nanba R, Kuroda S, Ishikawa T, Houkin K, Iwasaki Y. Increased expression of hepatocyte growth factor in cerebrospinal fluid and intracranial artery in moyamoya disease. Stroke 2004;35(12):2837–2842
15. Soriano SG, Cowan DB, Proctor MR, Scott RM. Levels of soluble adhesion molecules are elevated in the cerebrospinal fluid of children with moyamoya syndrome. Neurosurgery 2002;50(3):544–549
16. Ueno M, Kira R, Matsushima T, et al. Moyamoya disease and transforming growth factor-beta1. J Neurosurg 2000;92(5):907–908
17. Hojo M, Hoshimaru M, Miyamoto S, et al. Role of transforming growth factor-beta1 in the pathogenesis of moyamoya disease. J Neurosurg 1998;89(4):623–629
18. Yoshimoto T, Houkin K, Takahashi A, Abe H. Angiogenic factors in moyamoya disease. Stroke 1996;27(12):2160–2165
19. Kang HS, Kim SK, Cho BK, Kim YY, Hwang YS, Wang KC. Single nucleotide polymorphisms of tissue inhibitor of metalloproteinase genes in familial moyamoya disease. Neurosurgery 2006;58(6):1074–1080, discussion 1074–1080
20. Mineharu Y, Liu W, Inoue K, et al. Autosomal dominant moyamoya disease maps to chromosome 17q25.3. Neurology 2008;70(24 Pt 2):2357–2363
21. Roder C, Peters V, Kasuya H, et al. Analysis of ACTA2 in European Moyamoya disease patients. Eur J Paediatr Neurol 2011;15(2):117–122
22. Hervé D, Touraine P, Verloes A, et al. A hereditary moyamoya syndrome with multisystemic manifestations. Neurology 2010;75(3):259–264
23. Milewicz DM, Kwartler CS, Papke CL, Regalado ES, Cao J, Reid AJ. Genetic variants promoting smooth muscle cell proliferation can result in diffuse and diverse vascular diseases: evidence for a hyperplastic vasculomyopathy. Genet Med 2010;12(4):196–203
24. Shimojima K, Yamamoto T. ACTA2 is not a major disease-causing gene for moyamoya disease. J Hum Genet 2009;54(11):687–688
25. Guo DC, Papke CL, Tran-Fadulu V, et al. Mutations in smooth muscle alpha-actin (ACTA2) cause coronary artery disease, stroke, and Moyamoya disease, along with thoracic aortic disease. Am J Hum Genet 2009;84(5):617–627
26. Ikeda H, Sasaki T, Yoshimoto T, Fukui M, Arinami T. Mapping of a familial moyamoya disease gene to chromosome 3p24.2-p26. Am J Hum Genet 1999;64(2):533–537
27. Nanba R, Tada M, Kuroda S, Houkin K, Iwasaki Y. Sequence analysis and bioinformatics analysis of chromosome 17q25 in familial moyamoya disease. Childs Nerv Syst 2005;21(1):62–68
28. Inoue TK, Ikezaki K, Sasazuki T, Matsushima T, Fukui M. Linkage analysis of moyamoya disease on chromosome 6. J Child Neurol 2000;15(3):179–182
29. Han H, Pyo CW, Yoo DS, Huh PW, Cho KS, Kim DS. Associations of Moyamoya patients with HLA class I and class II alleles in the Korean population. J Korean Med Sci 2003;18(6):876–880
30. Sakurai K, Horiuchi Y, Ikeda H, et al. A novel susceptibility locus for moyamoya disease on chromosome 8q23. J Hum Genet 2004;49(5):278–281

31. Scott RM, Smith JL, Robertson RL et al. Long-term outcome in children with moyamoya syndrome after cranial revascularization by pial synangiosis. J Neurosurg 2004 February;100(2 Suppl Pediatrics):142–9

32. Tanghetti B, Capra R, Giunta F, Marini G, Orlandini A. Moyamoya syndrome in only one of two identical twins. Case report. J Neurosurg 1983;59(6):1092–1094

33. Wakai K, Tamakoshi A, Ikezaki K, et al. Epidemiological features of moyamoya disease in Japan: findings from a nationwide survey. Clin Neurol Neurosurg 1997; 99(Suppl 2):S1–S5

34. Nagaraja D, Verma A, Taly AB, Kumar MV, Jayakumar PN. Cerebrovascular disease in children. Acta Neurol Scand 1994;90(4):251–255

35. Baba T, Houkin K, Kuroda S. Novel epidemiological features of moyamoya disease. J Neurol Neurosurg Psychiatry 2008;79(8):900–904

36. Yonekawa Y, Ogata N, Kaku Y, Taub E, Imhof HG. Moyamoya disease in Europe, past and present status. Clin Neurol Neurosurg 1997;99(Suppl 2):S58–S60

37. Uchino K, Johnston SC, Becker KJ, Tirschwell DL. Moyamoya disease in Washington State and California. Neurology 2005;65(6):956–958

38. Caldarelli M, Di Rocco C, Gaglini P. Surgical treatment of moyamoya disease in pediatric age. J Neurosurg Sci 2001;45(2):83–91

39. Suzuki J, Kodama N. Moyamoya disease—a review. Stroke 1983;14(1):104–109

40. Han DH, Nam DH, Oh CW. Moyamoya disease in adults: characteristics of clinical presentation and outcome after encephalo-duro-arterio-synangiosis. Clin Neurol Neurosurg 1997;99(Suppl 2):S151–S155

41. Han DH, Kwon OK, Byun BJ, et al; Korean Society for Cerebrovascular Disease. A co-operative study: clinical characteristics of 334 Korean patients with moyamoya disease treated at neurosurgical institutes (1976–1994). Acta Neurochir (Wien) 2000;142(11):1263–1273, discussion 1273–1274

42. Hankinson TC, Bohman LE, Heyer G, et al. Surgical treatment of moyamoya syndrome in patients with sickle cell anemia: outcome following encephaloduroarteriosynangiosis. J Neurosurg Pediatr 2008;1(3): 211–216

43. Ullrich NJ, Robertson R, Kinnamon DD, et al. Moyamoya following cranial irradiation for primary brain tumors in children. Neurology 2007;68(12):932–938

44. Jea A, Smith ER, Robertson R, Scott RM. Moyamoya syndrome associated with Down syndrome: outcome after surgical revascularization. Pediatrics 2005;116(5): e694–e701

45. Codd PJ, Scott RM, Smith ER. Seckel syndrome and moyamoya. J Neurosurg Pediatr 2009;3(4):320–324

46. Qaiser R, Scott RM, Smith ER. Identification of an association between Robinow syndrome and moyamoya. Pediatr Neurosurg 2009;45(1):69–72

47. Bober MB, Khan N, Kaplan J, et al. Majewski osteodysplastic primordial dwarfism type II (MOPD II): expanding the vascular phenotype. Am J Med Genet A 2010;152A(4):960–965

48. Smith ER, McClain CD, Heeney M, Scott RM. Pial synangiosis in patients with moyamoya syndrome and sickle cell anemia: perioperative management and surgical outcome. Neurosurg Focus 2009;26(4):E10

49. Seol HJ, Wang KC, Kim SK, Hwang YS, Kim KJ, Cho BK. Headache in pediatric moyamoya disease: review of 204 consecutive cases. J Neurosurg 2005;103(5, Suppl)439–442

50. Nishimoto AUK, Onbe H. Cooperative study on moyamoya disease in Japan. Cooperative study on moyamoya disease in Japan. 1981. p. 53–8.

51. Hallemeier CL, Rich KM, Grubb RL Jr, et al. Clinical features and outcome in North American adults with moyamoya phenomenon. Stroke 2006;37(6): 1490–1496

52. Massaro M, Thorarensen O, Liu GT, Maguire AM, Zimmerman RA, Brodsky MC. Morning glory disc anomaly and moyamoya vessels. Arch Ophthalmol 1998;116(2):253–254

53. Roach ES, Golomb MR, Adams R, et al; American Heart Association Stroke Council; Council on Cardiovascular Disease in the Young. Management of stroke in infants and children: a scientific statement from a Special Writing Group of the American Heart Association Stroke Council and the Council on Cardiovascular Disease in the Young. Stroke 2008;39(9):2644–2691

54. Yamada I, Suzuki S, Matsushima Y. Moyamoya disease: comparison of assessment with MR angiography and MR imaging versus conventional angiography. Radiology 1995;196(1):211–218

55. Katz DA, Marks MP, Napel SA, Bracci PM, Roberts SL. Circle of Willis: evaluation with spiral CT angiography, MR angiography, and conventional angiography. Radiology 1995;195(2):445–449

56. Takanashi JI, Sugita K, Niimi H. Evaluation of magnetic resonance angiography with selective maximum intensity projection in patients with childhood moyamoya disease. Eur J Paediatr Neurol 1998;2(2):83–89

57. Yamada I, Matsushima Y, Suzuki S. Moyamoya disease: diagnosis with three-dimensional time-of-flight MR angiography. Radiology 1992;184(3):773–778

58. Fujiwara H, Momoshima S, Kuribayashi S. Leptomeningeal high signal intensity (ivy sign) on fluid-attenuated inversion-recovery (FLAIR) MR images in moyamoya disease. Eur J Radiol 2005;55(2):224–230

59. Robertson RL, Chavali RV, Robson CD, et al. Neurologic complications of cerebral angiography in childhood moyamoya syndrome. Pediatr Radiol 1998;28(11): 824–829

60. Kodama N, Aoki Y, Hiraga H, Wada T, Suzuki J. Electroencephalographic findings in children with moyamoya disease. Arch Neurol 1979;36(1):16–19

61. Lee M, Zaharchuk G, Guzman R, Achrol A, Bell-Stephens T, Steinberg GK. Quantitative hemodynamic studies in moyamoya disease: a review. Neurosurg Focus 2009; 26(4):E5

62. Kirkham FJ, DeBaun MR. Stroke in Children with Sickle Cell Disease. Curr Treat Options Neurol 2004;6(5): 357–375

63. Roach ES. Etiology of stroke in children. Semin Pediatr Neurol 2000;7(4):244–260

64. Rosser TL, Vezina G, Packer RJ. Cerebrovascular abnormalities in a population of children with neurofibromatosis type 1. Neurology 2005;64(3):553–555

65. Smith ER, Scott RM. Progression of disease in unilateral moyamoya syndrome. Neurosurg Focus 2008; 24(2):E17

66. Imaizumi T, Hayashi K, Saito K, Osawa M, Fukuyama Y. Long-term outcomes of pediatric moyamoya disease monitored to adulthood. Pediatr Neurol 1998; 18(4):321–325

67. Choi JU, Kim DS, Kim EY, Lee KC. Natural history of moyamoya disease: comparison of activity of daily living in surgery and non surgery groups. Clin Neurol Neurosurg 1997;99(Suppl 2):S11–S18

68. Kurokawa T, Chen YJ, Tomita S, Kishikawa T, Kitamura K. Cerebrovascular occlusive disease with and without the moyamoya vascular network in children. Neuropediatrics 1985;16(1):29–32

69. Ezura M, Takahashi A, Yoshimoto T. Successful treatment of an arteriovenous malformation by chemical embolization with estrogen followed by conventional radiotherapy. Neurosurgery 1992;31(6):1105–1107, discussion 1107

70. Kuroda S, Ishikawa T, Houkin K, Nanba R, Hokari M, Iwasaki Y. Incidence and clinical features of disease progression in adult moyamoya disease. Stroke 2005; 36(10):2148–2153

71. Fung LW, Thompson D, Ganesan V. Revascularisation surgery for paediatric moyamoya: a review of the lite wd rature. Childs Nerv Syst 2005;21(5):358–364

72. Bowen MD, Burak CR, Barron TF. Childhood ischemic stroke in a nonurban population. J Child Neurol 2005; 20(3):194–197

73. Scott RM. Moyamoya syndrome: a surgically treatable cause of stroke in the pediatric patient. Clin Neurosurg 2000;47:378–384

74. Ganesan V. Moyamoya: to cut or not to cut is not the only question. A paediatric neurologist's perspective. Dev Med Child Neurol 2010;52(1):10–13

75. Ikezaki K. Rational approach to treatment of moyamoya disease in childhood. J Child Neurol 2000;15(5): 350–356

76. Kim SK, Wang KC, Kim IO, Lee DS, Cho BK. Combined encephaloduroarteriosynangiosis and bifrontal encephalogaleo (periosteal) synangiosis in pediatric moyamoya disease. Neurosurgery 2008;62(6, Suppl 3) 1456–1464

77. Matsushima T, Inoue T, Katsuta T, et al. An indirect revascularization method in the surgical treatment of moyamoya disease—various kinds of indirect procedures and a multiple combined indirect procedure. Neurol Med Chir (Tokyo) 1998;38(Suppl): 297–302

78. Kawaguchi S, Okuno S, Sakaki T. Effect of direct arterial bypass on the prevention of future stroke in patients with the hemorrhagic variety of moyamoya disease. J Neurosurg 2000;93(3):397–401

79. Houkin K, Kamiyama H, Abe H, Takahashi A, Kuroda S. Surgical therapy for adult moyamoya disease. Can surgical revascularization prevent the recurrence of intracerebral hemorrhage? Stroke 1996;27(8): 1342–1346

80. Sencer S, Poyanli A, Kiriş T, Sencer A, Minareci O. Recent experience with Moyamoya disease in Turkey. Eur Radiol 2000;10(4):569–572

81. Houkin K, Kuroda S, Nakayama N. Cerebral revascularization for moyamoya disease in children. Neurosurg Clin N Am 2001;12(3):575–584, ix ix

82. Dauser RC, Tuite GF, McCluggage CW. Dural inversion procedure for moyamoya disease. Technical note. J Neurosurg 1997;86(4):719–723

83. Soriano SG, Sethna NF, Scott RM. Anesthetic management of children with moyamoya syndrome. Anesth Analg 1993;77(5):1066–1070

84. Drazin D, Calayag M, Gifford E, Dalfino J, Yamamoto J, Boulos AS. Endovascular treatment for moyamoya disease in a Caucasian twin with angioplasty and Wingspan stent. Clin Neurol Neurosurg 2009;111(10): 913–917

85. Khan N, Dodd R, Marks MP, Bell-Stephens T, Vavao J, Steinberg GK. Failure of primary percutaneous angioplasty and stenting in the prevention of ischemia in Moyamoya angiopathy. Cerebrovasc Dis 2011;31(2): 147–153

86. El-Hakam LM, Volpi J, Mawad M, Clark G. Angioplasty for acute stroke with pediatric moyamoya syndrome. J Child Neurol 2010;25(10):1278–1283

87. Yang S, Yu JL, Wang HL, Wang B, Luo Q. Endovascular embolization of distal anterior choroidal artery aneurysms associated with moyamoya disease. A report of two cases and a literature review. Interv Neuroradiol 2010;16(4):433–441

88. Kelly ME, Bell-Stephens TE, Marks MP, Do HM, Steinberg GK. Progression of unilateral moyamoya disease: A clinical series. Cerebrovasc Dis 2006;22(2-3): 109–115

11

Endovascular Therapy for Moyamoya Disease

Michael P. Marks

◆ Introduction

Moyamoya disease is manifest as a progressive stenosis involving the distal portions of the internal carotid arteries with concomitant involvement of the anterior and middle cerebral arteries. Angiographically, these areas of stenosis, which often progress to occlusion, are often indistinguishable from other intracranial angiopathies including atherosclerosis and vasculitis. However, unlike patients with atherosclerotic or vasculitic stenosis, patients with moyamoya disease usually manifest a network of collateral blood supply, which appears as a proliferation or hypertrophy of small arteries in the region of the perforating vessels.[1] Typically, there are two peak age groups for presentation: the earlier one during childhood and the later peak in middle-aged adults.[2] Patients may have a variety of symptoms that are commonly attributed to brain ischemia or hemorrhage. Both children and adults present with ischemic symptoms, but hemorrhage most often manifests in adult patients.[3,4]

No medical therapy that improves or slows the progressive angiopathic changes has been identified. The mainstay of therapy for ischemic symptoms is surgical revascularization to increase blood flow to the ischemic brain.[5–8] Experience with angioplasty and/or stenting to increase blood flow to the patient with moyamoya via endovascular means is limited. Furthermore, endovascular therapy has been used in only a few cases to treat angiographically identifiable aneurysms considered responsible for hemorrhagic complications of the disease. This chapter reviews these endovascular therapeutic approaches to the treatment of ischemic and hemorrhagic conditions in patients with moyamoya disease.

◆ Pathophysiologic Considerations

The pathogenesis of moyamoya disease remains unclear. Infection may play a role as may genetic factors.[9] Moyamoya disease has also been associated with other conditions such as radiotherapy to the head or neck, Down syndrome, neurofibromatosis type 1, and sickle cell disease.[10]

Pathologic analysis of the steno-occlusive sites shows no evidence of the changes associated with other angiopathies affecting the intracranial vasculature such as arteriosclerosis and vasculitis. Rather, the stenosed arteries in patients with moyamoya disease demonstrate thickened intima marked by proliferation of smooth muscle cells.[11,12] The collateral vessels that develop in response to acquired stenosis show evidence of thinning in the media with fragmentation of the elastic lamina and the formation of microaneurysms.[12,13] These features are thought to represent the probable site for the hemorrhagic changes that occur in patients with moyamoya disease.

◆ Endovascular Therapy for Stenotic Arteries

Angioplasty, stenting, or both have been used most extensively to treat refractory, symptomatic intracranial stenosis related to arteriosclerosis. These techniques have been suggested as a means to increase cerebral blood flow and to reduce the risk of recurrent ischemic symptoms in symptomatic patients. Surgical bypasses, as evaluated in the Extracranial-to-Intracranial Bypass Study and more recently in the Carotid Occlusion Surgery Study, have not proven to be beneficial in this group of patients.[14] In contrast, surgical treatment of patients with moyamoya disease with indirect or direct bypasses has a demonstrated benefit.

Endovascular therapy with angioplasty and/or stenting is potentially attractive because it is less invasive than surgical revascularization. However, there is little documented evaluation of this alternative, and the durability of the outcomes in this progressive disease is not clearly established. To date, endovascular techniques have been used to treat moyamoya disease in 10 patients.[15-20] As with endovascular therapy for intracranial atherosclerosis, patients have been treated with angioplasty alone or with angioplasty and stenting.

Kornblihtt et al[15] reported the first such case, implanting a stent in the intracranial portion of the internal carotid artery in an 18-year-old girl with transient ischemic attacks involving the left hemisphere. Clinical and angiographic follow-up at 46 months showed that the stent was fully patent, and the patient had no recurrent symptoms. Rodriguez et al[16] treated a 37-year-old man with bilateral disease and left hemisphere symptoms referable to the left hemisphere. They performed balloon angioplasty, which significantly improved blood flow to the left hemisphere. They followed the patient for 2 years with no angiographic evidence of restenosis. The patient remained asymptomatic during these 2 years of follow-up.

Drazin et al[17] reported endovascular treatment of moyamoya disease in a Caucasian twin. The 40-year-old woman initially presented with left hemispheric symptoms, suggesting an acute stroke. She underwent emergent angioplasty of her left middle cerebral artery (MCA) with good improvement of blood flow. Within 3 months, however, she developed a new aphasia from a stroke involving the left MCA territory. Imaging demonstrated occlusion of the angioplasty site. Twenty-two months later, she presented with a new right hemispheric stroke and underwent placement of a Wingspan stent (Boston Scientific, Natick, MA) after angioplasty in the supraclinoid carotid artery. At 3 months, she had recurrent stenosis. Further angioplasty was performed without complications. She was followed for 2 years clinically and for 15 months after the second angioplasty. She demonstrated no symptoms or radiographic change at that time.

El-Hakam et al[18] reported the youngest patient to undergo endovascular therapy for the treatment of moyamoya disease. A 3-year-old girl had diffuse narrowing of the supraclinoid segments of both internal carotid arteries that extended into the anterior MCAs. She presented to the hospital with transient left leg weakness. During hospitalization, she became densely hemiplegic on the left side. She underwent emergent angioplasty of the supraclinoid right internal carotid artery within 6 hours of the onset of her symptoms. After the procedure, her blood flow was significantly improved through the vessels of the right hemisphere and her strength rapidly improved. Two weeks later, she underwent a right dural inversion revascularization. Two years later, angiography showed that the right internal carotid artery had been completely occluded, but transdural collaterals had developed. The authors used angioplasty to relieve acute symptoms from what they described as an impending carotid occlusion, affording some time for a surgical procedure to be performed.

Khan et al[19] reported the largest experience: six endovascular procedures performed in five patients (**Fig. 11.1**). Two patients underwent internal carotid artery angioplasty and Wingspan stenting in three arterial territories. Angioplasty alone was performed in one patient, and two patients underwent angioplasty and placement of a Wingspan stent in

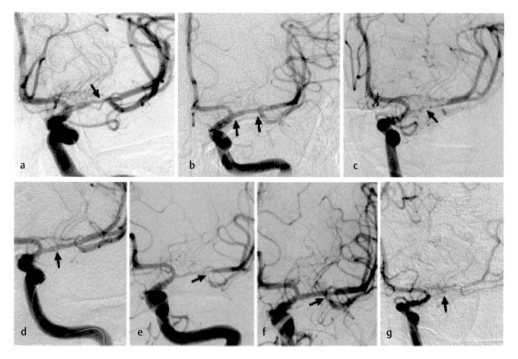

Fig. 11.1a–g Anteroposterior angiograms of the left internal carotid artery. (**a**) Initial M1 stenosis (*arrow*). (**b**) Angioplasty and stenting showing increased M1 diameter (*arrows*). (**c**) Recurrence of stenosis at 6 months (*arrow*). (**d**) Reangioplasty at 6 months (*arrow*). (**e**) Repeat angiography 2 months later reveals recurrent high-grade M1 and proximal M2 stenoses (*arrow*). (**f**) Reangioplasty of both M1 and M2 (*arrow*). (**g**) Occlusion of M1 segment prior to revascularization surgery (*arrow*). Source: Used with permission from Khan N, Dodd R, Marks MP, Bell-Stephens T, Vavao J, Steinberg GK. Failure of primary percutaneous angioplasty and stenting in the prevention of ischemia in moyamoya angiopathy. (Courtesy of Cerebrovascular Dis 2011;31:147–153.)

the MCA. All five patients developed recurrent ischemic symptoms with transient ischemic attacks. At a mean of 4 months, three patients underwent repeat endovascular treatment for restenosis. Because of their recurrent symptoms, all five patients ultimately underwent surgical revascularization. The authors point out a potential bias in this reported series, which represents patients referred to a center that performs a high number of surgical revascularization procedures for patients with moyamoya disease. Therefore, their patients may represent a select group who have failed angioplasty and stenting.

Santirso et al[20] reported the single case of a woman with bilateral ischemic lesions and evidence of bilateral moyamoya disease who presented with a sudden episode of aphasia and paresis of her right arm. She underwent revascularization with angioplasty and Wingspan stenting in the left MCA. Subsequently, her speech improved as did her arm strength, but neither normalized completely. After 13 months follow-up, arteriography showed mild interval restenosis, but she had experienced no recurrent events at this follow-up.

None of the cases reported to date have demonstrated complications, but the rate of restenosis and/or recurrent symptoms has been high, and the durability of endovascular therapy is questionable. In this limited experience of treating 12 vascular territories (in 10 patients), restenosis and/or recurrent symptoms occurred in 9 territories. Three territories were treated with angioplasty alone, two of which showed subsequent occlusion. Nine territories were treated with stenting, seven of which showed restenosis or recurrent symptoms. Eight of the nine stent cases were performed with the Wingspan stent. High rates of restenosis in the treatment of atherosclerotic disease have been found with this stent, particularly in the anterior circulation (internal carotid arteries and MCAs) in younger patients.[21–23] Some authors have speculated that these lesions behave differently because they may have an inflammatory component or may represent moyamoya angiopathy.[23]

◆ Treatment of Aneurysms in Patients with Moyamoya Disease

Hemorrhage associated with moyamoya disease has been thought to be directly related to bleeding from collateral vessels under hemodynamic stress. Pathologic evaluation of these vessels has demonstrated evidence of vessel wall thinning and microaneurysym formation thought to predispose the vessel to rupture.[12,13] Relatively high rates of rebleeding with an increased incidence of mortality and lower rates of good clinical outcomes have been associated with these rebleeding episodes.[24] Surgical revascularization has been proposed as a way to reduce the risk of bleeding by reducing the hemodynamic demands on the collateral vessels.[24,25] In some cases, sequential angiography after revascularization has shown obliteration of peripheral aneurysms.[26] Long-term follow-up of patients with hemorrhagic moyamoya disease that have undergone surgical revascularization suggests that the procedure reduces but does not eliminate rehemorrhage.[24–27] In addition to surgical bypass, direct surgical treatment of collateral vessel aneurysms is possible. Surgical interventions have included aneurysmectomy and neck clipping.[27,28] However, there is significant concern about the surgical approach because of the deep location of these aneurysms and the hemodynamic stresses created by surgery in a patient with a significantly compromised circulation.

Several case reports have documented endovascular treatment of small aneurysms on lenticulostriate or choroidal arteries thought to be responsible for patient hemorrhage.[29–33] Kim et al[30] reported eight patients with moyamoya disease who were treated by endovascular means after presenting with intracerebral or intraventricular hemorrhage. Seven of the patients had aneurysms that were successfully occluded without complications. One procedure failed due to an inability to navigate the catheter into the small posterior choroidal artery. No further bleeding occurred in the patients. Six patients recovered completely from their hemorrhage. The patients in this series were all embolized with n-butyl cyanoacrylate.

Harreld and Zomorodi[31] reported a single patient with moyamoya disease who underwent embolization of a lenticulostriate artery. The authors pointed out that with a microcatheter positioned somewhat proximal in the lenticulostriate artery feeding the aneurysm, the patient developed left facial palsy after sodium amytal testing. The catheter was advanced more distally in the lenticulostriate artery, and repeat testing showed no neurologic deficit. Subsequent embolization with n-butyl cyanoacrylate obliterated the aneurysm, and the patient had no neurologic symptoms from the procedure.

Yang et al[29] reported two patients with moyamoya disease who underwent successful endovascular treatment of aneurysms in the distal segment of the anterior choroidal artery. One patient had hemorrhaged and the other patient had not. The patient with bleeding was treated with cyanoacrylate, but the patient with the unruptured aneurysm was treated with coil embolization. The authors stressed that endovascular embolization may be safe in the more distal portion of the anterior choroidal circulation, beyond the cisternal segment of the artery.

◆ Conclusion

Based on the limited experience with angioplasty or stenting of stenosed arteries in patients with moyamoya disease, these procedures do not appear to be durable. High rates of restenosis or continued symptoms have been encountered in the few cases reported. Endovascular treatment of distal artery aneurysms may be beneficial in select patients with moyamoya disease who present with hemorrhage. Although these aneurysms may regress after bypass procedures, rates of rebleeding in these patients are relatively high and more immediate endovascular treatment may be beneficial.

References

1. Scott RM, Smith ER. Moyamoya disease and moyamoya syndrome. N Engl J Med 2009;360(12):1226–1237

2. Achrol AS, Guzman R, Lee M, Steinberg GK. Pathophysiology and genetic factors in moyamoya disease. Neurosurg Focus 2009;26(4):E4

3. Han DH, Nam DH, Oh CW. Moyamoya disease in adults: characteristics of clinical presentation and outcome after encephalo-duro-arterio-synangiosis. Clin Neurol Neurosurg 1997;99(Suppl 2):S151–S155

4. Scott RM, Smith JL, Robertson RL et al. Long-term outcome in children with moyamoya syndrome after cranial revascularization by pial synangiosis. J Neurosurg 2004 February;100(2 Suppl Pediatrics):142–9

5. Fung LW, Thompson D, Ganesan V. Revascularisation surgery for paediatric moyamoya: a review of the literature. Childs Nerv Syst 2005;21(5):358–364

6. Veeravagu A, Guzman R, Patil CG, Hou LC, Lee M, Steinberg GK. Moyamoya disease in pediatric patients: outcomes of neurosurgical interventions. Neurosurg Focus 2008;24(2):E16

7. Matsushima T, Inoue T, Ikezaki K, et al. Multiple combined indirect procedure for the surgical treatment of children with moyamoya disease. A comparison with single indirect anastomosis and direct anastomosis. Neurosurg Focus 1998;5(5):e4

8. Guzman R, Lee M, Achrol A, et al. Clinical outcome after 450 revascularization procedures for moyamoya disease. Clinical article. J Neurosurg 2009;111(5):927–935

9. Yamada H, Deguchi K, Tanigawara T, et al. The relationship between moyamoya disease and bacterial infection. Clin Neurol Neurosurg 1997;99(Suppl 2): S221–S224

10. Kuroda S, Houkin K. Moyamoya disease: current concepts and future perspectives. Lancet Neurol 2008; 7(11):1056–1066

11. Fukui M, Kono S, Sueishi K, Ikezaki K. Moyamoya disease. Neuropathology 2000;20(Suppl):S61–S64

12. Yamashita M, Oka K, Tanaka K. Histopathology of the brain vascular network in moyamoya disease. Stroke 1983;14(1):50–58

13. Burke GM, Burke AM, Sherma AK, Hurley MC, Batjer HH, Bendok BR. Moyamoya disease: a summary. Neurosurg Focus 2009;26(4):E11

14. The EC/IC Bypass Study Group. Failure of extracranial-intracranial arterial bypass to reduce the risk of ischemic stroke. Results of an international randomized trial. N Engl J Med 1985;313(19):1191–1200

15. Kornblihtt LI, Cocorullo S, Miranda C, Lylyk P, Heller PG, Molinas FC. Moyamoya syndrome in an adolescent with essential thrombocythemia: successful intracranial carotid stent placement. Stroke 2005;36(8): E71–E73

16. Rodriguez GJ, Kirmani JF, Ezzeddine MA, Qureshi AI. Primary percutaneous transluminal angioplasty for early moyamoya disease. J Neuroimaging 2007;17(1): 48–53

17. Drazin D, Calayag M, Gifford E, Dalfino J, Yamamoto J, Boulos AS. Endovascular treatment for moyamoya disease in a Caucasian twin with angioplasty and Wingspan stent. Clin Neurol Neurosurg 2009;111(10): 913–917

18. El-Hakam LM, Volpi J, Mawad M, Clark G. Angioplasty for acute stroke with pediatric moyamoya syndrome. J Child Neurol 2010;25(10):1278–1283

19. Khan N, Dodd R, Marks MP, Bell-Stephens T, Vavao J, Steinberg GK. Failure of primary percutaneous angioplasty and stenting in the prevention of ischemia in Moyamoya angiopathy. Cerebrovasc Dis 2011;31(2): 147–153

20. Santirso D, Oliva P, González M, et al. Intracranial stent placement in a patient with moyamoya disease. J Neurol 2012;259(1):170–171

21. Albuquerque FC, Levy EI, Turk AS, et al. Angiographic patterns of Wingspan in-stent restenosis. Neurosurgery 2008;63(1):23–27, discussion 27–28

22. Levy EI, Turk AS, Albuquerque FC, et al. Wingspan in-stent restenosis and thrombosis: incidence, clinical presentation, and management. Neurosurgery 2007; 61(3):644–650, discussion 650–651

23. Turk AS, Levy EI, Albuquerque FC, et al. Influence of patient age and stenosis location on wingspan in-stent restenosis. AJNR Am J Neuroradiol 2008;29(1): 23–27

24. Yoshida Y, Yoshimoto T, Shirane R, Sakurai Y. Clinical course, surgical management, and long-term outcome of moyamoya patients with rebleeding after an episode of intracerebral hemorrhage: An extensive follow-Up study. Stroke 1999;30(11):2272–2276

25. Saeki N, Nakazaki S, Kubota M, et al. Hemorrhagic type moyamoya disease. Clin Neurol Neurosurg 1997; 99(Suppl 2):S196–S201

26. Kuroda S, Houkin K, Kamiyama H, Abe H. Effects of surgical revascularization on peripheral artery aneurysms in moyamoya disease: report of three cases. Neurosurgery 2001;49(2):463–467, discussion 467–468

27. Kawaguchi S, Okuno S, Sakaki T. Effect of direct arterial bypass on the prevention of future stroke in patients with the hemorrhagic variety of moyamoya disease. J Neurosurg 2000;93(3):397–401

28. Sakai K, Mizumatsu S, Terasaka K, Sugatani H, Higashi T. Surgical treatment of a lenticulostriate artery aneurysm. Case report. Neurol Med Chir (Tokyo) 2005; 45(11):574–577

29. Yang S, Yu JL, Wang HL, Wang B, Luo Q. Endovascular embolization of distal anterior choroidal artery aneurysms associated with moyamoya disease. A report of two cases and a literature review. Interv Neuroradiol 2010;16(4):433–441

30. Kim SH, Kwon OK, Jung CK, et al. Endovascular treatment of ruptured aneurysms or pseudoaneurysms on the collateral vessels in patients with moyamoya disease. Neurosurgery 2009;65(5):1000–1004, discussion 1004

31. Harreld JH, Zomorodi AR. Embolization of an unruptured distal lenticulostriate aneurysm associated with moyamoya disease. AJNR Am J Neuroradiol 2011;32(3): E42–E43

32. Larrazabal R, Pelz D, Findlay JM. Endovascular treatment of a lenticulostriate artery aneurysm with N-butyl cyanoacrylate. Can J Neurol Sci 2001;28(3): 256–259

33. Gandhi CD, Gilad R, Patel AB, Haridas A, Bederson JB. Treatment of ruptured lenticulostriate artery aneurysms. J Neurosurg 2008;109(1):28–37

12

Indirect Revascularization Procedures for Moyamoya Disease

John E. Wanebo, Gregory J. Velat, Joseph M. Zabramski, Peter Nakaji, and Robert F. Spetzler

◆ Introduction

Indirect surgical revascularization techniques for moyamoya disease have evolved over the past five decades; their variety is a reflection of surgical ingenuity and advances in modern medicine. Vascularized donor tissues such as the superficial temporal artery (STA), galea, dura, muscle, and omentum have been used alone and in combination to augment intracranial blood flow. Indirect procedures avoid many potential technical pitfalls of direct anastomosis, including ischemia from temporary arterial occlusion, extended anesthesia time, and the relatively small caliber of extra- and intracranial arteries. The assumption underlying indirect procedures is that the tissues will grow together over time, bringing with them collateral vasculature, which will gradually provide the brain with additional blood flow. Adult patients with moyamoya with advanced disease and maximal arterial vasodilation may be candidates for indirect revascularization. The rationale for this strategy is that patients will thereby avoid a potential hyperperfusion syndrome associated with the sudden increase in blood flow provided by direct anastomosis.[1] However, patients undergoing indirect anastomosis must await the uncertain and gradual ingrowth of vessels to receive additional flow.

It should be stressed that patients undergoing indirect bypass are at the same anesthetic risk as patients undergoing direct bypass. Therefore, the same attention must be paid to the use of antiplatelet agents, avoidance of hypotension, and maintenance of normocapnia.

This chapter reviews the most common indirect anastomosis operations: encephalodurosynangiosis (EDS), encephalomyosynangiosis (EMS), encephaloduroarteriosynangiosis (EDAS), encephaloduroarteriomyosynangiosis (EDAMS), omental transposition and transplantation, multiple cranial bur holes, pericranial transfer, and galeal procedures. We specifically address variations of techniques using artery, muscle, dura, pericranium, and galea as donor tissues. The combinations of indirect procedures with and without direct bypass are also reviewed.

◆ Anatomic Considerations for Indirect Revascularization

Donor tissues for indirect revascularization include temporalis muscle, galea, pericranium, and dura. All are served by branches of the external carotid artery (**Fig. 12.1a**). The external carotid artery terminates in the STA and internal maxillary artery. The internal maxillary artery has three ascending collateral branches: the anterior deep temporal artery, the posterior deep temporal artery, and the middle meningeal artery. The anterior deep temporal and posterior deep temporal arteries interconnect with the middle deep temporal artery, a branch of the proximal STA, and serve

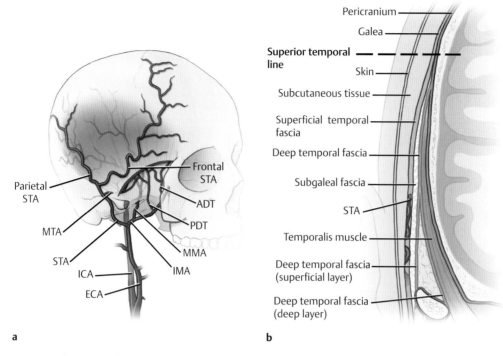

a   b

Fig. 12.1a, b **(a)** Branches of the superficial temporal artery (STA) and the internal maxillary artery (IMA) are the terminal branches of the external carotid artery (ECA), which irrigate the temporal parietal scalp and the temporalis muscle. The anterior deep temporal artery (ADT), the posterior deep temporal artery (PDT), and the middle meningeal artery (MMA) branch off of the IMA. The middle temporal artery (MTA) to the temporalis muscle is a proximal branch of the superficial temporal artery. ICA, internal carotid artery. **(b)** Cross-sectional view demonstrating galeal relationships relative to the superior temporal line. Below the superior temporal line, the galea becomes the superficial temporal fascia. (Used with permission from Barrow Neurological Institute.)

the temporalis muscle. The middle meningeal artery is a terminal branch of the internal maxillary artery. It penetrates the base of the temporal bone through the foramen spinosum and divides into anterior, middle (temporal), and posterior branches. The temporal branch of the middle meningeal artery anastomoses with the deep temporal arteries in the temporal bone, and the middle meningeal artery anastomoses with the STA in the parietal bone.

These arteries can form anastomotic networks in both the vertical and horizontal plane.[2] The STA divides into frontal and parietal branches 2 to 4 cm above the zygoma. The STA lies 2 cm in front of the external auditory canal, and its diameter ranges from 2 to 5 mm (mean, 3.24 mm) at this level. The frontal STA anastomoses with the supraorbital and supratrochlear arteries anteriorly, whereas the parietal STA joins with the occipital artery posteriorly. In cadaveric studies, the STA branches

anastomose to the contralateral side at the vertex in all normal cases. A single STA provides sufficient blood flow to vascularize the entire scalp. When indirect revascularization is being considered, it is critical to be aware of the anatomic layers and vascular supply. The well-known pneumonic SCALP, which denotes *s*kin, subcutaneous tissue, *a*poneurosis, *l*oose areolar tissue, and *p*ericranium, provides a basic description. The STA and occipital artery carry the primary vascular supplies for the galea, whereas the supraorbital and supratrochlear arteries serve the pericranium. As well described by Matsushima and Inaba, a series of natural collaterals develops in the setting of cerebral ischemia with moyamoya disease.[3]

The galea is part of the subcutaneous muscular aponeurosis system (**Fig. 12.1b**). The galea above the superior temporal line is the robust layer deep to the epidermis and dermal fat, and it joins the frontalis and occipitalis muscles.

It is difficult to separate the galea from the fat and dermal layer above it because no clear plane exists. Plastic surgeons describe sharply elevating the galea from the subcutaneous fat in a subfollicular plane by keeping the hair follicles superficial. Below the superior temporal line, the galeal layer is less well defined and is part of the temporal parietal fascia. The STA runs in the temporal parietal fascia. The superficial temporal vein is always superficial to the temporal parietal fascia and posterior superior to the STA. Other terms for the temporal parietal fascia are the superficial temporal fascia or galea extension. At the level of the zygoma, the galea is loosely connected to the subdermal fat; it becomes more adherent at the vertex. The temporalis muscle is covered by the deep temporal fascia, a thick, firm layer that connects to periosteum in all directions.

◆ Encephalodurosynangiosis

The description of EDS is credited to Tsubokawa et al who reported laying a vascularized dural graft onto the surface of the brain to treat a patient with cerebral ischemia secondary to thrombosis in 1964.[4] This procedure was later applied to the treatment of moyamoya disease. The rationale for this form of indirect anastomosis is that the dura itself has a robust blood supply that is predominantly available through its outer leaflet. Applying the outer surface of the dura to the brain creates an opportunity for an extracranial-to-intracranial anastomosis to form. EDS is seldom performed as a standalone operation today.

The technique for EDS is as follows. The patient is positioned supine with the head turned to the contralateral side and secured in a rigid head holder. Either a curvilinear or linear scalp incision is made following the course of the STA (**Fig. 12.2a**). The STA and its associated branches should be preserved. A craniotomy centered over the Sylvian fissure is performed (**Fig. 12.2b**). The size of the craniotomy is tailored to the extent of the ischemic brain territory.

Under microscopic guidance, the dura is opened in cruciate fashion, preserving large middle meningeal branches. The dural leaflets are inverted underneath the craniotomy edges to promote neovascularization to the underlying cortex (**Fig. 12.2c**). When the dura is opened, great care should be taken to preserve the middle meningeal artery. The middle meningeal artery often traverses the central portion of the dural opening. In these cases, the dura should be opened around the middle meningeal artery. The resulting island of dura containing the middle meningeal artery may then be inverted using two nonabsorbable sutures sewn to either the patient's native skull using small bur holes or to the edge of the tucked dural leaflets. The bone flap is replaced (**Fig. 12.2d, e**), and the incision is closed in the usual fashion.

◆ Encephalomyosynangiosis

In 1950, Henschen first reported EMS when he used the temporalis muscle as a donor graft to revascularize the brain of a patient with bilateral internal carotid artery occlusions and refractory seizures.[5] The surgery reduced seizure frequency in the patient. This technique was popularized in the late 1970s when surgeons experimented with new techniques to provide collateral circulation for affected patients with moyamoya. In 1977, Karasawa et al subsequently performed EMS procedures on 10 patients with moyamoya disease with good results.[6] Temporalis muscle was sutured directly to the underlying dura. Matsushima et al recommended a larger craniotomy flap and also added suturing the frontalis muscle to the dura.[7] This operation provided surgeons with an alternative strategy for treating patients who had failed direct anastomosis or who lacked good donor and/or recipient vessels. The contemporary definition of the EMS procedure deviates slightly from Karasawa's technique in that the dura is typically opened along the extent of the craniotomy to allow direct apposition of muscle to the underlying cerebral cortex.

EMS is a straightforward procedure. The patient is positioned supine with the head turned to the contralateral side and supported in a rigid head holder. A linear or curvilinear incision is demarcated over the temporalis muscle (**Fig. 12.3a**). In subperiosteal fashion, the temporalis muscle is carefully dissected from the underlying cranium to preserve the blood supply. A large craniotomy is fashioned to accommodate the temporalis muscle. The dura is opened widely, sparing the middle meningeal artery, and then inverted. The muscle is

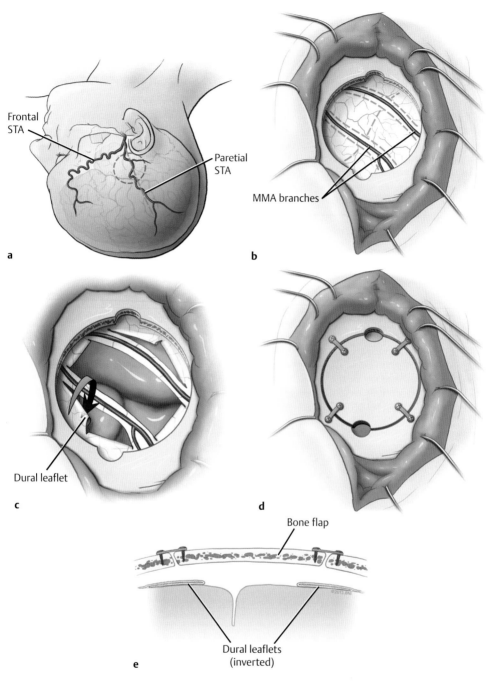

Frontal STA

Paretial STA

MMA branches

Dural leaflet

Bone flap

Dural leaflets (inverted)

Fig. 12.2a–e Encephalodurosynangiosis. (**a**) Craniotomy (*dashed circle*) and scalp incision (*blue dashed line*) along parietal branch of superficial temporal artery (STA). (**b**) Craniotomy deep to temporalis muscle with cruciate dural incision (*blue dashed lines*), which preserves the two middle meningeal artery (MMA) branches visible in this image. (**c**) Leaflets of dura inverted and tucked under (*arrow*). (**d**) Replacement of bone flap. (**e**) Cross-sectional view of inverted dura. (Used with permission from Barrow Neurological Institute.)

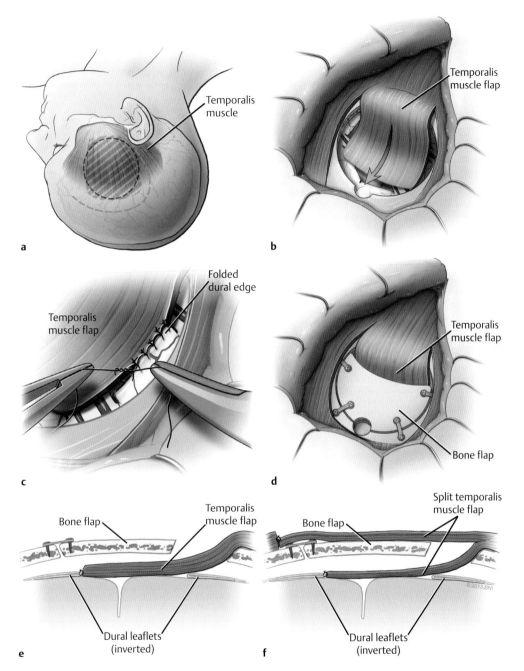

Fig. 12.3a–f Encephalomyosynangiosis. (**a**) Frontotemporal incision (*blue dashed line*) and frontotemporal craniotomy (*dashed circle*). (**b**) Flap of temporalis muscle and overlying fascia cut on three sides. (**c**) Temporalis muscle flap sutured to superior, anterior, and posterior edges of cruciate dural opening. (**d**) Craniotomy flap reconstructed with plates keeping a sufficient gap inferiorly to accommodate the temporalis muscle. (**e**) Cross-sectional view of temporalis muscle under the edge of the craniotomy flap. (**f**) Cross-sectional view of alternative split-thickness temporalis muscle graft with the external layer placed over the bone and the internal layer sutured to dura under the bone. (Used with permission from Barrow Neurological Institute.)

placed directly on top of the underlying brain (**Fig. 12.3b**). Nonabsorbable sutures are often placed to secure the muscle to the dural edges (**Fig. 12.3c**). The bone flap is carefully replaced over the muscle and secured using titanium plates (**Fig. 12.3d**). A horizontal section of bone is usually shaved off the inferior aspect of the temporal bone flap to avoid compromising perfusion to the temporalis muscle (**Fig. 12.3e**).

Major disadvantages of EMS include the obvious cosmetic deformity created by transposing the temporalis muscle as well as the potential for intracranial mass effect to develop. A split-thickness temporalis muscle graft may reduce the poor cosmetic effect of the muscle defect while also decreasing the bulk of muscle tissue in the epidural space. Tu et al described using a frontotemporal incision and splitting the temporalis muscle into external and internal layers, placing the internal layer on the brain surface and the external layer over the bone flap.[8] This technique reduces mass effect on the brain and aids in cosmesis and mastication. Yoshida et al also mentioned the split temporalis muscle technique (**Fig. 12.3f**).[9] Alternative sources of muscle graft, including latissimus dorsi and serratus anterior free flaps, have also been used.[10] Cosmetic deformity may be minimized by using alternative muscle sources. However, their use is more technically challenging because of the arterial and venous anastomoses required to preserve flap perfusion.

Several case series have detailed good outcomes of the EMS procedure in patients with moyamoya disease. Takeuchi et al treated 10 pediatric patients with moyamoya using the EMS technique and local temporalis muscle grafts.[11] Seven patients experienced either complete resolution ($n = 4$) or improvement ($n = 3$) in their ischemic symptoms. The intelligence quotients of several patients improved, as had cerebral blood flow at follow-up. Postoperative cerebral angiography demonstrated significant collateralization of the middle cerebral artery (MCA) territory from the overlying temporalis muscle grafts in most patients with reduction in the size of abnormally dilated arteries in the region of the basal ganglia.

Irikura et al reviewed their series of 13 pediatric patients with moyamoya who underwent EMS using temporalis muscle on a total of 24 sides.[12] Cerebral angiography was performed 6 to 88 months after surgery. Significant revascularization, defined as more than one-third of the MCA territory, was observed in 18 sides (75%). The remaining six sides all showed evidence of some collateralization. Abnormal basal ganglia vasculature was reduced in 94% of the treated sides.

Yoshioka and Tominaga performed the EMS procedure on three adult patients with moyamoya using latissimus dorsi ($n = 2$) or serratus anterior ($n = 1$) muscle free flaps.[10] At postoperative follow-up intervals ranging from 8 to 42 months, neurological symptoms had resolved in all patients. Postoperative angiography confirmed vessel collateralization in two of the patients. Complications of EMS include postoperative seizures and mass effect from the muscle graft.[13,14] Touho reported symptomatic brain compression from a hypertrophied and ossified temporalis muscle graft in a young girl who presented with contralateral lower facial paralysis and arm weakness 6 years after undergoing EMS.[13] Xenon-enhanced computed tomography showed that the patient had decreased cerebral blood flow underneath the muscle flap. She improved neurologically after intravenous hydration on several occasions.

◆ Encephaloduroarterio-synangiosis

In 1981, Matsushima et al first described the technique of transplanting a branch of the STA intracranially through an opening in the dura, leaving the distal and proximal artery intact.[15] Since this initial publication, EDAS has been used by Matsushima's group alone and in combination with other indirect and direct techniques to supplement vascular supply to the cerebral cortex with good results.[7,16–19] This technique has been adopted by many surgeons, particularly for the treatment of pediatric moyamoya disease (**Fig. 12.4a–f**).

Similar to the direct bypass procedure, the STA is carefully microdissected through a skin incision that approximates the course of the most robust STA branch (usually the parietal branch) (**Fig. 12.4a**). The STA branch is dissected free of the surrounding temporalis fascia. The anterior STA branch should be preserved because it may provide potential

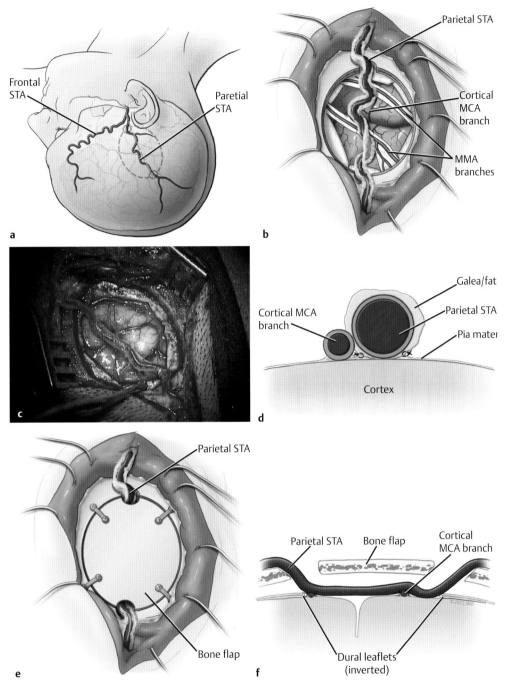

Fig. 12.4a–f Encephaloduroarteriosynangiosis. (**a**) Incision along parietal superficial temporal artery (STA). Oval-shaped craniotomy (*dashed line*) under the incision, with bur holes at top and bottom to accommodate the STA en passage. (**b**) Dura opened in cruciate fashion, preserving middle meningeal artery (MMA) branches and with the parietal STA dissected free. MCA, middle cerebral artery. (**c**) Photograph of prepared encephalo-duroarteriosynangiosis field in a 35-year-old male patient. (**d**) Cross-sectional view of 10–0 suture anchoring the galea and fat of the STA to the pia adjacent to the cortical MCA branch. (**e**) Reconstruction of bone flap with STA travelling en passage under the bone flap through the expanded bur holes. (**f**) Cross-sectional view of STA under bone flap. (Used with permission from Barrow Neurological Institute.)

collateral blood supply to the underlying cortex. The senior author (R.F.S.) recommends removing adherent adventitia around the entire length of the arterial branch that may impede angiogenesis. Two bur holes are fashioned: one at the floor of the middle fossa and another just superior to the superficial temporal line. The diameters of the holes must be large enough to accommodate the STA donor vessel. As previously described, a craniotomy is centered over the Sylvian fissure.

The dura is opened in cruciate fashion to preserve large middle meningeal artery branches (**Fig. 12.4b**). The STA branch is placed in direct opposition to the underlying cortex. In 1980, Spetzler et al first described a modification to the EDAS procedure in which the arachnoid overlying the cortex is opened to allow direct contact between the STA donor branch and cortical arteries.[20] Using this technique, more commonly referred to as pial synangiosis, the STA branch is sutured to the dissected arachnoid using several interrupted 10–0 nylon stitches to approximate the donor artery over several cortical arteries along the length of the STA branch (**Fig. 12.4c, d**). The STA branch is left intact to allow blood to flow en passage. The dural leaflets, usually four to six total, are inverted and folded underneath the native skull.

Some surgeons have advocated a watertight closure in which the dura is sutured directly to the galeal flap attached to the STA branch.[21,22] In our experience, we have had no complications related to cerebrospinal fluid leakage over the course of many cases. The dural inversion provides an additional source of blood flow for cortical neovascularization. After meticulous hemostasis is achieved, the craniotomy flap is carefully beveled and secured in place using titanium plates and screws (**Fig. 12.4e, f**). The scalp is closed in the usual fashion taking care not to harm the STA.

Clinical outcomes after EDAS tend to be good. Matushima and coworkers' initial description of the procedure detailed the improved clinical results of a 9-year-old patient with moyamoya who had presented with hemiparesis, seizures, and behavioral disorder. At the 6-month follow-up examination, the patient showed remarkable clinical improvement that corresponded to improved brain revascularization on the treated side.[15] Likewise,

Tripathi et al performed the EDAS procedure on eight children diagnosed with moyamoya disease.[23] At 2 years of follow-up, all patients remained asymptomatic of their moyamoya disease without strokes or transient ischemic attacks.

Fujita et al compared the EDAS and EMS procedures in 10 patients with moyamoya.[24] Seven patients underwent the EDAS procedure on one side and the EMS surgery on the other, while three patients were treated with the EDAS procedure bilaterally. Postoperative angiography confirmed increased vascularity on the EDAS-treated sides compared with the sides treated by EMS. Regional cerebral blood flow studies further confirmed increased blood flow to the EDAS-treated sides.

In 2002, Isono's group compared the EDAS, EDAMS, and EMS procedures in a cohort of 11 children diagnosed with moyamoya disease.[25] Ten patients underwent the EDAS procedure on 16 sides. The EDAMS technique was performed on four patients (total of four sides), while EMS was used on only one side. Postoperatively, patients were followed for more than 100 months. A total of 92% of sides treated by EDAS showed significant neovascularization compared with 50% of sides treated either by EDAMS or EMS. In 2004, Scott et al reported the largest clinical series of patients treated with the EDAS procedure.[26] The 143 pediatric patients with moyamoya who received a modification of pial synangiosis during the EDAS operation over a 17-year period were reviewed retrospectively. Preoperatively, 68% of the patients had suffered a stroke and 43% had a history of transient ischemic attacks. Altogether, 271 EDAS procedures were performed on the study group, and 30-day morbidity rates were low. Eleven strokes (7.7% per patient or 4% per treated side) and three transient ischemic attacks (2.1% per patient) occurred in the perioperative period. Clinical follow-up was available in 126 patients more than 12 months from the time of surgery. Four patients (3.2%) suffered delayed strokes, one patient (0.7%) experienced reversible transient ischemic attacks, and two patients (1.4%) suffered persistent transient ischemic attacks. The group later reported only one postoperative cerebrospinal fluid leak in more than 200 patients who underwent the modified EDAS pial synangiosis procedure.[27]

◆ Posterior Circulation Encephaloduroarterio-synangiosis

Matsushima and Inaba first described posterior circulation indirect revascularization using the occipital artery as a donor source for moyamoya disease.[22] After insonating the occipital artery course with Doppler ultrasonography, a sigmoid incision is made over the course of the occipital artery (**Fig. 12.5a**). The occipital artery with a strip of attached galea is dissected free from subcutaneous fat, pericranium, and muscle. After a supratentorial occipital bone flap is created, an H-shaped dural incision is made (**Fig. 12.5b**). The dura is folded into the subdural space under the edges of the craniotomy. The arachnoid membrane is opened widely, and the galeal cuff around the occipital artery is sutured to the dural edge (**Fig. 12.5c**). Hayashi et al reported the successful treatment of three patients with recurrent ischemic symptoms after revascularization surgery using occipital artery EDAS.[28] Ischemia involving the distribution of the posterior

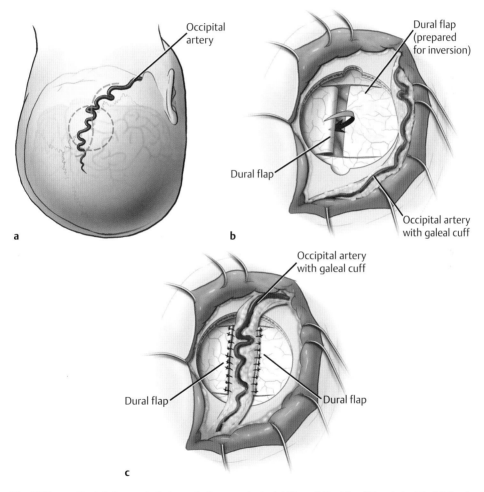

Fig. 12.5a–c Occipital encephaloduroarteriosynangiosis. (**a**) Sigmoid incision (*blue dashed line*) following the course of the occipital artery and parietal occipital craniotomy (*dashed circle*). (**b**) Prepared occipital encephaloduroarteriosynangiosis field with occipital artery isolated with fascia on side, occipital muscle retracted, bone flap elevated, and dura opened in the shape of a wide H. (**c**) Galea around edges of occipital artery sutured to edges of dura. (Used with permission from Barrow Neurological Institute.)

cerebral artery (PCA) is increasingly recognized in patients with moyamoya disease. In a prospective Korean series of 410 surgically treated patients, 10% underwent indirect revascularization of the posterior circulation.[29]

◆ Encephaloduroarterio-myosynangiosis

EDAMS combines aspects of all major indirect revascularization procedures. Dural leaflets are inverted onto the underlying cortex, an arterial donor (typically the STA), and muscle flap (typically a portion of the temporalis muscle). In 1984, Kinugasa et al first proposed this procedure.[30]

The EDAMS procedure is performed in a manner similar to the other indirect bypass procedures described previously. A traditional pterional incision is usually performed to expose a sufficient amount of temporalis muscle (**Fig. 12.6a**). Nakashima et al advocate a question mark–shaped incision large enough to accommodate preserving both STA branches en passage.[31] The STA may be left attached to the facial cuff or dissected to the outer adventitial layer as recommended by the senior author (R.F.S.). A large craniotomy is performed to allow sufficient room to apply the STA vessel en passage as well as the temporalis muscle graft. Ishii et al reported making the bone flap 8 cm by 10 cm.[32]

The dural leaflets are opened in cruciate fashion. The middle meningeal artery should be preserved within the dural leaflets and inverted onto the underlying cortex using nonabsorbable sutures as previously described (see **Fig. 12.4d**). The arachnoid is opened sharply over large cortical arterial branches, and a pial synangiosis may be performed using 10–0 nylon suture and the STA branch. Alternatively, the STA may be left attached to a facial cuff and sutured to the inverted dural leaflets. The temporalis muscle is placed over the remaining exposed brain and secured in place in a similar fashion (**Fig. 12.6b**). Ozgur et al reported a variation in which the cuff of both parietal and frontal STA branches is sewn to edges of the temporalis muscle on the inside and to edges of dura on the outside (**Fig. 12.6c**).[33] The temporalis muscle can be accommodated by removing the inferior edge of the bone flap (**Fig. 12.6d, e**) or by plating the

bone flap in an elevated position.[32] If the STA has been harvested with a galeal flap, the edges of the scalp flap may be quite tenuous; the surgeon must grab sufficient tissue with the interrupted sutures for scalp closure.

In the original series by Kinugasa et al, the EDAMS procedure was performed in 17 patients with moyamoya (13 children) on 28 sides.[30] Ten patients presented with transient ischemic attacks and seven presented with strokes. At a mean follow-up of more than 3 years after the EDAMS procedure, 13 patients showed clinical improvement. Postoperatively, one patient who underwent bilateral EDAMS worsened. Three additional patients failed to change clinically. Postoperative cerebral angiograms were obtained from 10 patients (16 sides). The angiographic results were compared with patients who previously underwent EDAS procedures at the same institution. The ratio of extensive vessel collateralization was higher in patients who underwent the EDAMS surgery compared with those who underwent EDAS.

Houkin et al treated 35 adult patients with moyamoya with combined direct STA-to-MCA anastomosis and EDAMS procedures on 51 sides.[34] The results from this cohort were compared retrospectively to the same procedure performed in 12 pediatric patients with moyamoya on 22 sides. Of 53 sides, 47 (89%) were studied with cerebral angiography after surgery. Revascularization was qualified as good or poor. In adult patients, 90% of the sides (42/47) were found to have good revascularization of the vascular territory supplied by the STA-to-MCA anastomosis compared with only 38% of sides (18/47) where the EDAMS procedure had been performed. Interestingly, the STA-to-MCA anastomosis provided good revascularization in only 68% of sides (15/22) in pediatric patients compared with in 100% of sides treated with the EDAMS operation. The interval between surgery and follow-up angiography was not reported. It is possible that the adult patients who underwent the EDAMS procedure were evaluated too early after surgery to provide sufficient time for revascularization.

Kim et al retrospectively compared the revascularization results of the EDAS and EDAMS procedures in 24 pediatric patients with moyamoya.[35] Twelve patients underwent EDAS on 16 sides, five patients received the EDAMS procedure on 8 sides, and seven patients underwent

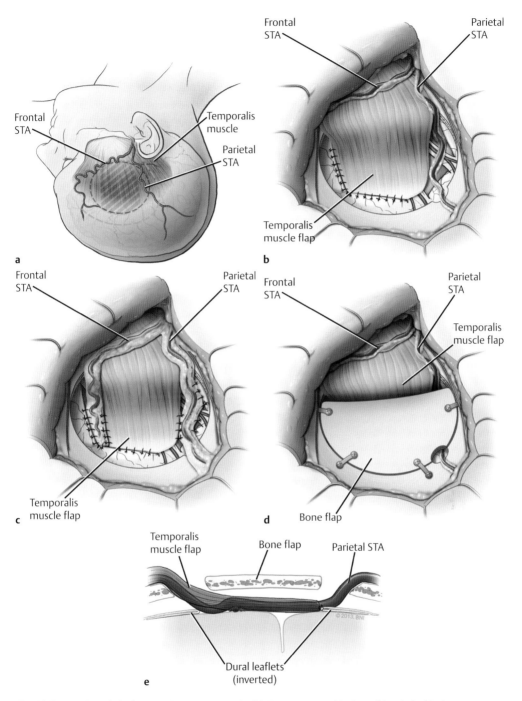

Fig. 12.6a–e Encephaloduroarteriomyosynangiosis. (**a**) Frontotemporal incision (*blue dashed line*) encompassing the parietal superficial temporal artery (STA) and temporalis muscle. The craniotomy is indicated by the *dashed circle*. (**b**) Cut temporalis muscle sutured to anterior and superior dural edges with parietal STA on surface of brain. (**c**) Variation of encephaloduroarteriomyosynangiosis where both frontal and parietal STA are dissected free and sutured to edges of dura and of temporalis muscle as shown. (**d**) Reconstruction of bone flap with generous opening inferiorly to accommodated passage of arteries and muscle. (**e**) Cross-sectional view of temporalis muscle and STA branches under the bone flap. (Used with permission from Barrow Neurological Institute.)

combined STA-to-MCA direct anastomosis combined with EDAMS on 12 sides. Based on cerebral angiography performed 4 months to 5 years postoperatively, EDAMS significantly improved the extent of vessel collateralization compared with the EDAS procedure ($p < 0.05$). This observation held true regardless of the combined STA-to-MCA direct anastomosis. Excellent or good clinical outcomes were more common after the EDAMS procedure alone or in combination with an STA-to-MCA bypass compared with EDAS.

◆ Omental Transposition and Transplantation

The first intracranial omental transposition for moyamoya disease is credited to Karasawa et al in 1978.[36] A large segment of omentum was anastomosed to the STA and superficial temporal vein via end-to-end anastomosis with the gastroepiploic vascular tree in a patient with advanced bilateral moyamoya disease. Clinical function improved after the transplanted omentum was placed directly on the brain. Previously, omentum had been shown to function as a viable source of reserve blood supply in experimental animal and human surgical procedures.[37–39] Advantages of omental transplantation include relative plasticity of the graft material and the capability of covering a large surface area. Several groups have advocated this technique for indirect treatment of moyamoya disease that primarily affects the posterior and anterior cerebral artery (ACA) territories.[40–42] Potential disadvantages of omental transplantation include intracranial mass effect and potential wound infection in the setting of a necrotic omental flap.[42]

Omentum may be transposed or transplanted as a vascular free flap to provide blood flow to the cerebral cortex. The greater omentum is harvested through a midline abdominal incision. The gastroepiploic vessels are dissected and preserved. A large craniotomy is fashioned on the affected side. For transplantation of an omental free flap, the STA and superficial temporal vein branches should be identified and preserved (**Fig. 12.7**). The gastroepiploic vessels are dissected for additional length along their attachment to the omentum

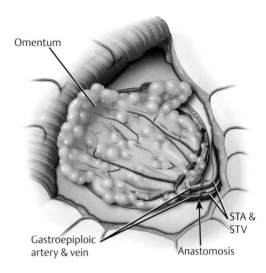

Fig. 12.7 Omental transplant. Segment of omentum isolated and placed directly on the cortex in a frontotemporal exposure. The dura is resected or inverted under the bone. The gastroepiploic artery and vein of the omentum are anastomosed to the parietal superficial temporal artery (STA) and superficial temporal vein (STV). (Used with permission from Barrow Neurological Institute.)

and divided. Heparinized saline is used to flush the gastroepiploic artery and vein in preparation of anastomosis.

Direct end-to-end or end-to-side anastomoses are performed between the STA and gastroepiploic artery followed by the superficial temporal vein and gastroepiploic vein using 10–0 nylon suture (**Fig. 12.7**). The arterial anastomosis is usually performed first to confirm adequate flow through the graft on the venous end. Alternatively, indocyanine green fluoroscopy can be used to verify arterial patency. A cortical vein may be used in place of the superficial temporal vein if it is unsuitable for anastomosis. The vascularized graft is placed directly in contact with the cerebral cortex after the dura is widely opened.

Omental transposition may be performed instead of transplantation. The harvested omentum is left attached to its vascular supply and lengthened through a series of relaxing cuts. It is tunneled subcutaneously to the cranium and placed in direct contact with the cerebral cortex. Care must be taken to avoid postoperative constriction of the transposed graft as well as abdominal hernia formation. A nasogastric tube is typically left in place for several days after surgery to provide prophylaxis against gastric stasis, which may occur following division of the gastric blood supply. Postoperative seizure prophylaxis may be considered.

Omental transplantation and transposition have been associated with promising results, particularly in patients with recurrent symptoms after direct or other indirect bypass procedures. Havlik et al reported successful resolution of ischemic symptoms after omental transposition in a woman with moyamoya disease who had previously undergone an STA-to-MCA anastomosis.[43] In the largest clinical series published to date, Karasawa et al treated 30 pediatric patients with moyamoya with omental transplantation to symptomatic ACA and/or PCA territories.[40] At a mean follow-up of 3.8 years, all patients who received omental transplantation to the affected ACA circulation and 11 of 13 patients (85%) with PCA territory symptoms showed signs of clinical improvement, most within 1 month of surgery. No procedural complications occurred in this series. Touho et al reported significant reductions in transient ischemic attacks in five pediatric patients with moyamoya following omental transplantation as salvage therapy.[44] These patients suffered persistent neurological symptoms (e.g., paraparesis, urinary incontinence, and mental slowing) despite previous revascularization procedures, including EDAS and direct STA-to-MCA anastomosis. In four patients, the transient ischemic symptoms completely resolved following omental transplantation. The transient ischemic attacks of the remaining patient decreased.

◆ Multiple Cranial Bur Holes

Cranial bur holes may promote neovascularization as a standalone operation or in combination with either indirect or direct bypass procedures. Endo et al first described fortuitous neovascularization in a child with moyamoya disease who was treated with a frontal bur hole for placement of a ventricular drain following an intraventricular hemorrhage.[45] Three-month follow-up angiography demonstrated marked neovascularization at the bur hole site. The patient subsequently underwent bilateral

EMS procedures with good angiographic and clinical results. Multiple small case series support the role of multiple cranial bur holes to augment intracranial blood supply.[45–48] This technique is particularly useful for watershed and ACA territories that may not receive sufficient revascularization following either direct or indirect bypass techniques due to the small size of the STA distally.

The procedure is straightforward, but several considerations must be made before multiple cranial bur holes are made. The location and number of bur holes should be tailored to cortical territories at risk of infarction. Preoperative perfusion imaging and/or cerebral angiography should be performed to help identify at-risk territories as well as collateral vessels at risk for disruption by the approach. Attempts should be made to avoid incising the scalp over branches of the external carotid artery and occipital artery, which may provide vital collateral blood supply to the underlying brain. A handheld Doppler may be used to identify the underlying scalp arteries and to avoid interruption.

One of two basic incisions is usually made, either a bicoronal incision or a midline sagittal incision. A zig-zag retrocoronal incision provides a nice cosmetic result (**Fig. 12.8a**).[49] The midline sagittal incision avoids external carotid branches and can facilitate posterior circulation bur holes (**Fig. 12.8b**). A subgaleal saline injection can help preserve the underlying pericranium. Generous bur holes should be fashioned using either a high-speed drill or Hudson brace to facilitate dural inversion onto the underlying cortex. In some instances, a small craniotomy may be turned to connect two adjacent bur holes to improve dural exposure.

The dura is opened in cruciate fashion, and the underlying arachnoid is incised sharply. The dural leaflets are inverted underneath the native skull to promote neovascularization. The pericranium can be dissected in a triangular shape over the bur hole, preserved, and then inserted onto the cortex to further augment blood supply (**Fig. 12.8c**).[49–51] Single, titanium, dog-bone–shaped plates may be placed over the holes to prevent potential scalp dimpling and to minimize impedance of neovascularization.[52] The scalp is reapproximated. Postoperative imaging is limited to plain computed tomography to rule out the presence of

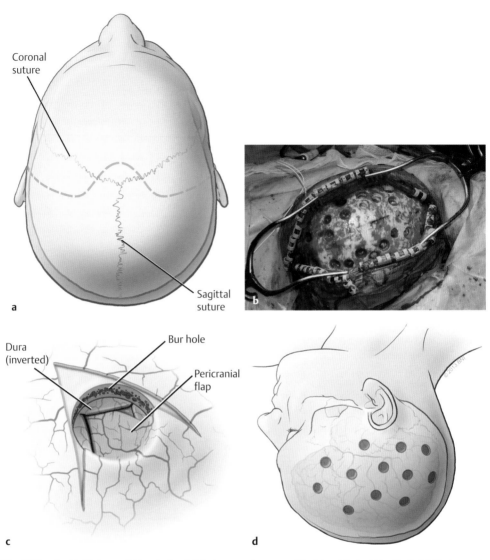

Fig. 12.8a–d Multiple cranial bur holes. (**a**) A zig-zag retrocoronal incision (*dashed blue line*). (**b**) Photograph of multiple cranial bur holes performed through a sagittal incision, which preserves the superficial temporal artery region bilaterally. (**c**) Pericranium opened in a triangular-shaped fashion over the individual bur hole and placed on surface of cortex after the dura and arachnoid have been opened. (**d**) View of multiple cranial bur holes (10 to 24) placed in frontal parietal and occipital regions of affected hemisphere. (Used with permission from Barrow Neurological Institute.)

a hematoma. Subsequent imaging to reassess perfusion should be performed after an interval of at least 3 to 6 months.

The positioning and number of bur holes used for this technique vary. In general, placement of bur holes should coincide with the patient's symptomatology and/or cerebral perfusion imaging studies. Multiple bur holes have the potential to revascularize the ACA, MCA, and PCA distributions. Endo et al placed multiple cranial bur holes in five pediatric patients with moyamoya following the incidental discovery of neovascularization at a ventricular bur hole site in a patient with moyamoya disease.[45] Bilateral frontal bur holes were performed in all patients centered between the hairline and coronal suture, ~3 to 5 cm off midline. Two patients underwent simultaneous EMS procedures at the time of bur hole placement, while the other three patients had multiple cranial bur holes placed months after bilateral EMS procedures. Either dynamic computed tomography imaging or conventional cerebral angiography showed improved vascularization in all cases.

Kawaguchi et al placed multiple cranial bur holes (one to four bur holes over each cerebral hemisphere) in 10 adult patients with moyamoya.[47] Eight patients presented with transient ischemic symptoms, while two patients suffered infractions before surgical intervention. Altogether, 43 bur holes were placed: 36 centered over the MCA territory and 7 over the ACA territory. An EDAS procedure was performed simultaneously in one patient. At a mean follow-up of 34.7 months, 41 of 43 bur holes (95%) demonstrated neovascularization. Transient ischemic symptoms resolved or decreased in all patients.

Sainte-Rose et al treated 14 pediatric patients with moyamoya using the multiple cranial bur holes technique.[49] Between 10 and 24 bur holes were placed in the fronto-temporo-parieto-occipital areas of each treated hemisphere (**Fig. 12.8d**). Ten children underwent bilateral procedures, and four underwent unilateral bur holes on the more severely affected side (one patient received a prior EDAMS operation). No postoperative ischemic events occurred. Two patients experienced delayed seizures (one at 2 weeks and the other 5 months postoperatively). Subcutaneous fluid collections resolved after five procedures following treatment with tapping and compressive head dressings.

◆ Galeal Procedures

Several authors have described using galea as a donor tissue. The galea aponeurotica is the strength layer of the scalp just deep to the subcutaneous fat and contains the STA below the superior temporal line (**Figs. 12.9a, 12.1b**). Matsushima and Inaba described using the cuff

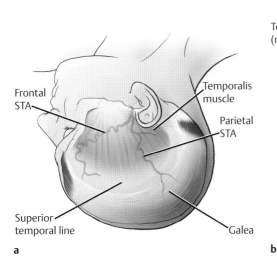
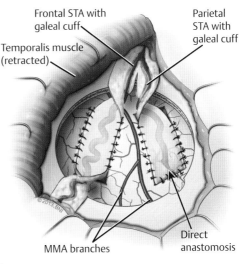

Fig. 12.9a, b Galeal procedures. (**a**) The galea below the superior temporal line is split into the superficial temporal fascia, in which the superficial temporal artery (STA) lies, and the deep temporal fascia, which covers the temporalis muscle. Above the superior temporal line, the galea is very adherent to the dermal layer above it; it can be isolated by dissecting just deep to the hair follicles. (**b**) A wide cuff of the galea is kept with the STA branches and rotated to place the artery on the cortex. It is then sutured to the adjacent dura. The frontal STA branch is used for encephaloduroarteriosynangiosis and the parietal STA is used for direct anastomosis to the middle cerebral artery. MMA, middle meningeal artery. (Used with permission from Barrow Neurological Institute.)

of galea adjacent to the STA and suturing it to the dura as part of the EDAS procedure.[22] Kim et al left a 2- to 3-cm cuff of galea attached to both branches of the STA and then inverted the STA-galeal flap and sewed it to edges of dura. Direct STA-to-MCA bypass was also performed with the parietal STA branch (**Fig. 12.9b**).[53] Shirane et al reported the encephalogaleomyosynangiosis procedure where the temporalis muscle and the galea of the skin were peeled to make a thin monolayer flap that is sutured to the cut edges of the dura.[54] Kawamoto and coworkers described galeoduroencephalosynangiosis in which a half circle of galea approximately half of the size of the semicircular skin flap is dissected over a bur hole and then sutured to dura.[50,51] With the use of the strength layer of the scalp for revascularization, attention to detail with skin closure is critical to avoid wound breakdown.

◆ Pericranial Flap

An additional source of tissue to supply blood that can be added to any of the previously described procedures is placement of the pericranium in contact with the brain.[55] Several authors describe the galea as a component of an indirect procedure when actually the pericranium is being utilized. The pericranium is a layer of periosteum on the skull that has variable vascularity. It has the major advantages of being highly anastomotic, easily mobilized, and present over the entire scalp wherever muscle is not present, including the convexities where other vascularized tissues for indirect bypass are sparse. Yoshioka and Rhoton noted the classic anatomy of the pericranium served by branches of the supraorbital artery (**Fig. 12.10a**).[56]

Several variations of techniques use the pericranium. In 1994, Kinugasa et al described the ribbon technique of using a combination of pericranium and galea to revascularize the ACA territory in eight pediatric patients with moyamoya (**Fig. 12.10b–d**).[57] In this technique, an 8-cm incision is made 2 cm anterior and parallel to the coronal suture (**Fig. 12.10b**) through the subcutaneous fat but not through the galea, which is exposed in a broad region anterior and posterior to the incision. A long triangular strip of galea is cut with the apex as far lateral

as possible. For bilateral procedures, a second long triangular strip of dura is cut either anterior or posterior to the other strip but with its apex on the contralateral side. Cauterization applied down to the bone allows the galea and pericranium to be cut at the same time. This triangular flap of galea and pericranium is elevated from the bone.

Bur holes are placed adjacent to the sagittal sinus allowing a small bifrontal craniotomy to be elevated (**Fig. 12.10c**). A 1×1-cm square of dura is resected adjacent to the sagittal sinus, and the arachnoid membrane is incised. The galeal-pericranial strips are inserted into the interhemispheric fissure (**Fig. 12.10d**). The small bone flap is replaced allowing the galeal grafts through the bur holes, and the skin is closed. This skin incision can be joined with a frontotemporal incision and combined with the EDAMS procedure unilaterally or bilaterally. In their small series, transient ischemic attacks resolved in six patients and improved in the other two patients. Revascularization was extensive in the six patients with follow-up angiography. Kim et al described success with encephalogaleopericraniosynangiosis, a variation of the ribbon procedure using an S-shaped bicoronal incision 2 cm in front of the coronal suture and using both pericranium and galea when possible for ACA revascularization.[21]

As a component of a combined procedure, Kuroda et al reported using a pericranial graft without galea to cover the ACA territory and emphasized the importance of basing the flap anteriorly on the supratrochlear and supraorbital arteries (see Combined Indirect Procedures).[55] Pericranium also can be used as a donor tissue in the bur hole procedures discussed previously in the chapter.[49]

◆ Dural Variations

Multiple techniques use dura as a donor tissue. An essential tenet for using dura is that the blood flow to the dura derives from meningeal arteries on its external surface while the internal surface of the dura remains relatively avascular. With the dural inversion technique, the flaps or leaves of dura are folded under the bone to allow the vascular surface to oppose the brain surface (see **Fig. 12.2c**). It is critical not to cut the major meningeal

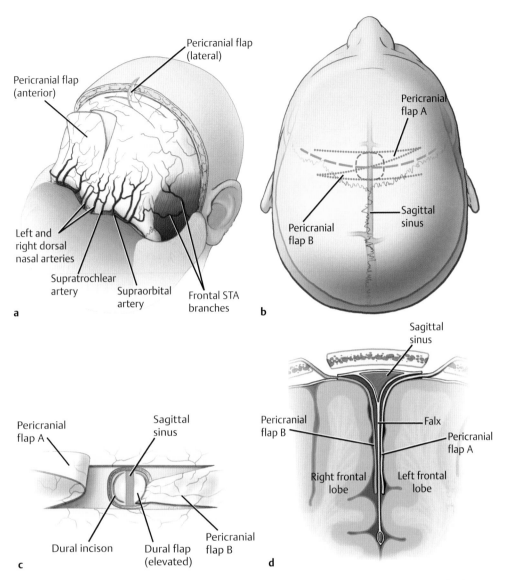

Fig. 12.10a–d Pericranial procedures. (**a**) Pericranial flaps can be based anteriorly off of supraorbital arteries or can be based laterally. STA, superficial temporal artery. (**b**) Encephalogaleopericranial synangiosis with two flaps of pericranium based laterally (*green line*) elevated via a bicoronal incision (*dashed blue line*). The craniotomy is indicated by the *dashed circle*. (**c**) Small bifrontal craniotomy elevated over sagittal sinus and mesial frontal lobes. (**d**) Pericranial flaps placed over frontal lobes and inserted into interhemispheric fissure. (Used with permission from Barrow Neurological Institute.)

arterial branches that can be identified on preoperative angiography and also visualized directly. In fact, King et al used superselective angiography to study 18 hemispheres in pediatric patients with moyamoya who underwent EDAS and demonstrated that the contribution of the middle meningeal artery exceeded or equaled that of the STA in 78% of cases.[58] Some advocate resecting windows of dura, preserving meningeal arteries and allowing muscle or galea to contact the cortex directly. Others support resecting the inner

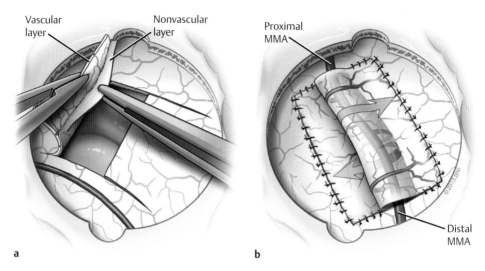

Fig. 12.11a, b Dural variations. (**a**) Resection of inner, nonvascular layer of dura. (**b**) Rotation of dural flap about axis of middle meningeal artery and sutured to adjacent dural edge. MMA, middle meningeal artery. (Used with permission from Barrow Neurological Institute.)

nonvascular layer of dura and then inverting it (**Fig. 12.11a**).[52] Shirane et al cut dura into ribbon pedicles and inserted them into sulci after opening the arachnoid.[54] Others have placed dura deep into the interhemispheric fissure. Dauser et al rotated a 2-cm cuff of dura around the middle meningeal artery and sutured it to other dural edges in the inverted position (**Fig. 12.11b**).[59] One concern with this technique is compromising the blood flow from the rotation.

◆ Combined Indirect Procedures

In an effort to maximize indirect revascularization, many authors have combined several different techniques during the same procedure. At least two authors have reported that the extent of indirect revascularization depends on the amount of brain exposed, although this point is not yet proven. Combined procedures can be performed as a single operation or as sequential operations. Combined procedures use combinations of the various donor tissues such as dura, dural artery (middle meningeal artery), large

external carotid artery branches (STA or occipital artery), pericranium, muscle, or galea. These donor tissues can cover the MCA, ACA, or PCA distributions.

Several combined indirect procedures have been reported. Unsatisfied with the results of EDAS alone, Matsushima and coworkers reported the outcomes of several procedures combined to treat pediatric patients with moyamoya.[7,16–18] Three indirect bypass procedures are performed via two ipsilateral craniotomies with EDAS and EMS being done through a frontotemporal craniotomy to cover the temporoparietal region (**Fig. 12.12a–c**). The frontal STA and frontalis muscle assist with medial frontal coverage. An incision is made along the posterior STA and then extended anteriorly. After a temporoparietal craniotomy is performed, the dura is resected around the borders of the middle meningeal artery and the galeal cuff around the STA is sewn to the dura. The temporalis muscle is laid over the brain surface, and the bone flap is replaced. The combined procedures of Matsushima and coworkers mapped the course of both branches of the STA (**Fig. 12.12a–c**).[7] Two horseshoe incisions are made, each with one limb based on a branch of the STA

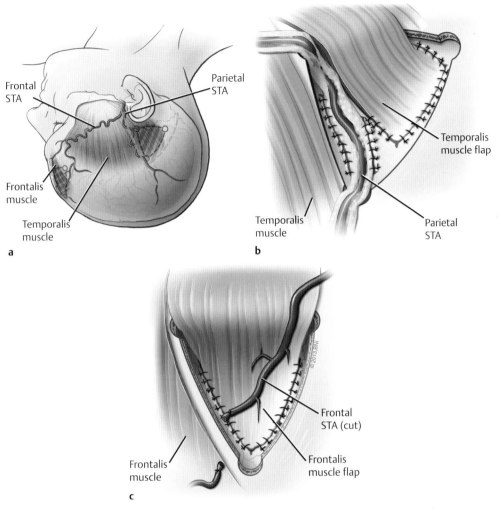

Frontal STA

Parietal STA

Frontalis muscle

Temporalis muscle

a

Temporalis muscle flap

Temporalis muscle

Parietal STA

b

Frontal STA (cut)

Frontalis muscle

Frontalis muscle flap

c

Fig. 12.12a–c Combined indirect procedures. (**a**) Incisions (*dashed blue lines*) and craniotomy sites (*dashed lines*) for combined temporoparietal encephalomyosynangiosis (EMS) and encephaloduroarteriosynangiosis (EDAS) with frontal EMS procedures. (**b**) Temporoparietal EMS and EDAS. Temporoparietal incision with preservation of parietal superficial temporal artery (STA) for use with EDAS and posterior temporalis muscle for EMS. (**c**) Frontal EMS using frontalis muscle flap based on frontal STA is sutured to the adjacent dura. (Used with permission from Barrow Neurological Institute.)

(**Fig. 12.12a**). For the temporoparietal EMS and EDAS procedures, a cut down over the posterior STA serves as the posterior limb of the horseshoe incision (**Fig. 12.12b**). For frontal "EMS," a cut down over the anterior STA serves as the posterior branch of a horseshoe incision (**Fig. 12.12c**). A small medial frontal craniotomy flap is elevated, the dura is resected, and the frontalis muscle and cut

end of the STA are sutured to the dural edges. Matsushima reported good revascularization of two-thirds or more of the MCA distribution in 56% of the patients.[7] Symptoms disappeared in 56% compared with 41% of patients undergoing EDAS alone.

Tu et al described multiple indirect revascularization variations by combining EAS using both anterior and posterior branches of the

STA with a cuff of galea and temporalis muscle for EMS.[8] In their variation, a frontotemporal incision is made to accommodate dissecting the frontal and parietal STA branches. The temporalis muscle is bivalved into two flaps, which are rotated so that the arteries are adjacent to the brain surface. The middle meningeal artery is preserved by opening the dura and arachnoid widely. Half of the temporalis muscle is sutured to dural edges while the other half is reattached to the outside of the bone after the cranioplasty is completed.

Several authors described combining parietal EDAS with multiple cranial bur holes in one or more stages.[52,60] In both adults and pediatric age groups, bur holes are placed in the distribution of the ACA, PCA, or both to augment MCA revascularization from parietal EDAS.

The group from Seoul National University Children's Hospital is a proponent of multiple combined indirect procedures.[21,29,50] Recently, 410 consecutive patients underwent relatively uniform revascularization procedures, and 81% had good or excellent clinical outcomes.[29] In most cases, the procedure was performed in stages with the symptomatic hemodynamically affected hemisphere treated first. One or more additional stages could be used to address the contralateral side and ischemia of the ACA and PCA. In brief, a parietal STA EDAS is performed in the usual fashion. A modified ribbon procedure is added. Contralateral parietal EDAS and occipital artery EDAS can be added as needed.

Multiple EDAS procedures offer another option for multiple combined indirect procedures. Tenjin and Ueda described a small series of pediatric patients in which EDAS was performed on any combination of frontal STA, parietal STA, and occipital artery on one or both sides.[61] Approximately 5 cm of STA with a cuff of galea is sutured to adjacent dura. The frontal STA or occipital artery was added sequentially in the setting of unsteady gait, persistent urinary incontinence, or cognitive decline, all of which improved with additional surgery.

◆ Combined Indirect and Direct Procedures

Using both direct and indirect procedures benefits from the immediate and large caliber of revascularization from a direct procedure and the broad anatomic coverage afforded by indirect procedures. Houkin et al combined a direct STA-to-MCA bypass with EDAMS in children (**Fig. 12.13a**).[62] Specific points of this combined procedure include making a frontotemporal incision encompassing the parietal STA and maximizing the size of the bone flap. Three bur holes and temporal craniectomy help preserve the middle meningeal artery and dura. The frontal branch of the STA is anastomosed directly with a frontal branch of the MCA to address frontal lobe revascularization. The parietal STA is kept intact for the STA onlay component of EDAMS, and the temporalis

Fig. 12.13a–f Combined direct and indirect procedures. (**a**) Layout of a direct superficial temporal artery (STA)-to-middle cerebral artery (MCA) bypass (*arrowhead* indicates anastomosis) using the frontal STA branch and an indirect encephaloduroarteriosynangiosis using the parietal STA combined with application of temporalis muscle to the brain surface to complete an encephaloduroarteriomyosynangiosis. (**b**) The incision (*dashed blue lines*) for the STA-to-MCA bypass combined with an encephaloduromyoarteriopericranios ynangiosis (EDMAPS) courses just posterior to the parietal STA up to midline then travels forward to the hairline. This exposure allows one to perform both a frontal temporal craniotomy under the temporalis muscle and a parasagittal frontal craniotomy. The frontal pericranium and both STA branches are preserved. The craniotomies are indicated by the *dashed lines*. (**c**) EDMAPS utilizing the parietal STA for an encephaloduroarteriosynangiosis indirect bypass and the frontal STA branch for a direct anastomotic bypass. The anastomosis is indicated by the *arrowhead*. (**d**) EDMAPS variation where both frontal and parietal STA branches are sewn to cortical MCA branches (*arrowheads*). (**e**) Encephaloduroarteriomyosynangiosis combined with direct STA-to-MCA and direct STA-to-anterior cerebral artery bypasses (anastomoses are indicated by *arrowheads*). The frontal STA passes over a strip of bone between frontal and temporal craniotomies. (**f**) Pericranium and temporalis muscle sutured to adjacent dura in parasagittal and frontotemporal craniotomies. (Used with permission from Barrow Neurological Institute.)

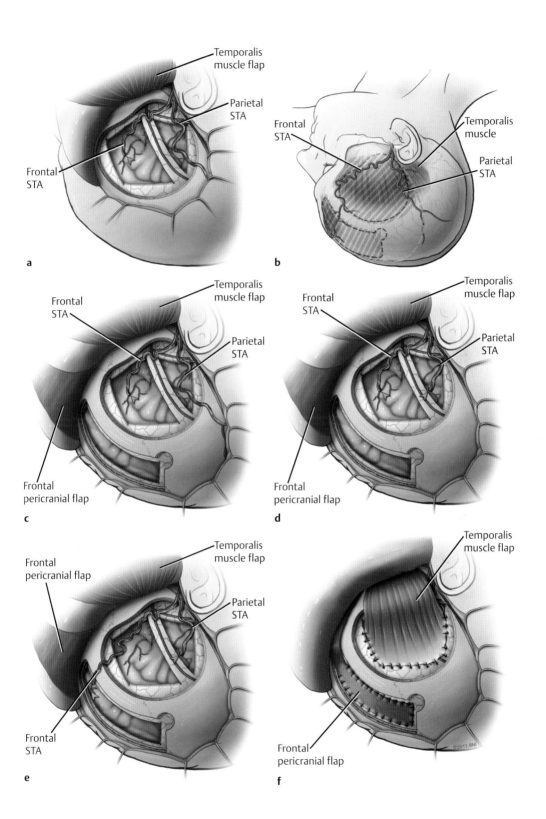

a

b

c

d

e

f

muscle is flattened with relaxing incisions and sewn to the adjacent dura to complete the EDAMS procedure.

Kim et al combined STA-to-MCA bypass with large inverted galeal strips based on STA branch pedicles (see **Fig. 12.9c**).[53] In this procedure, a frontotemporal incision posterior to the parietal STA is carried forward to the anterior superior extent of the frontal STA. After the galeal scalp flap is elevated off the temporalis muscle, an incision is made in the galea 2 cm in front of and 2 cm behind each STA branch, forming a Y-shaped galeal pedicle based on both STA branches. The frontal STA is maintained in continuity while the parietal STA is divided as distally as possible. The galeal flap is retracted, and a linear incision is made in the temporalis muscle. Three bur holes are placed over the proximal and distal STA branches, and a frontotemporal craniotomy is elevated. A temporal craniectomy is performed piecemeal to preserve the middle meningeal artery branches. The dura is opened in a cruciate fashion, preserving the middle meningeal artery branches, and then rolled under the bone edges. A parietal STA-to-MCA bypass is performed. Both galeal pedicles are rotated so that the external galea apposes the cortical surface and the edges of the galea are sutured to the dural edges. The bone is plated back into position using bur hole gaps to accommodate the STA-galeal pedicles. The temporalis muscle and skin are closed.

Kuroda et al reported 47 adult and 28 pediatric patients with moyamoya who underwent STA-to-MCA direct bypass in addition to encephaloduromyoarterioperipcraniosynangiosis (**Fig. 12.13b–d**).[55] This study reflects the addition of pericraniosynangiosis in the ACA distribution to ameliorate mesial frontal ischemia. The skin incision follows the parietal STA superior to the bregma and passes forward in the midline to the hairline (**Fig. 12.13b**). The parietal STA is dissected and kept in continuity. The temporalis muscle is dissected widely. The frontal STA is also dissected as distally as possible. An anteriorly based medial frontal pericranial graft is dissected with care to preserve the venous and arterial supply from the supratrochlear and supraorbital vessels. The pericranial graft is based on a wide pedicle. Ideally, it is large enough to cover the exposed brain. First, a frontotemporal craniotomy is elevated under the temporalis muscle. The dura is opened, preserving the middle meningeal artery. A frontal STA-to-MCA bypass is performed using the frontal STA branch (**Fig. 12.13c**). Kuroda describes indirect parietal STA-to-MCA bypass as a primary method (**Fig. 12.13c**), though the double barrel method of adding the parietal STA-to-MCA anastomoses remains an option (**Fig. 12.13d**).[55] A mesial anterofrontal craniotomy is elevated. The dural is incised in a crucial fashion and leaflets are inverted under the bone. The pericranial graft is placed over cortex with its edges sewn to the dural border (**Fig. 12.13f**).

Like others, Ishikawa et al called for revascularization of the ACA distribution to improve cognitive symptoms associated with medial frontal ischemia (**Fig. 12.13b, e**).[63] In an effort to reduce the risk of postoperative ACA infarction while waiting for indirect revascularization to mature and to achieve immediate pansynangiosis, they treated 16 patients, half children and half adults, who underwent simultaneous STA-to-ACA and STA-to-MCA direct bypass surgery in addition to EDAMS and encephalogaleoarteriosynangiosis. For this procedure, the skin incision extends along the parietal STA, continues to the bregma, and extends forward in the midline to the hairline (**Fig. 12.13b**). The frontal STA branch is dissected as far as possible to allow for an STA-ACA end-to-side anastomosis to an A4 cortical branch via an anterior parasagittal strip craniotomy (**Fig. 12.13e**). A frontal-based rectangular strip of galeal is also inserted into the parasagittal craniotomy. The parietal STA is dissected and used for an STA-to-MCA direct bypass through a second frontotemporal craniotomy. Care is taken to preserve the main middle meningeal artery branches with the dural opening, and the temporalis muscle is to complete the EDAMS. Both bone flaps are replaced with sufficient room to accommodate both STA branches, the temporalis muscle, and galea flap.

This group performed bilateral procedures in 10 cases. Transient ischemic attacks resolved in all but two cases, and improved IQ scores were documented in three patients, including two adults with only one infarct. Although the indications for these complex procedures are vague and the 16 patients were chosen from a group of 22 whose results are not reported, the feasibility and general success of pansynangiosis, including simultaneous ACA and MCA direct anastomosis, is documented.

◆ Conclusion

Various indirect bypass options are available depending on the anatomy and needs of any given patient with moyamoya disease. A combination of onlay tissues is most commonly chosen. At present, all rely on ingrowth over time to achieve improvements in cerebral perfusion. Lack of good donor or recipient vessels, or concern over sudden hyperperfusion, constitute the main indications for their use.

References

1. Fujimura M, Kaneta T, Mugikura S, Shimizu H, Tominaga T. Temporary neurologic deterioration due to cerebral hyperperfusion after superficial temporal artery-middle cerebral artery anastomosis in patients with adult-onset moyamoya disease. Surg Neurol 2007;67(3):273–282

2. Casanova R, Cavalcante D, Grotting JC, Vasconez LO, Psillakis JM. Anatomic basis for vascularized outertable calvarial bone flaps. Plast Reconstr Surg 1986; 78(3):300–308

3. Matsushima Y, Inaba Y. The specificity of the collaterals to the brain through the study and surgical treatment of moyamoya disease. Stroke 1986;17(1):117–122

4. Tsubokawa T, Kikuchi H, Asano S. Surgical treatment for intracranial thrombosis. Case report of "duropexia." Neurol Med Chir (Tokyo) 1964;6:48–49

5. Henschen C. [Surgical revascularization of cerebral injury of circulatory origin by means of stratification of pedunculated muscle flaps]. Langenbecks Arch Klin Chir Ver Dtsch Z Chir 1950;264:392–401

6. Karasawa J, Kikuchi H, Furuse S, Sakaki T, Yoshida Y. A surgical treatment of "moyamoya" disease "encephalomyo synangiosis". Neurol Med Chir (Tokyo) 1977; 17(1 Pt 1):29–37

7. Matsushima T., Inoue T., Ikezaki K. et al. Multiple combined indirect procedure for the surgical treatment of children with moyamoya disease. A comparison with single indirect anastomosis and direct anastomosis. Neurosurg Focus 1998; 5, 5:e4

8. Tu YK, Liu HM, Kuo MF, Wang PJ, Hung CC. Combined encephalo-arterio-synangiosis and encephalo-myosynangiosis in the treatment of moyamoya disease. Clin Neurol Neurosurg 1997;99(Suppl 2):S118–S122

9. Yoshida YK, Shirane R, Yoshimoto T. Non-anastomotic bypass surgery for childhood moyamoya disease using dural pedicle insertion over the brain surface combined with encephalogaleomyosynangiosis. Surg Neurol 1999;51(4):404–411

10. Yoshioka N, Tominaga S. Cerebral revascularization using muscle free flap for ischemic cerebrovascular disease in adult patients. Neurol Med Chir (Tokyo) 1998;38(8):464–468, discussion 467–468

11. Takeuchi S, Tsuchida T, Kobayashi K, et al. Treatment of moyamoya disease by temporal muscle graft 'encephalomyo-synangiosis'. Childs Brain 1983;10(1):1–15

12. Irikura K, Miyasaka Y, Kurata A, et al. The effect of encephalo-myo-synangiosis on abnormal collateral vessels in childhood moyamoya disease. Neurol Res 2000;22(4):341–346

13. Touho H. Cerebral ischemia due to compression of the brain by ossified and hypertrophied muscle used for encephalomyosynangiosis in childhood moyamoya disease. Surg Neurol 2009;72(6):725–727

14. Zipfel GJ, Fox DJ Jr, Rivet DJ. Moyamoya disease in adults: the role of cerebral revascularization. Skull Base 2005;15(1):27–41

15. Matsushima Y, Fukai N, Tanaka K, et al. A new surgical treatment of moyamoya disease in children: a preliminary report. Surg Neurol 1981;15(4):313–320

16. Matsushima T, Fujiwara S, Nagata S, et al. Surgical treatment for paediatric patients with moyamoya disease by indirect revascularization procedures (EDAS, EMS, EMAS). Acta Neurochir (Wien) 1989;98, 3–4:135–140

17. Matsushima T, Inoue T, Katsuta T, et al. An indirect revascularization method in the surgical treatment of moyamoya disease—various kinds of indirect procedures and a multiple combined indirect procedure. Neurol Med Chir (Tokyo) 1998;38(Suppl):297–302

18. Matsushima T, Inoue T, Suzuki SO, Fujii K, Fukui M, Hasuo K. Surgical treatment of moyamoya disease in pediatric patients—comparison between the results of indirect and direct revascularization procedures. Neurosurgery 1992;31(3):401–405

19. Matsushima Y, Aoyagi M, Fukai N, Tanaka K, Tsuruoka S, Inaba Y. Angiographic demonstration of cerebral revascularization after encephalo-duro-arteriosynangiosis (EDAS) performed on pediatric moyamoya patients. Bull Tokyo Med Dent Univ 1982;29(1):7–17

20. Spetzler RF, Roski RA, Kopaniky DR. Alternative superficial temporal artery to middle cerebral artery revascularization procedure. Neurosurgery 1980;7(5): 484–487

21. Kim SK, Wang KC, Kim IO, Lee DS, Cho BK. Combined encephaloduroarteriosynangiosis and bifrontal encephalogaleo(periosteal)synangiosis in pediatric moyamoya disease. Neurosurgery 2002;50(1):88–96

22. Matsushima Y, Inaba Y. Moyamoya disease in children and its surgical treatment. Introduction of a new surgical procedure and its follow-up angiograms. Childs Brain 1984;11(3):155–170

23. Tripathi P, Tripathi V, Naik RJ, Patel JM. Moya Moya cases treated with encephaloduroarteriosynangiosis. Indian Pediatr 2007;44(2):123–127

24. Fujita K, Tamaki N, Matsumoto S. Surgical treatment of moyamoya disease in children: which is more effective procedure, EDAS or EMS? Childs Nerv Syst 1986; 2(3):134–138

25. Isono M, Ishii K, Kamida T, Inoue R, Fujiki M, Kobayashi H. Long-term outcomes of pediatric moyamoya disease treated by encephalo-duro-arterio-synangiosis. Pediatr Neurosurg 2002;36(1):14–21

26. Scott RM, Smith JL, Robertson RL, et al. Long-term outcome in children with moyamoya syndrome after cranial revascularization by pial synangiosis. J Neurosurg 2004;100, 2 Suppl Pediatrics:142–149

27. Smith ER, Scott RM. Surgical management of moyamoya syndrome. Skull Base 2005;15(1):15–26

28. Hayashi T, Shirane R, Tominaga T. Additional surgery for postoperative ischemic symptoms in patients

with moyamoya disease: the effectiveness of occipital artery-posterior cerebral artery bypass with an indirect procedure: technical case report. Neurosurgery 2009;64(1):E195–E196, discussion E196

29. Kim SK, Cho BK, Phi JH, et al. Pediatric moyamoya disease: An analysis of 410 consecutive cases. Ann Neurol 2010;68(1):92–101

30. Kinugasa K, Mandai S, Kamata I, Sugiu K, Ohmoto T. Surgical treatment of moyamoya disease: operative technique for encephalo-duro-arterio-myo-synangiosis, its follow-up, clinical results, and angiograms. Neurosurgery 1993;32(4):527–531

31. Nakashima H, Meguro T, Kawada S, Hirotsune N, Ohmoto T. Long-term results of surgically treated moyamoya disease. Clin Neurol Neurosurg 1997; 99(Suppl 2):S156–S161

32. Ishii K, Morishige M, Anan M, et al. Superficial temporal artery-to-middle cerebral artery anastomosis with encephalo-duro-myo-synangiosis as a modified operative procedure for moyamoya disease. Acta Neurochir Suppl (Wien) 2010;107:95–99

33. Ozgur BM, Aryan HE, Levy ML. Indirect revascularisation for paediatric moyamoya disease: the EDAMS technique. J Clin Neurosci 2006;13(1):105–108

34. Houkin K, Kamiyama H, Abe H, Takahashi A, Kuroda S. Surgical therapy for adult moyamoya disease. Can surgical revascularization prevent the recurrence of intracerebral hemorrhage? Stroke 1996;27(8):1342–1346

35. Kim DS, Kang SG, Yoo DS, Huh PW, Cho KS, Park CK. Surgical results in pediatric moyamoya disease: angiographic revascularization and the clinical results. Clin Neurol Neurosurg 2007;109(2):125–131

36. Karasawa J, Kikuchi H, Kawamura J, Sakai T. Intracranial transplantation of the omentum for cerebrovascular moyamoya disease: a two-year follow-up study. Surg Neurol 1980;14(6):444–449

37. Goldsmith HS, Chen WF, Duckett SW. Brain vascularization by intact omentum. Arch Surg 1973; 106(5):695–698

38. Goldsmith HS, Duckett S, Chen WF. Spinal cord vascularization by intact omentum. Am J Surg 1975; 129(3):262–265

39. Yaşargil MG, Yonekawa Y, Denton I, Piroth D, Benes I. Experimental intracranial transplantation of autogenic omentum majus. J Neurosurg 1974;40(2):213–217

40. Karasawa J, Touho H, Ohnishi H, Miyamoto S, Kikuchi H. Cerebral revascularization using omental transplantation for childhood moyamoya disease. J Neurosurg 1993;79(2):192–196

41. Yoshioka N, Tominaga S, Suzuki Y, et al. Cerebral revascularization using omentum and muscle free flap for ischemic cerebrovascular disease. Surg Neurol 1998;49(1):58–65, discussion 65–66

42. Yoshioka N, Tominaga S, Suzuki Y, et al. Vascularized omental graft to brain surface in ischemic cerebrovascular disease. Microsurgery 1995;16(7):455–462

43. Havlik RJ, Fried I, Chyatte D, Modlin IM. Encephalo-omental synangiosis in the management of moyamoya disease. Surgery 1992;111(2):156–162

44. Touho H, Karasawa J, Tenjin H, Ueda S. Omental transplantation using a superficial temporal artery previously used for encephaloduroarteriosynangiosis. Surg Neurol 1996;45(6):550–558, discussion 558–559

45. Endo M, Kawano N, Miyaska Y, Yada K. Cranial burr hole for revascularization in moyamoya disease. J Neurosurg 1989;71(2):180–185

46. Kawaguchi T, Fujita S, Hosoda K, Shibata Y, Komatsu H, Tamaki N. [Usefulness of multiple burr-hole operation for child Moyamoya disease]. No Shinkei Geka 1998; 26(3):217–224

47. Kawaguchi T, Fujita S, Hosoda K, et al. Multiple burr-hole operation for adult moyamoya disease. J Neurosurg 1996;84(3):468–476

48. Oliveira RS, Amato MC, Simão GN, et al. Effect of multiple cranial burr hole surgery on prevention of recurrent ischemic attacks in children with moyamoya disease. Neuropediatrics 2009;40(6):260–264

49. Sainte-Rose C, Oliveira R, Puget S, et al. Multiple bur hole surgery for the treatment of moyamoya disease in children. J Neurosurg 2006;105(6, Suppl)437–443

50. Kawamoto H, Inagawa T, Ikawa F, Sakoda E. A modified burr-hole method in galeoduroencephalosynangiosis for an adult patient with probable moyamoya disease-case report and review of the literature. Neurosurg Rev 2001;24, 2–3:147–50

51. Kawamoto H, Kiya K, Mizoue T, Ohbayashi N. A modified burr-hole method 'galeoduroencephalosynangiosis' in a young child with moyamoya disease. A preliminary report and surgical technique. Pediatr Neurosurg 2000;32(5):272–275

52. Dusick JR, Gonzalez NR, Martin NA. Clinical and angiographic outcomes from indirect revascularization surgery for Moyamoya disease in adults and children: a review of 63 procedures. Neurosurgery 2011;68(1):34–43, discussion 43

53. Kim DS, Yoo DS, Huh PW, Kang SG, Cho KS, Kim MC. Combined direct anastomosis and encephaloduro-arteriogaleosynangiosis using inverted superficial temporal artery-galeal flap and superficial temporal artery-galeal pedicle in adult moyamoya disease. Surg Neurol 2006;66(4):389–394, discussion 395

54. Shirane R, Yoshida Y, Takahashi T, Yoshimoto T. Assessment of encephalo-galeo-myo-synangiosis with dural pedicle insertion in childhood moyamoya disease: characteristics of cerebral blood flow and oxygen metabolism. Clin Neurol Neurosurg 1997; 99(Suppl 2):S79–S85

55. Kuroda S, Houkin K, Ishikawa T, Nakayama N, Iwasaki Y. Novel bypass surgery for moyamoya disease using pericranial flap: its impacts on cerebral hemodynamics and long-term outcome. Neurosurgery 2010;66(6):1093–1101, discussion 1101

56. Yoshioka N, Rhoton AL Jr. Vascular anatomy of the anteriorly based pericranial flap. Neurosurgery 2005; 57(1, Suppl)11–16, discussion 11–16

57. Kinugasa K, Mandai S, Tokunaga K, et al. Ribbon enchephalo-duro-arterio-myo-synangiosis for moyamoya disease. Surg Neurol 1994;41(6):455–461

58. King JA, Armstrong D, Vachhrajani S, Dirks PB. Relative contributions of the middle meningeal artery and superficial temporal artery in revascularization surgery for moyamoya syndrome in children: the results of superselective angiography. J Neurosurg Pediatr 2010;5(2):184–189

59. Dauser RC, Tuite GF, McCluggage CW. Dural inversion procedure for moyamoya disease. Technical note. J Neurosurg 1997;86(4):719–723

60. Abla AA, Gandhoke G, Clark JC, et al. Surgical outcomes for Moyamoya angiopathy at Barrow Neurological Institute with comparison of adult indirect STA-MCA bypass, adult direct STA-MCA bypass and pediatric STA-MCA bypass. 154 revascularization surgeries in 140 affected hemispheres. Neurosurgery in press

61. Tenjin H, Ueda S. Multiple EDAS (encephalo-duro-arterio-synangiosis). Additional EDAS using the frontal branch of the superficial temporal artery (STA) and the occipital artery for pediatric moyamoya patients in whom EDAS using the parietal branch of STA was insufficient. Childs Nerv Syst 1997;13(4):220–224

62. Houkin K, Kamiyama H, Takahashi A, Kuroda S, Abe H. Combined revascularization surgery for childhood moyamoya disease: STA-MCA and encephalo-duro-arterio-myo-synangiosis. Childs Nerv Syst 1997;13(1): 24–29

63. Ishikawa T, Kamiyama H, Kuroda S, Yasuda H, Nakayama N, Takizawa K. Simultaneous superficial temporal artery to middle cerebral or anterior cerebral artery bypass with pan-synangiosis for Moyamoya disease covering both anterior and middle cerebral artery territories. Neurol Med Chir (Tokyo) 2006;46(9): 462–468

13

Direct Revascularization Procedures for Moyamoya Disease

John E. Wanebo, Gregory J. Velat, Joseph M. Zabramski, Peter Nakaji, and Robert F. Spetzler

◆ Introduction

Surgical treatment of moyamoya disease is designed to augment cerebral blood flow to reduce the risk of stroke. Both direct and indirect bypass techniques have been attempted. These interventions typically involve the redirection of blood flow from the external to internal carotid artery circulations. This chapter focuses on indications for direct surgical anastomosis and the surgical nuances and techniques to optimize revascularization.

◆ Patient Selection

No standardized guidelines exist for the selection of potential bypass candidates suffering from moyamoya disease. Typically, patients present to the neurosurgeon after hemorrhage or the onset of ischemic symptoms. It is unclear, however, if bypass affects the natural history of hemorrhage once it has already occurred, although it may reduce the risk of initial hemorrhage.[1–3] Ideally, bypass should be performed prior to development of permanent cerebral infarction, which typically occurs in watershed arterial territories. In cases where patients present prior to ischemic symptoms, prophylactic bypass procedures ameliorate the risk of stroke. Most physicians agree that surgical intervention should not be undertaken in the acute period following an ischemic stroke or hemorrhage.

◆ Bypass Selection

Once a patient is deemed a surgical candidate, multiple issues must be considered before a bypass is performed. Imaging studies to assess cerebral perfusion and potential areas of cerebral infarction are needed to detail the extent of the disease. Computed tomography (CT) perfusion angiography is readily available at most centers. Magnetic resonance imaging (MRI) perfusion has been shown to be effective in the diagnosis of moyamoya disease, but its availability is limited to select tertiary care institutions. Single photon emission computed tomography or CT perfusion with acetazolamide challenge provides valuable information about cerebrovascular reserve.

Cerebral angiography is the gold standard diagnostic modality for moyamoya disease because it allows both the internal and external carotid artery circulations to be examined. From this study, the size of potential donor arteries and the extent of collateralization can be estimated, as can disease chronicity by examining cortical arteries. In the early stages of moyamoya disease, the caliber of affected vessels remains relatively normal and cortical collateralization is not yet extensive. These vessels are ideal for direct anastomosis. In contrast, distal small cortical vessels with significant dilatation and larger vessels with reduced vessel diameter and collateralization indicative of chronic disease should be considered less attractive for direct bypass due to the increased perioperative risk of infarction or hyperperfusion syndrome. A patient's individual anatomy is also important in the selection of bypass. The small diameter of potential donor grafts and cortical recipient vessels often precludes direct bypass in children.

◆ Direct Anastomosis

Direct anastomosis has several potential advantages over indirect techniques. Direct bypass provides immediate revascularization, thereby avoiding the hysteretic effect of indirect procedures, which typically require several months to mature. Direct bypass may more reliably reduce hemodynamic stress to affected moyamoya vessels. Direct surgical intervention for moyamoya disease is typically performed using a superficial temporal artery (STA)-to-middle cerebral artery (MCA) end-to-side anastomosis; however, occipital artery[4] and interposition vein grafts have also been used for revascularization.[5] In 1972, Yasargil performed the first successful STA-to-MCA bypass for moyamoya disease,[6] ~15 years after Takeuchi and Shimizu's initial description of the disease.[7] Yasargil performed an end-to-end anastomosis in a 4-year-old child with progressive hemiparesis and speech difficulty. At the child's 2-year follow-up examination, motor function and speech had improved. Angiography confirmed flow through the bypass with improved cerebral circulation.[8]

Numerous reports in the pediatric and adult literature have documented successful cerebral revascularization after direct anastomosis with or without adjunctive indirect procedures for the treatment of moyamoya disease.[1,2,6,8-27] Although technically challenging, direct anastomosis has been reported to produce favorable outcomes in pediatric patients.[12,21,26,28] Other groups have modified the traditional STA-to-MCA direct anastomosis to include branches of the anterior cerebral artery (ACA)

for select patients.[29-32] In Japan, a prospective trial is under way to evaluate patient outcomes after direct anastomosis in the treatment of moyamoya disease.[33]

Anesthesia Considerations

During the perioperative period, several important factors must be considered to reduce the risk of iatrogenic ischemic complications. An experienced neuroanesthesia team is critical to achieving surgical operative success. Patients should be maintained on aspirin or other antiplatelet agents prior to and after surgery. Somatosensory-evoked potentials and electroencephalography are monitored routinely to help avoid potential intraoperative deficits. Blood pressure should be maintained within the patient's baseline range throughout the procedure. Hyperventilation must be avoided to minimize cerebral vasoconstriction. During the perioperative period, volume status is usually expanded using crystalloid (typically 1.25 to 1.5 times maintenance through postoperative day 1), especially in children. After surgery, arterial blood pressure should be monitored carefully in the intensive care unit to avoid both hypertensive and hypotensive events. Pressors are occasionally required and may be weaned over several days.

Surgical Technique

It is worth mentioning again that patients should be started on daily aspirin or another antiplatelet agent prior to bypass surgery. The patient is positioned supine on the operating table, and the head is secured in place using a Mayfield head holder. The head should be rotated 60 degrees contralateral to the side of surgery with the zygoma positioned at the highest point. Using a handheld Doppler probe, the course of the STA and its frontal and parietal branches are marked on the patient's scalp from the root of the zygoma as far distally as possible above the superficial temporal line (usually 9 to 10 cm). No local anesthetic is used, because injection into the subcutaneous tissue may inadvertently injure the STA.

The skin incision is made with a no. 15 blade directly over the STA with the aid of the

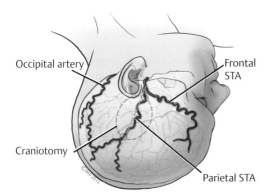

Fig. 13.1 Illustration showing direct superficial temporal artery (STA)-to–middle cerebral artery bypass. The incision (*blue dashed line*) follows the parietal branch of the STA and allows for a 5-cm temporal craniotomy (*dashed circle*). (Used with permission from Barrow Neurological Institute.)

operating microscope (**Fig. 13.1**). Microdissection of the STA can be started at the level of the superficial temporal line and proceed toward the zygoma, or be performed in the reverse direction. Working from superior to inferior is usually technically easier because it is a more natural direction for the hands. Care must be taken during the dissection because the course of the STA is typically tortuous and becomes more superficial near the zygoma. The superficial temporal vein rests in the tissue layer superficial to the STA, which runs within the galea. The superficial temporal vein is usually posterior and superior to the STA. If it is difficult to identify the artery, a handheld intraoperative Doppler probe can be used to verify arterial pulsations. The vessel should be dissected from the underlying temporalis fascia, and the adventitia should be cleared from the distal portion of the donor artery. Both STA branches should be preserved if at all possible. In some instances, a double-barrel bypass may be required to provide sufficient collateral blood flow. Once mobilized, the STA should be kept moist and under minimal tension. A papaverine-soaked sponge may be used to vasodilate the STA before anastomosis.

The temporalis muscle is sharply divided in a linear fashion using a scalpel. Subperiosteal dissection is used to mobilize the temporalis muscle, which is held back using low-profile

fishhooks. The STA is kept outside of the fishhooks. A single bur hole is placed near the floor of the middle fossa. The bur hole should be large enough to allow the STA to pass freely beneath the planned craniotomy.

A craniotomy centered over the Sylvian fissure is turned to expose the underlying frontal and temporal lobes. During the craniotomy, great care should be taken to preserve the underlying middle meningeal artery, which may provide important collateral vessels to the underlying cortex. The inner table of the craniotomy should be beveled to create additional room when the bone flap is replaced after the bypass is completed. The dura is opened under microscopic guidance in a cruciate fashion to expose the underlying brain. The dural cuts should be made to avoid interruption of large middle meningeal dural arteries (**Fig. 13.2**). Cauterization of dural bleeders should be minimized to optimize potential collateralization. The dural leaflets are tucked under the bone edges to provide additional collateralization by encephaloduroarteriosynangiosis (EDAS).

Superficial Temporal Artery–to–Middle Cerebral Artery Anastomosis Technique

Experience has proven that absolute attention to detail when performing each step of the anastomosis maximizes the chance of a durable, robust connection and reduces the

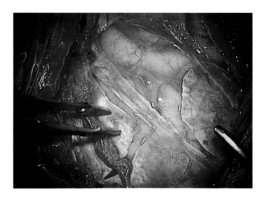

Fig. 13.2 Intraoperative photograph showing the dura opened in a cruciate fashion, allowing preservation of one or more middle meningeal artery branches. (Used with permission from Barrow Neurological Institute.)

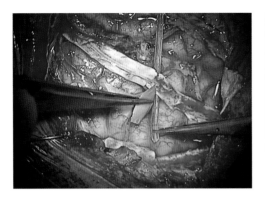

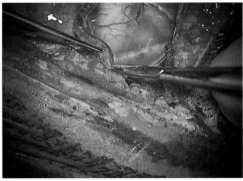

Fig. 13.3 Intraoperative photograph showing placement of microvacuum suction (3 French) under rubber backing. (Used with permission from Barrow Neurological Institute.)

Fig. 13.4 Intraoperative photograph showing removal of adventitia from distal superficial temporal artery while the superficial temporal artery remains in situ. (Used with permission from Barrow Neurological Institute.)

ischemic time related to use of temporary vessel occlusion. The techniques described have worked well at our institution.[34] Other experienced centers have their own equally effective preferences.

The site is carefully inspected to identify a suitable recipient artery, typically an M4 branch. The ideal recipient artery is about the same caliber as the donor STA branch. It has a relatively straight course and is located superficially. A recipient vessel in the center of the surgical field is easier to work with than one near the edge. If there are no suitable recipient arteries on the cortical surface, the Sylvian fissure may be split to find an appropriate M3 branch. Technically, such vessels are more difficult to anastomose.

Once an appropriate recipient vessel has been identified, the surrounding arachnoid is dissected free and mobilized carefully to preserve any collateral vessels supplying the underlying cortex. If possible, 10 mm of MCA should be mobilized. This length provides sufficient room for temporary clip application without distorting the MCA. At times, small perforating vessels entering directly into the cortex from the MCA anastomotic site must be divided to maintain a blood-free field. A small piece of latex or plastic is placed beneath the recipient vessel to secure it and provide a colored background for improved visualization (**Fig. 13.3**). A 5-French malleable suction catheter can be placed beneath the colored background or under the dependent bone edge to

maintain a clear field at the site of the planned anastomosis.

To prepare the STA, 10 mm of adventitia is removed from the STA while it is still intact (**Fig. 13.4**). The STA is then cut obliquely at a length that will allow it to be mobilized back and forth during the anastomosis. A temporary aneurysm clip is used to occlude blood flow, and the vessel is flushed with heparinized saline. Additional adventitia is dissected from the distal 10 mm of the STA, and the cut end is fish-mouthed to allow an anastomosis two to three times the width of the recipient vessel (usually 2.5 to 3.0 mm) (**Fig. 13.5**). Mini temporary aneurysm clips (2 or 3 mm) are placed

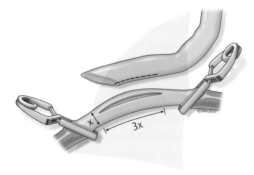

Fig. 13.5 Illustration showing superficial temporal artery fish-mouthed to match the 3-mm opening in the adjacent middle cerebral artery. Mini-AVM 2-mm clips are placed on the middle cerebral artery proximal and distal to the anastomosis site. (Used with permission from Barrow Neurological Institute.)

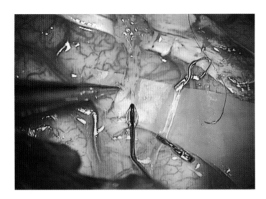

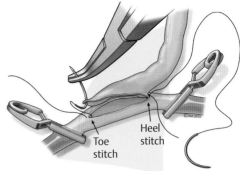

Fig. 13.6 Intraoperative photograph showing fully prepared anastomotic field. The superficial temporal artery and middle cerebral artery are irrigated with pure heparin using a 27-gauge blunt ophthalmic needle. (Used with permission from Barrow Neurological Institute.)

Fig. 13.7 Illustration showing the placement of proximal and distal middle cerebral artery–superficial temporal artery sutures into the heel and toe of the superficial temporal artery fish-mouth, with the suture passing from the outside in on the middle cerebral artery and from the inside out on the superficial temporal artery. (Used with permission from Barrow Neurological Institute.)

obliquely on either end of the recipient MCA segment (**Figs. 13.5** and **13.6**). Ideally, temporary clips are chosen for the delicate M4 branch so that they are just strong enough to occlude flow but gentle enough to minimize endothelial injury to the MCA. The anesthesiologist must be informed before temporary clipping so that systolic blood pressure is maintained at or slightly above baseline levels to help prevent ischemic complications.

A no. 11 blade or miniophthalmic no. 11 blade arachnoid knife is used to perform the arteriotomy in the recipient MCA segment. This arteriotomy can be extended with microscissors, and then the MCA is flushed with pure heparin using a 27-gauge blunt ophthalmic catheter (**Fig. 13.6**). An anastomosis two to three times the diameter of the typical 1-mm diameter M4 branch helps maximize inflow. A matched STA opening and MCA arteriotomy minimize any dog ears in the anastomoses. The arteriotomy site of the MCA can be marked with dye to further facilitate visualization of the delicate arterial walls during the anastomoses. A curved needle 3.5 to 3.8 mm long with nylon suture (10–0) is used to perform the end-to-side anastomosis.

If possible, the anastomosis should be performed so that flow from the STA is directed into the proximal MCA, maximizing the flow to surrounding MCA territory. The heel of the STA is tacked to the MCA so that it faces the surgeon (**Fig. 13.7**). This configuration makes it easier to sew this component of the anastomosis where the angle between the STA and MCA is closed down.

After the toe and heel of the STA are tacked to the MCA, the anastomosis can be completed in a running or interrupted fashion (**Fig. 13.8**). The more difficult side is usually done first. If a running technique is used, 6 to 12 small loops ~3 to 5 mm in diameter are made. The lumen is inspected before each loop is sequentially tightened and finally tied to the tail end of the other suture. The second side of the running closure is performed in the same way with careful inspection of the lumen before each loop is tightened to ensure that the opposite wall of the anastomosis has not been inadvertently included in the suture line (**Fig. 13.9**). Interrupted sutures are an equally effective option, particularly in areas more difficult to reach or in training circumstances. Interrupted sutures may also have the theoretical advantage of allowing the anastomosis size to expand over time. If a running suture is used, the footprint of the anastomosis should be large enough (2.5 to 3.5 times the diameter of the vessels being sutured) that the anastomosis is not itself a source of resistance.

Once the anastomosis is completed, the distal MCA clip is opened and the degree and exact location of any bleeding from the anastomosis is assessed. The proximal clip

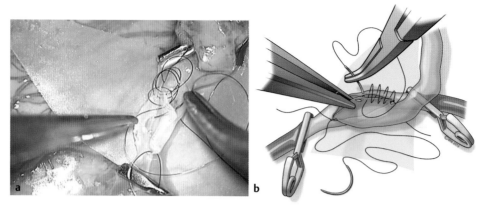

Fig. 13.8a, b Intraoperative photograph (**a**) and illustration (**b**) showing a series of continuous loops, 3 to 5 mm in diameter, in both superficial temporal artery and middle cerebral artery, allowing for visualization of both arterial walls. (Used with permission from Barrow Neurological Institute.)

is maintained in position. Additional interrupted sutures may be placed at any briskly bleeding sites, and minor bleeding points can usually be controlled with Surgicel (Ethicon 360, Somerville, NJ). Removal of the proximal MCA clip allows flow across the bypass. To reduce the risk of embolus or thrombus, an attempt should be made to flush the vessels in the direction from the MCA, out the unused frontal branch of the STA (**Fig. 13.10a–e**). If a proximal STA branch has been cut, back bleeding can be allowed from this vessel; otherwise, the proximal STA clip is removed and the anastomosis is inspected again for hemostasis (**Fig. 13.11**). An indocyanine

green angiogram and/or Doppler ultrasonogram can be used to assess flow through the anastomosis (**Fig. 13.12**). A compromised anastomosis is usually addressed by replacement of any suboptimal sutures, by milking any small amount of clot, or by making a small arteriotomy in the adjacent STA segment to flush the obstruction with pure heparin followed by simple closure with interrupted suture. The use of burst suppression anesthesia and back flow from distal M4 branches affords the surgeon ample time to make a revision safely. A bypass can fail because of technical factors or potentially because of reduced hemodynamic demand by the recipient artery.

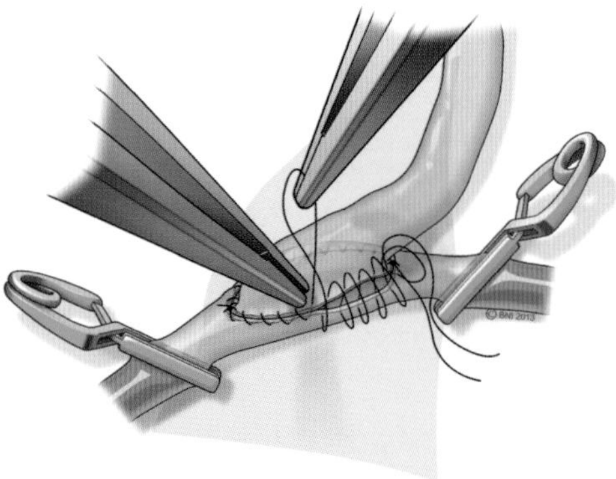

After adequate hemostasis is attained, the bone flap is carefully replaced and the temporalis muscle is loosely reapproximated to prevent constriction of the bypass. The wound is closed using galeal stitches and staples. Patients should be maintained on aspirin or other antiplatelet agents indefinitely to prevent thrombosis of the bypass.

Superficial Temporal Artery–to–Anterior Cerebral Artery Bypass Technique

Although revascularization of the ACA distribution usually involves indirect techniques such as bur holes or pericranial and/or galeal flaps, a direct STA-to-ACA bypass has been reported in several small series of patients with

Fig. 13.9 Illustration showing controlled tightening of each loop of the second side of the anastomosis, as performed on the first side. (Used with permission from Barrow Neurological Institute.)

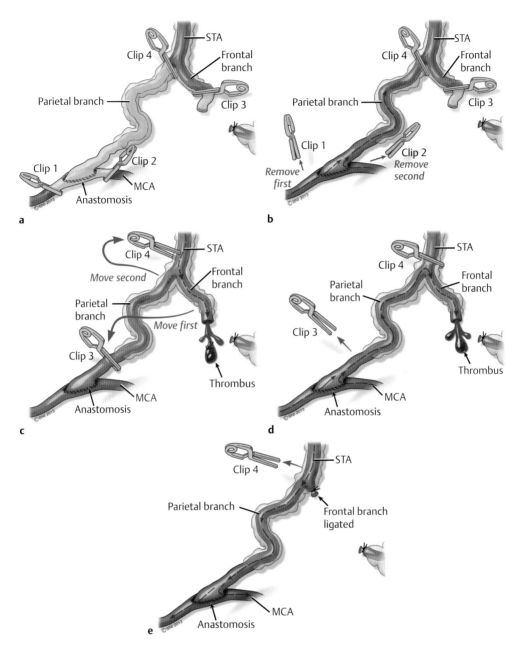

Fig. 13.10a–e Illustrations showing the clip removal sequence when a superficial temporal artery (STA) side branch is used for flushing the vessels. (**a**) Clip arrangement used when the frontal branch is divided and clipped, and clips are placed on the parietal branch of the STA and the proximal and distal middle cerebral artery (MCA). Potential thrombus near clips shown. (**b**) The clip on the distal MCA (clip 1) is removed and the clip on the proximal MCA (clip 2) is removed, flushing thrombus into the STA. (**c**) The clip on the frontal STA (clip 3) is moved to the distal parietal branch of the STA. The clip on the proximal parietal branch (clip 4) is removed and placed on the main trunk of the STA, allowing flushing of any main STA thrombus out the frontal STA while protecting the MCA. (**d**) The clip on the distal parietal branch (clip 3) is removed, allowing flushing from the MCA into the frontal STA and out. (**e**) The frontal branch of the STA is ligated and the clip on the main trunk of the STA (clip 4) is removed. (Used with permission from Barrow Neurological Institute.)

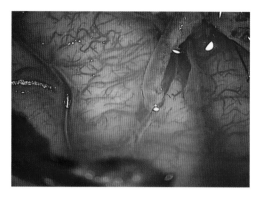

Fig. 13.11 Intraoperative photograph of the completed anastomosis. (Used with permission from Barrow Neurological Institute.)

moyamoya disease.[18,31,32] The STA-to-ACA anastomosis has been criticized for its limited flow augmentation related to the small distal donor and recipient vessels; nevertheless, several authors have described success with this technique, although they acknowledge that the procedure is not always technically feasible.[18,31,32]

Kawashima et al performed both STA-to-MCA and STA-to-ACA bypasses in seven patients with moyamoya disease, including one child.[32] Symptoms resolved completely in five of their patients. There are four salient features of this technique: using a long STA branch (frontal or parietal branch),

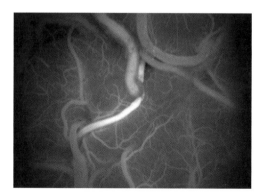

Fig. 13.12 Indocyanine green angiography documenting the patency of the anastomosis. (Used with permission from Barrow Neurological Institute.)

identifying a recipient ACA branch near the bregma, using a separate craniotomy for the MCA and ACA procedures, and using a small number of interrupted sutures for the ACA anastomoses. In this technique, a frontotemporal incision is made, and the parietal STA is dissected from the back of the incision. The frontal STA branch is dissected from the galeal side. One of the two STA branches, usually the frontal branch, is dissected for 10 cm or as long as possible. A 4-cm medial frontal craniotomy and a 4-cm frontotemporal craniotomy are fashioned. The long STA branch is passed subdurally under the bone bridge between the two craniotomies and up to the recipient ACA branch, which is usually in a sulcus at the level of the coronal suture. For the ACA anastomoses, a wide interstitch interval is used with only three interrupted 10–0 sutures per side. Hemostasis is provided by applying gentle pressure with a Cottonoid (Johnson & Johnson, New Brunswick, NJ) after declamping.

Iwama et al reported an STA-to-ACA bypass series for moyamoya disease.[31] They used an interposition graft of another STA branch to achieve the length needed to reach the ACA in four of five patients.[31] The interposition STA conduit is first sewn end-to-side to the ACA recipient and then end-to-end to the proximal STA feeding graft.

Other Direct Bypass Techniques

In addition to the STA, several other external branches can be used for direct revascularization for the treatment of moyamoya disease. The occipital artery has been used as a donor artery for direct revascularization of the MCA or posterior cerebral artery branches.[4,35] The posterior auricular artery has also been prepared as a donor artery to the recipient angular branch of the MCA (0.6 mm diameter).[36] Taniguchi et al used the distal stump of the STA for additional revascularization after the proximal stump of the same STA branch had been used for a more proximal MCA anastomosis.[37] In the setting of moyamoya disease, the use of a high-flow venous interposition graft has essentially been abandoned due to increased risk of reperfusion hemorrhage.[35]

Direct Bypass Imaging Techniques

High-resolution CT angiography of the brain can be used effectively to delineate the location and size of STA donor branches and MCA recipient branches. Three-dimensional digital subtraction angiography has also been advocated for preoperative planning of the craniotomy.[38] Digital subtraction angiography remains the gold standard for assessing bypass patency and progression of moyamoya disease. CT angiography serves as an accurate tool for assessing postoperative patency of a bypass.[39]

Surgical Outcomes

The major benefit of direct revascularization is immediate restoration of blood flow to the affected brain to ameliorate ischemic signs and symptoms. Multiple surgical series have demonstrated improved clinical outcomes after direct anastomosis in adults. Kobayashi et al performed 10 STA-to-MCA bypasses in seven adult patients with moyamoya, and angiographic results improved in six of the treated patients.[20] The patient who failed to demonstrate angiographic benefit suffered a fatal stroke after surgery.

Khan et al performed 44 direct revascularization procedures in 23 European patients with moyamoya disease.[18] All patients underwent an STA-to-MCA bypass. Ten patients were treated with a supplemental STA-to-ACA bypass. Three patients received supplemental indirect arteriosynangiosis using the occipital artery to the affected territories. There was one fatal postoperative complication in this series: an ischemic MCA territory infarction on the nonoperated side.

In another series, 39 patients with impaired preoperative cerebral blood flow and/or vasomotor reserve underwent 65 revascularization procedures.[22] Direct STA-to-MCA anastomosis was performed in 56 procedures. Saphenous vein interposition grafts were used in three procedures and EDAS was used in six additional procedures. Three perioperative deaths followed STA-to-MCA anastomosis. The perioperative morbidity rate was 12.3%, and seven complications

occurred in the direct revascularization cohort. Approximately 3 months after surgery, cerebral blood flow improved in 15 patients who underwent unilateral direct STA-to-MCA anastomosis.

Steinberg's group recently published their results of 450 revascularization procedures performed on 264 patients with moyamoya.[12] Direct revascularization was used in the majority of cases (95% of adults and 76% of children). At a mean follow-up of 4.9 years, low surgical morbidity (3.5%) and mortality (0.7%) rates were observed per treated hemisphere. The 5-year risk of perioperative or delayed stroke or death was 5.5%. Based on the modified Rankin scale, the authors reported significant improvement in the patients' quality of life ($p < 0.0001$).

Matsushima et al compared single indirect revascularization procedures to direct STA-to-MCA anastomosis performed on 72 hemispheres in 50 pediatric patients with moyamoya.[28] Direct bypass was performed in 16 patients in 19 sides, whereas EDAS was used on 18 sides in 12 patients. A modified combined indirect revascularization technique (encephalomyosynangiosis over the frontotemporoparietal region) was performed on 35 sides in 22 patients. Patients underwent cerebral angiography 4 to 25 months after surgery. The direct bypass procedure yielded the most robust collateralization and improved clinical outcomes compared with the indirect procedures. Two patients undergoing STA-to-MCA anastomosis had postoperative strokes. One minor stroke occurred in a patient after EDAS. Two symptomatic epidural hematomas developed after the combined indirect procedure.

Sakamoto et al performed a double-barrel STA-to-MCA anastomosis combined with encephalomyosynangiosis on 19 hemispheres in 10 pediatric patients with moyamoya.[26] Postoperative angiography confirmed revascularization to the affected MCA and watershed territories. The frequency of transient ischemic attacks decreased after surgery, only occurring in four patients at short-term follow-up. At a mean long-term follow-up of 4 years, no ischemic episodes were induced in the patients by hyperventilation, and no late neurological deterioration was documented.

Hemodynamic evaluation of brain perfusion using positron emission tomography has demonstrated elevated regional cerebral blood volume in the basal ganglia of patients with moyamoya disease with corresponding reductions in cerebral blood flow and elevations in oxygen extraction in the MCA territories indicating misery cortical perfusion. Following direct STA-to-MCA anastomosis, improvements in misery perfusion and improvements of blood flow in the basal ganglia have been observed on positron emission tomography.[40] This redistribution of blood flow may reduce hemodynamic stress on diseased moyamoya vessels, potentially reducing the risk of hemorrhage.

Several studies have demonstrated reduced hemorrhagic complications after direct revascularization. Houkin et al observed a 25% reduction in moyamoya vessels in 24 patients who presented with hemorrhagic moyamoya disease after undergoing combined STA-to-MCA direct revascularization and encephaloduroarteriomyosynangiosis.[1] At a mean follow-up of 6.4 years, only 3 of 24 patients (12.5%) who had initially presented with hemorrhage suffered an additional bleed. In a retrospective review of 43 patients with moyamoya who presented with intracranial hemorrhage and who underwent direct bypass, diseased moyamoya vessels decreased by 60% and the postoperative hemorrhage rate was 20% at a mean follow-up of 3.7 years.[2]

Fujii et al retrospectively reviewed the hemorrhage rate of 290 patients with moyamoya disease treated at multiple centers.[11] In 152 patients who underwent direct bypass, the hemorrhage rate was 19.1% compared with 28.3% in 138 patients managed conservatively. Okada et al performed direct STA-to-MCA anastomosis in 15 patients who presented with intracranial hemorrhage.[25] The perioperative hemorrhage rate was 6.7%. Reduced moyamoya vessels were observed in 60% of patients. A 20% spontaneous rebleed rate was observed at a mean follow-up of 7.8 years. Three patients suffered fatal intracranial hemorrhages. Preoperative regional cerebral blood flow improved significantly after surgery, and the perioperative hemorrhage rate was 6.7%.

Another study analyzed the recurrent hemorrhage rate associated with 22 patients with hemorrhagic moyamoya disease.[17] Six patients underwent direct bypass whereas five underwent EDAS. Eleven patients were treated conservatively. At a mean follow-up of 8 years, patients who underwent direct revascularization suffered no additional hemorrhagic strokes compared with 60% of the patients who underwent EDAS and 54% of patients managed conservatively, suggesting that direct revascularization may work more effectively than indirect revascularization for hemorrhagic moyamoya disease.

Complications

Multifactorial ischemic complications may occur after direct anastomosis. Any temporary reduction in cerebral perfusion may result in perioperative stroke. It is imperative to discuss the intraoperative management of these cases with anesthesia prior to beginning the procedure. In contrast to most neurosurgical procedures, it is critical to maintain the patient's baseline systolic blood pressure throughout the entire operation and avoid hyperventilation. Temporary cortical vessel occlusion is unique to direct bypass and increases the perioperative risk of stroke. Adequate burst suppression and minimization of clamp time may reduce, but cannot eliminate, this inherent risk.

Horn et al analyzed the risk of intraoperative ischemia related to temporary vessel occlusion in 20 consecutive adults who suffered transient ischemic attacks related to occlusive cerebrovascular disease.[41] All patients underwent direct STA-to-MCA bypasses. Postoperative MRIs were obtained within 48 hours of surgery. Two patients (20%) were found to have diffusion disturbances without permanent clinical sequela. The duration of temporary vessel occlusion ranged from 25 to 42 minutes (mean 33 ± 7 minutes).

Mesiwala et al reported a perioperative stroke rate of 7.7% (5/65 procedures) after STA-to-MCA bypass.[22] All infarctions were detected on routine postoperative MRI and were clinically silent. Guzman et al observed a procedural ischemic stroke rate of 1.7% (8/450 procedures) after revascularization surgery for moyamoya disease.[12] Direct STA-to-MCA anastomosis was performed in seven of these procedures. The ipsilateral side was affected in half of the cases.

Bypass occlusion may also cause postoperative ischemic complications. Mesiwala et al observed a delayed bypass occlusion rate of 4.6% (3/65 procedures: 2 STA-to-MCA bypasses and 1 STA-to-MCA bypass with an interposition saphenous venous graft) on follow-up angiography.[22] Hemorrhagic complications can also follow direct revascularization.

Several factors may play important roles in the development of postoperative hemorrhage. Revascularization of previously ischemic tissue is the most likely culprit similar to hemorrhagic transformation of infarcted brain parenchyma after acute ischemic stroke. Autoregulatory mechanisms are usually dampened in diseased moyamoya vessels. Furthermore, patients are typically maintained on aspirin perioperatively. Mesiwala et al observed a fatal postoperative intracerebral hemorrhage rate of 3.1% (2/65 procedures) at locations remote from the STA-to-MCA anastomosis.[22] Guzman's group reported that the rate of procedural intracerebral hemorrhage was 1.8% (8/450 procedures) after direct revascularization.[12] All hemorrhage occurred in previous ischemic territory ipsilateral to the surgical side.

Hyperperfusion syndrome resulting in transient neurological deterioration has also been reported after direct bypass. Fujimura et al observed symptomatic cerebral hyperperfusion in 27.5% of treated sides after direct STA-to-MCA bypass on postoperative MRI.[42] All neurological symptoms attributable to hyperperfusion eventually resolved. Kim et al estimated cerebral hyperperfusion to be responsible for transient neurological deterioration in 17% of their cases who underwent direct bypass.[43] The peak of increased cerebral perfusion, as measured by single photon emission computed tomography, occurred on the third postoperative day. Other complications have included delayed intracerebral hemorrhage,[44] chronic subdural hematoma formation,[45] and rupture of an intracranial MCA aneurysm related to altered hemodynamics[46] after STA-to-MCA anastomosis.

◆ Conclusion

Although technically more challenging than indirect bypass, STA-to-MCA and other direct bypass procedures provide an immediate improvement in cerebral blood flow to the patient suffering ischemic symptoms secondary to moyamoya disease, and may be more effective in decreasing the risk of recurrent hemorrhage in those presenting with hemorrhagic stroke.

References

1. Houkin K, Kamiyama H, Abe H, Takahashi A, Kuroda S. Surgical therapy for adult moyamoya disease. Can surgical revascularization prevent the recurrence of intracerebral hemorrhage? Stroke 1996;27(8): 1342–1346

2. Iwama T, Hashimoto N, Murai BN, Tsukahara T, Yonekawa Y. Intracranial rebleeding in moyamoya disease. J Clin Neurosci 1997;4(2):169–172

3. Iwama T, Morimoto M, Hashimoto N, Goto Y, Todaka T, Sawada M. Mechanism of intracranial rebleeding in moyamoya disease. Clin Neurol Neurosurg 1997;99(Suppl 2):S187–S190

4. Spetzler R, Chater N. Occipital artery–middle cerebral artery anastomosis for cerebral artery occlusive disease. Surg Neurol 1974;2(4):235–238

5. Lougheed WM, Marshall BM, Hunter M, Michel ER, Sandwith-Smyth H. Common carotid to intracranial internal carotid bypass venous graft. Technical note. J Neurosurg 1971;34(1):114–118

6. Donaghy RM. Neurologic surgery. Surg Gynecol Obstet 1972;134(2):269–270

7. Takeuchi K, Shimizu K. Hypogenesis of bilateral internal carotid arteries. No To Shinkei 1957;9:37–43

8. Krayenbühl HA. The Moyamoya syndrome and the neurosurgeon. Surg Neurol 1975;4(4):353–360

9. Amine AR, Moody RA, Meeks W. Bilateral temporalmiddle cerebral artery anastomosis for Moyamoya syndrome. Surg Neurol 1977;8(1):3–6

10. Boone SC, Sampson DS. Observations on moyamoya disease: a case treated with superficial temporal-middle cerebral artery anastomosis. Surg Neurol 1978; 9(3):189–193

11. Fujii K, Ikezaki K, Irikura K, Miyasaka Y, Fukui M. The efficacy of bypass surgery for the patients with hemorrhagic moyamoya disease. Clin Neurol Neurosurg 1997;99(Suppl 2):S194–S195

12. Guzman R, Lee M, Achrol A, et al. Clinical outcome after 450 revascularization procedures for moyamoya disease. Clinical article. J Neurosurg 2009;111(5): 927–935

13. Hänggi D, Mehrkens JH, Schmid-Elsaesser R, Steiger HJ. Results of direct and indirect revascularisation for adult European patients with Moyamoya angiopathy. Acta Neurochir Suppl (Wien) 2008;103:119–122

14. Holbach KH, Wassmann H, Wappenschmidt J. Superficial temporal-middle cerebral artery anastomosis in Moyamoya disease. Acta Neurochir (Wien) 1980; 52, 1–2:27–34

15. Houkin K, Kuroda S, Ishikawa T, Abe H. Neovascularization (angiogenesis) after revascularization in moyamoya disease. Which technique is most useful for moyamoya disease? Acta Neurochir (Wien) 2000;142(3):269–276

16. Karasawa J, Kikuchi H, Furuse S, Kawamura J, Sakaki T. Treatment of moyamoya disease with STA-MCA anastomosis. J Neurosurg 1978;49(5):679–688

17. Kawaguchi S, Okuno S, Sakaki T. Effect of direct arterial bypass on the prevention of future stroke in patients with the hemorrhagic variety of moyamoya disease. J Neurosurg 2000;93(3):397–401

18. Khan N, Schuknecht B, Boltshauser E, et al. Moyamoya disease and Moyamoya syndrome: experience in Europe; choice of revascularisation procedures. Acta Neurochir (Wien) 2003;145(12):1061–1071, discussion 1071

19. Kikuchi H, Karasawa J. [STA-cortical MCA anastomosis for cerebrovascular occlusive disease.] No Shinkei Geka 1973;1:15–19

20. Kobayashi H, Hayashi M, Handa Y, Kabuto M, Noguchi Y, Aradachi H. EC-IC bypass for adult patients with moyamoya disease. Neurol Res 1991;13(2):113–116

21. Matsushima T, Inoue T, Suzuki SO, Fujii K, Fukui M, Hasuo K. Surgical treatment of moyamoya disease in pediatric patients—comparison between the results of indirect and direct revascularization procedures. Neurosurgery 1992;31(3):401–405

22. Mesiwala AH, Sviri G, Fatemi N, Britz GW, Newell DW. Long-term outcome of superficial temporal artery-middle cerebral artery bypass for patients with moyamoya disease in the US. Neurosurg Focus 2008;24(2):e15

23. Miyamoto S, Akiyama Y, Nagata I, et al. Long-term outcome after STA-MCA anastomosis for moyamoya disease. Neurosurg Focus 1998; 5, 5:e5

24. Miyamoto S, Nagata I, Hashimoto N, Kikuchi H. Direct anastomotic bypass for cerebrovascular moyamoya disease. Neurol Med Chir (Tokyo) 1998;38(Suppl):294–296

25. Okada Y, Shima T, Nishida M, Yamane K, Yamada T, Yamanaka C. Effectiveness of superficial temporal artery-middle cerebral artery anastomosis in adult moyamoya disease: cerebral hemodynamics and clinical course in ischemic and hemorrhagic varieties. Stroke 1998;29(3):625–630

26. Sakamoto H, Kitano S, Yasui T, et al. Direct extracranial-intracranial bypass for children with moyamoya disease. Clin Neurol Neurosurg 1997;99(Suppl 2):S128–S133

27. Sakamoto S, Ohba S, Shibukawa M, et al. Angiographic neovascularization after bypass surgery in moyamoya disease: our experience at Hiroshima University Hospital. Hiroshima J Med Sci 2007;56(3–4):29–32

28. Matsushima T, Inoue T, Ikezaki K, et al. Multiple combined indirect procedure for the surgical treatment of children with moyamoya disease. A comparison with single indirect anastomosis and direct anastomosis. Neurosurg Focus 1998;5(5):e4

29. Ishikawa T, Kamiyama H, Kuroda S, Yasuda H, Nakayama N, Takizawa K. Simultaneous superficial temporal artery to middle cerebral or anterior cerebral artery bypass with pan-synangiosis for Moyamoya disease covering both anterior and middle cerebral artery territories. Neurol Med Chir (Tokyo) 2006;46(9):462–468

30. Iwama T, Hashimoto N, Miyake H, Yonekawa Y. Direct revascularization to the anterior cerebral artery territory in patients with moyamoya disease: report of five cases. Neurosurgery 1998;42(5):1157–1161, discussion 1161–1162

31. Iwama T, Hashimoto N, Tsukahara T, Miyake H. Superficial temporal artery to anterior cerebral artery direct anastomosis in patients with moyamoya disease. Clin Neurol Neurosurg 1997;99(Suppl 2):S134–S136

32. Kawashima A, Kawamata T, Yamaguchi K, Hori T, Okada Y. Successful superficial temporal artery-anterior cerebral artery direct bypass using a long graft for moyamoya disease: technical note. Neurosurgery 2010; 67, 3 Suppl Operative:ons145–ons149

33. Miyamoto S; Japan Adult Moyamoya Trial Group. Study design for a prospective randomized trial of extracranial-intracranial bypass surgery for adults with moyamoya disease and hemorrhagic onset—the Japan Adult Moyamoya Trial Group. Neurol Med Chir (Tokyo) 2004;44(4):218–219

34. Wanebo JE, Zabramski JM, Spetzler RF. Superficial temporal artery-to-middle cerebral artery bypass grafting for cerebral revascularization. Neurosurgery 2004;55(2):395–398, discussion 398–399

35. Pandey P, Steinberg GK. Outcome of repeat revascularization surgery for moyamoya disease after an unsuccessful indirect revascularization. Clinical article. J Neurosurg 2011;115(2):328–336

36. Horiuchi T, Kusano Y, Asanuma M, Hongo K. Posterior auricular artery-middle cerebral artery bypass for additional surgery of moyamoya disease. Acta Neurochir (Wien) 2012;154(3):455–456

37. Taniguchi M, Taki T, Tsuzuki T, Tani N, Ohnishi Y. EC-IC bypass using the distal stump of the superficial temporal artery as an additional collateral source of blood flow in patients with Moyamoya disease. Acta Neurochir (Wien) 2007;149(4):393–398

38. Nakagawa I, Kurokawa S, Tanisaka M, Kimura R, Nakase H. Virtual surgical planning for superficial temporal artery to middle cerebral artery bypass using three-dimensional digital subtraction angiography. Acta Neurochir (Wien) 2010;152(9):1535–1540, discussion 1541

39. Besachio DA, Ziegler JI, Duncan TD, Wanebo JS. Computed tomographic angiography in evaluation of superficial temporal to middle cerebral artery bypass. J Comput Assist Tomogr 2010;34(3):437–439

40. Morimoto M, Iwama T, Hashimoto N, Kojima A, Hayashida K. Efficacy of direct revascularization in adult Moyamoya disease: haemodynamic evaluation by positron emission tomography. Acta Neurochir (Wien) 1999;141(4):377–384

41. Horn P, Scharf J, Peña-Tapia P, Vajkoczy P. Risk of intraoperative ischemia due to temporary vessel occlusion during standard extracranial-intracranial arterial bypass surgery. J Neurosurg 2008;108(3):464–469

42. Fujimura M, Mugikura S, Kaneta T, Shimizu H, Tominaga T. Incidence and risk factors for symptomatic cerebral hyperperfusion after superficial temporal artery-middle cerebral artery anastomosis in patients with moyamoya disease. Surg Neurol 2009;71(4):442–447

43. Kim JE, Oh CW, Kwon OK, Park SQ, Kim SE, Kim YK. Transient hyperperfusion after superficial temporal artery/middle cerebral artery bypass surgery as a

possible cause of postoperative transient neurological deterioration. Cerebrovasc Dis 2008;25(6):580–586

44. Fujimura M, Shimizu H, Mugikura S, Tominaga T. Delayed intracerebral hemorrhage after superficial temporal artery-middle cerebral artery anastomosis in a patient with moyamoya disease: possible involvement of cerebral hyperperfusion and increased vascular permeability. Surg Neurol 2009;71(2):223–227, discussion 227

45. Andoh T, Sakai N, Yamada H, et al. Chronic subdural hematoma following bypass surgery—report of three cases. Neurol Med Chir (Tokyo) 1992;32(9):684–689

46. Nishimoto T, Yuki K, Sasaki T, Murakami T, Kodama Y, Kurisu K. A ruptured middle cerebral artery aneurysm originating from the site of anastomosis 20 years after extracranial-intracranial bypass for moyamoya disease: case report. Surg Neurol 2005;64(3):261–265, discussion 265

14

Multiple Extracranial-Intracranial Bypass Surgery in Moyamoya Angiopathy

Nadia Khan and Yasuhiro Yonekawa

◆ Introduction

Neurosurgeons performing revascularization procedures to prevent strokes in patients with moyamoya must understand the progressive nature of the disease,[1–5] especially in children, and the extensive yet individual presentation of this angiopathy in each patient. To do so requires a meticulous and systematic preoperative evaluation of the patient and understanding the correlation among the clinical picture, angiographic stage, presence of old and new ischemia, and, most importantly, deficits in the patient's cerebral perfusion reserve. This information can help surgeons to individualize the revascularization procedure to optimize outcomes.

The direct superficial temporal artery (STA)–to–middle cerebral artery (MCA) bypass technique is the most common and universally performed revascularization technique for the treatment of moyamoya angiopathy.[6–8] However, moyamoya angiopathy is not limited to only the MCA. Its involvement usually extends to the anterior cerebral artery (ACA) and, to a lesser extent, to the posterior cerebral artery (PCA) uni- or bilaterally. Revascularization of these arterial territories must be entertained because global cerebral perfusion depends not only on the appearance and disappearance of the typical deep and transdural collaterals but also on the changing anatomy of the circle of Willis.

This chapter details our preoperative protocol for planning multiple direct bypasses and the types of revascularization procedures used to augment perfusion in the MCA, ACA, and PCA territories. When a direct bypass is not technically possible, multiple indirect revascularizations can be performed as a secondary treatment choice to augment impaired cerebral blood flow.

◆ Preoperative Evaluation and Choice of Single or Multiple Direct Bypasses

A preoperative evaluation includes clinical, neurological, and neuropsychological assessment; a magnetic resonance imaging stroke protocol study; six-vessel cerebral angiography; and, most importantly, a hemodynamic study evaluating deficits in the patient's regional perfusion reserve. Depending on the expertise available locally, the latter may be done by perfusion magnetic resonance imaging, xenon computed tomography, hexamethyl propylene amine oxime-single photon emission computed tomography, or $H_2{}^{15}O$-positron emission tomography (PET) with an acetazolamide challenge.

The choice of number and location of revascularization procedures is based primarily on the severity and extent of disease observed in the patient's clinical presentation, extent of previous ischemia/infarcts, presence of viable brain tissue, preoperative angiography, and

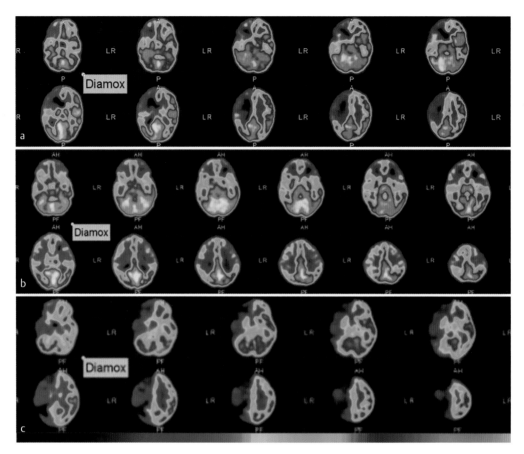

Fig. 14.1a–c Regional perfusion reserve deficits on $H_2^{15}O$-positron emission tomography after acetazolamide (Diamox) challenge in the anterior cerebral artery (ACA), middle cerebral artery (MCA), and posterior cerebral artery (PCA) distribution territories of three patients with moyamoya reiterate interpatient variations in cerebral perfusion and their effect on planning the type and location of cerebral revascularization needed. (**a**) A 2-year-old boy with symptomatic occlusion of right MCA, moyamoya collaterals, and bilateral stenosis of ACA on angiography with a correlating decrease in perfusion reserves in the right MCA and bilateral ACA territories. (**b**) A 10-year-old girl with symptomatic bilateral stenosis of the ACA and occlusion of MCA with moyamoya collaterals on angiography with a correlating decrease in perfusion in bilateral (left more than right) MCA and ACA territories. (**c**) A 1-year-old girl with symptomatic right MCA, ACA, and PCA stenosis and irregularities (i.e., disease begins at the carotid bifurcation on the left on angiography) with correlating decreased perfusion reserves in the right hemisphere and left ACA territories.

territorial decrease or absence of perfusion reserves on acetazolamide challenge studies.

Surgery is tailored to the perfusion territories of the MCA, ACA, or PCA (unilateral and/or bilateral). The aim is always to perform multiple direct anastomoses in the regions required (STA-to-MCA, STA-to-ACA, occipital artery [OA]-to-PCA). When the caliber of the donor or recipient vessels is too small, the vessels are too fragile, or they are unavailable at the desired site, indirect revascularization must suffice. Regardless of whether direct or indirect revascularization procedures are performed, it is important for

multiple revascularization procedures to be performed in every case (**Fig. 14.1**).

◆ Surgical Technique: Direct Revascularization

The Superficial Temporal Artery–to–Middle Cerebral Artery Bypass

A linear incision is placed over the parietal branch of the STA and the artery is dissected (8 to 10 cm of dissection and free preparation). A craniotomy follows. After a suitable MCA branch is identified, a direct anastomosis between the parietal branch of the STA and the branch of MCA is performed. Preoperative external carotid artery angiography and immediate preoperative Doppler ultrasonography are used to determine the presence of suitable donor vessels (STA, frontal and parietal branches, OA, posterior auricular artery). When the STA is hypoplastic, the OA or the posterior auricular artery can be used. Supra-Sylvian or infra-Sylvian cortical branches can be used as recipient vessels. The angular, posterior temporal, posterior parietal, anterior parietal, Rolandic, and pre-Rolandic branches are common choices. If the craniotomy must be extended because one of these branches is unavailable or its caliber is too small, the craniotomy can be extended anteriorly to locate the operculofrontal branch for a direct anastomosis.

The dura must be cut carefully without sacrificing the already present transdural arterial anastomosis. This goal can be achieved by avoiding a single large flap of dura, by limiting dural coagulation, and by using dural clips in case of bleeding. When further revascularization of the frontoparietal region is desired, double anastomoses can be performed. A frontoparietal skin flap must be prepared, and both the parietal and the frontal branches of the STA are dissected. The branches are used individually for the anastomosis in the fronto-opercular and parietal regions, respectively (**Fig. 14.2**).

The Superficial Temporal Artery–to–Anterior Cerebral Artery Bypass

The frontal branch of the STA is followed and dissected behind the hairline to the midline. If the frontal branch is not long enough and an STA-to-MCA bypass is not being performed at the same time, only indirect revascularization with encephalodurosynangiosis (EDS) and encephalogaleoperiosteal synangiosis (EGPS) can be performed. If an STA-to-MCA bypass is performed during the same setting, a curvilinear skin incision can be performed to dissect both the frontal and parietal branches of the STA followed by the respective craniotomies and anastomoses. Alternatively, two separate linear incisions following the course of the frontal and parietal branches can be used.

A problem arises only if the frontal branch fails to reach midline. In such cases, an interposition graft can be performed using the rest of the already prepared parietal branch. The craniotomy is usually placed anterior to the coronal suture and extends from the midline

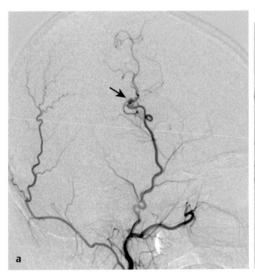
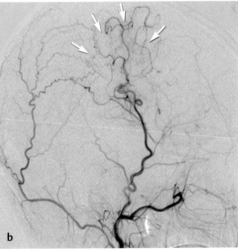

Fig. 14.2a, b Postoperative lateral view of external carotid artery (**a**) early and (**b**) late phase angiogram showing superficial temporal artery–to–middle cerebral artery bypass (*black arrow*) with good distal arterial filling (*white arrows*).

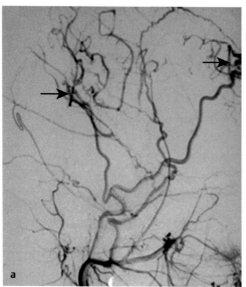
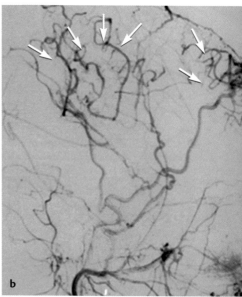

Fig. 14.3a, b Postoperative lateral view of external carotid artery (**a**) early and (**b**) late phase angiogram showing superficial temporal artery–to–middle cerebral artery and superficial temporal artery–to–anterior cerebral artery bypasses (*black arrows*) with good distal arterial filling (*white arrows*).

laterally. Distal cortical branches of the ACA (the middle internal frontal artery) can be located in the vicinity of the frontal bridging veins. In this region, the arachnoid membrane is usually thick. Only after this membrane is opened carefully may a cortical vessel be visible (**Figs. 14.3** and **14.4**).

The Occipital Artery–to–Posterior Cerebral Artery Bypass

This procedure is performed with the patient in the sitting or prone position. The OA is located and dissected. A suboccipital craniotomy is performed for a supracerebellar transtentorial route. Alternatively, a simple occipital craniotomy is performed, and a suitable cortical branch is located for the direct anastomosis. The recipient artery is usually located at the corner of the parahippocampal gyrus and the lingual gyrus in the supracerebellar transtentorial approach or anterior to the preoccipital notch in the latter. When a suitable cortical branch is not found, indirect encephaloduroarteriosynangiosis (EDAS) alone is performed with the OA.

◆ Surgical Technique: Indirect Revascularization

Encephalogaleoperiosteal Synangiosis, Encephalodurosynangiosis, Encephalomyosynangiosis, and Encephaloduroarteriosynangiosis

Larger craniotomies are performed by inverting several flaps of vascularized galeal-periosteal flaps (EGPS) or dural inversion flaps (EDS) onto the surface of the brain. This technique can be used in any region requiring revascularization: frontal, frontotemporal, frontoparietal, temporo-occipital, and occipital.

Either the frontal or parietal branch of the STA or the OA can be placed directly on the surface of the brain via a small frontal, temporal, or occipital craniotomy (EDAS), respectively, to stimulate growth of new vessels. These techniques can be used in combination with the classic STA-to-MCA bypass for revascularization of the motor area or in the frontal (ACA) and/or occipital (PCA) regions when a suitable donor or recipient vessel is unavailable for a direct anastomosis.

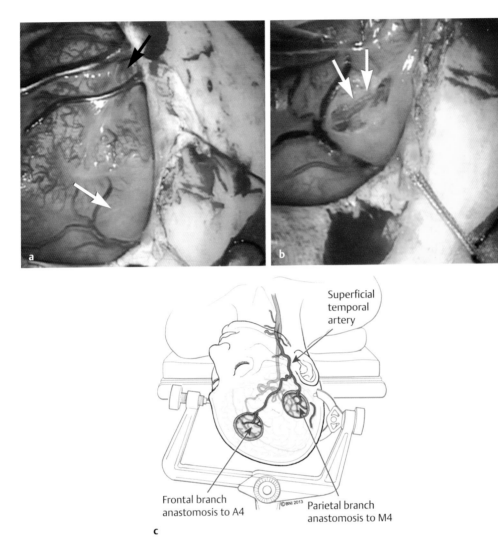

Superficial temporal artery

Frontal branch anastomosis to A4

©BNI 2013

Parietal branch anastomosis to M4

c

Fig. 14.4a–c (**a**) Intraoperative images of a frontal craniotomy prepared for a superficial temporal artery–to–anterior cerebral artery bypass just in front of the coronal suture. Note the hypervascularity on the cortical surface and the thickening of arachnoid membrane. A cortical artery (*white arrow*) is usually located posterior to the frontally bridging veins (*black arrow*) and observed (**b**) only after opening of the thickened arachnoid membrane (*white arrows*). (**c**) Schematic drawing showing patient positioning and locations of superficial temporal artery–to–middle cerebral artery and superficial temporal artery–to–anterior cerebral artery bypasses. (**Fig. 14.4b** used with permission from Barrow Neurological Institute.)

Increasingly, combined direct and indirect revascularizations are being performed (STA-to-MCA bypass with EGPS, EDS, and encephalomyosynangiosis). That is, after a direct STA-to-MCA anastomosis is performed, the dura is inverted and placed on the brain surface. Part of the temporalis muscle and the galea-periosteal flap, which is dissected before the craniotomy, are used to close the dural gap. In children undergoing this procedure, larger craniotomies are performed. The arachnoid membrane is then opened at several locations to allow widespread contact of the hypervascular tissue with the underlying brain to promote the desired neovascularization (**Fig. 14.5**).

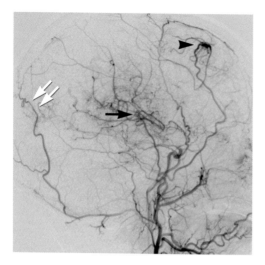

Fig. 14.5 Postoperative lateral view of external carotid artery angiogram showing superficial temporal artery–to–middle cerebral artery bypass (*black arrow*) and superficial temporal artery–to–anterior cerebral artery bypass (*black arrowhead*) with good direct distal arterial fillings, as well as occipital artery encephaloduroarteriosynangiosis, beginning with indirect revascularization (*white arrows*).

◆ Timing of Surgery and Staging of Multiple Revascularizations in a Single Patient

The following scenarios might be encountered in newly diagnosed, symptomatic patients: first diagnosis, symptomatic with previous stroke unilateral or bilateral; first diagnosis, symptomatic with acute unilateral stroke; bilateral disease but symptomatic on one side; bilateral disease and symptomatic on both sides; unilateral and symptomatic.

Surgery is always performed at the stage of clinical stabilization. In case of acute ischemic stroke, a minimum interval of 4 weeks from the onset of stroke is desirable. For unilateral and multiple revascularizations, a one-stage surgery is easily performed. For bilateral multiple revascularizations of the ACA, MCA, and/or PCA territories, staged surgery is beneficial. Usually an interval of 1 week is practical. When revascularization of the ACA and MCA territories is required in children, bilateral STA-to-MCA bypasses are performed first as a one-stage procedure. The side with the more progressive disease and symptoms is operated on first, followed by the other less symptomatic side. Bilateral STA-to-ACA bypasses are then performed.

One- or two-stage surgeries can be performed with no additional anesthesiological or surgical risk to the patient if adequate hydration and mean arterial blood pressure is maintained pre-, peri-, and postoperatively. Hypovolemia, hypotension, hypercapnia, and hypocapnia are to be avoided. The presence of an expert anesthesiological team as well as an intensivist is essential. Acetylsalicylic acid is administered before, during, and after surgery. Postoperative analgesia is important for the patient's comfort, especially in children (preventing crying in children prevents the resultant hypocapnia/hyperventilation). For children, the presence of a dedicated team within a pediatric hospital infrastructure (i.e., with a pediatric inpatient ward, operating room, anesthesia team, and intensive care unit) is crucial.

Asymptomatic patients with a clear, significant decrease in perfusion, deficits at baseline, and worsening in response to an acetazolamide challenge, especially on the dominant side (left side for right-handed patients), are also treated surgically.

◆ Clinical, Radiological, and Surgical Follow-up

Postoperative follow-up includes clinical, neurological, and neuropsychological assessments; magnetic resonance imaging stroke protocol study; six-vessel cerebral angiography; and a hemodynamic study (usually $H_2^{15}O$-PET with an acetazolamide challenge) 3 to 6 months after surgery. Depending on the patient's age (child or adult), these studies are repeated 1 to 3 years after treatment, at puberty, or at the time of maximum growth spurt in children. Patients with unilateral moyamoya angiopathy, especially in children younger than 5 years old, are followed closely for the occurrence of disease on the contralateral side when the disease can progress over a period of months.

The Zurich Experience

The previously discussed preoperative planning and multiple revascularization procedures have been performed since the early 1990s in more than 86 patients (26 adults, mean age 39 years; 60 children, mean age 4.9 years). In the majority of the children, bilateral multiple direct bypass procedures (mainly STA-to-MCA and STA-to-ACA) were the first choice for revascularization. Only when a recipient cortical branch of ACA was lacking was an indirect frontal EGPS, EDS, or EDAS performed. Due to the less frequent manifestation of the disease in the posterior circulation, only two adult patients underwent direct revascularization. Four children underwent EDAS using the OA. $H_2^{15}O$-PET has always been crucial in determining the extent of cerebral perfusion deficits and in individualizing surgery. Over the years, we have modified our strategy from two-stage to one-stage surgeries for both MCA territories. One-third of patients who were initially treated surgically underwent a two-staged revascularization procedure at an average time interval of 6 weeks between surgeries. All others with bilateral angiopathy, including the more recently diagnosed patients, underwent a one-staged revascularization procedure. In addition, in patients with only unilateral angiopathy and with involvement of more than one territory (MCA, ACA, PCA), all territories have successfully been revascularized in one sitting. In our experience, well-planned one-stage multiple procedures have not increased the morbidity rate. Adequate hydration before, during, and after surgery remains crucial. In terms of perioperative ischemia, immediate postoperative complications were observed in two earlier operated patients. One patient with postoperative ischemia of the frontoparietal region had recovered completely at 3 months of follow-up. One patient operated on in the early 1990s died after surgery from a massive infarction of the contralateral nonoperated side. At first follow-up 3 to 6 months after treatment and on an average after 5 years of follow-up, all other patients have been stroke free. On hemodynamic evaluation, cerebral perfusion had improved as had distal arterial filling on angiography in all patients.

◆ Discussion

Both children and adults with moyamoya disease have low cerebral perfusion, which when, in a state of decompensation, results in repeated ischemia and stroke. Performing cerebral revascularization procedures increases global cerebral perfusion after surgery, reinforcing the usefulness of surgery per se.[9-11]

Several revascularization procedures have been outlined extensively in the literature. Most of the literature stems from our Japanese colleagues who have reported their vast experience with the diagnosis and treatment of this angiopathy. The choice of revascularization technique depends on local understanding of the disease, the dedication of surgeons toward treating more adult patients than children and vice versa, and the surgical expertise and years of experience available.

A clear distinction is always made between direct and indirect methods of cerebral revascularization. Which procedure is more beneficial remains scientifically unproven because a randomized clinical trial is ethically impossible. Comparing periprocedural ischemia and reduction in long-term stroke rates between the two approaches is not possible. Factors such as correct diagnosis, correct surgical indication, age and gender of patient, presence of comorbid conditions, perioperative changes in hydration and blood pressure, and the surgeon's expertise and experience are usually not considered collectively.

Another factor never mentioned in the literature but that should be emphasized is the personal bias of individual neurosurgeons. The type of revascularization surgery selected depends on the surgeon's experience in performing a direct bypass. The surgical procedure of anastomosing extremely small caliber (< 1 mm) arteries (both donor and cortical arteries) can be cumbersome and require of years of experience to master. Indirect revascularization is technically easy and can be performed by a neurosurgeon with less experience in direct anastomosis.

The classic direct STA-to-MCA bypass procedure is commonly used to treat adults with moyamoya disease. It is less often used to treat the childhood form of the angiopathy, especially in children younger than 5 years of age. Induction of neovascularization depends on the condition of both the recipient (condition of brain, cerebrospinal fluid) and donor tissue (temporalis muscle; dural, galeal, and periosteal flap; donor arteries). Consequently, children fare far better with indirect procedures than adults because growth factors activating neovascularization are expected to be abundant in growing children. However, neovascularization after indirect anastomosis takes longer to establish than a direct anastomosis. In contrast, direct bypass immediately enhances blood flow. Yet when long-term follow-up after only indirect revascularization in both adults and children is considered, clinical outcomes have been comparable to those associated with a direct bypass.[12-14] Other groups suggest that direct anastomosis is the preferred revascularization technique in combination with indirect revascularization procedures in adults,[15-17] whereas single or multiple indirect revascularization[18,19] techniques are advocated for children. Most papers on choice of surgical techniques for the treatment of moyamoya disease describe revascularization of the motor areas (MCA territory), whereas only a few have described additional revascularization in other involved arterial territories.[20-26]

The cerebral perfusion status of the frontal region requires special attention. In children younger than 5 years old, moyamoya disease associated with repeated frontal ischemia can be devastating in terms of mental and cognitive development. Early revascularization can support normal childhood development and prevent severe mental retardation. In particular, when perfusion in the frontal region is severely decreased, an additional direct STA-to-ACA bypass is performed.[21-26] Despite the technical difficulties (preparation of a frontal craniotomy adequate to identify the appropriate recipient cortical vessel of the ACA, absence of a sufficiently long frontal branch of the STA for an additional end-to-end interposition graft), the direct STA-to-ACA bypass technique most improves revascularization of the ACA territory when performed by an experienced surgeon.

Less frequently seen in adults and more commonly observed in children is involvement of the posterior circulation with stenosis or occlusion of the PCA. In such cases,[27-30] a direct anastomosis can be performed between the OA and one of the cortical branches of the PCA. When technical limitations are present, indirect revascularization using dural carpeting EDS or EGPS after an occipital craniotomy or an arteriosynangiosis using OA-EDAS can easily be performed.

In our personal experience, the efficacy of multiple direct bypass procedures performed bilaterally has resulted in clinical improvements, and stabilization or improvement in the hemodynamic reserve capacities as observed on $H_2^{15}O$ PET studies. Postoperative angiography also shows an increase in focal perfusion in the region of the functional direct anastomoses.

A critical and systematic operative evaluative protocol is essential for planning the optimal surgical procedure. We advocate multiple direct revascularization procedures with modification of surgical planning (i.e., performing additional indirect revascularization procedures in regions where a direct bypass is technically infeasible).

◆ Conclusion

Choice of revascularization technique (i.e., direct or indirect) depends on a surgeon's personal surgical expertise and experience as well as on intraoperative anatomical and technical limitations. Given individual routine practice and bias, which technique is superior continues to be controversial.

References

1. Choi JU, Kim DS, Kim EY, Lee KC. Natural history of moyamoya disease: comparison of activity of daily living in surgery and non surgery groups. Clin Neurol Neurosurg 1997;99(Suppl 2):S11–S18
2. Imaizumi T, Hayashi K, Saito K, Osawa M, Fukuyama Y. Long-term outcomes of pediatric moyamoya disease monitored to adulthood. Pediatr Neurol 1998; 18(4):321–325
3. Kawano T, Fukui M, Hashimoto N, Yonekawa Y. Follow-up study of patients with "unilateral" moyamoya disease. Neurol Med Chir (Tokyo) 1994;34(11):744–747
4. Kim TW, Seo BR, Kim JH, Kim YO. Rapid progression of unilateral moyamoya disease. J Korean Neurosurg Soc 2011;49(1):65–67
5. Yeon JY, Shin HJ, Kong DS, et al. The prediction of contralateral progression in children and adolescents with unilateral moyamoya disease. Stroke 2011;42(10): 2973–2976
6. Karasawa J, Kikuchi H, Furuse S, Kawamura J, Sakaki T. Treatment of moyamoya disease with STA-MCA anastomosis. J Neurosurg 1978;49(5):679–688
7. Krayenbühl HA. The Moyamoya syndrome and the neurosurgeon. Surg Neurol 1975;4(4):353–360
8. Matsushima T, Inoue K, Kawashima M, Inoue T. History of the development of surgical treatments for moyamoya disease. Neurol Med Chir (Tokyo) 2012; 52(5):278–286
9. Horowitz M, Yonas H, Albright AL. Evaluation of cerebral blood flow and hemodynamic reserve in symptomatic moyamoya disease using stable Xenon-CT

blood flow. Surg Neurol 1995;44(3):251–261, discussion 262

10. Ikezaki K, Matsushima T, Kuwabara Y, Suzuki SO, Nomura T, Fukui M. Cerebral circulation and oxygen metabolism in childhood moyamoya disease: a perioperative positron emission tomography study. J Neurosurg 1994;81(6):843–850

11. Iwama T, Hashimoto N, Yonekawa Y. The relevance of hemodynamic factors to perioperative ischemic complications in childhood moyamoya disease. Neurosurgery 1996;38(6):1120–1125, discussion 1125–1126

12. Scott RM, Smith ER. Moyamoya disease and moyamoya syndrome. N Engl J Med 2009;360(12):1226–1237

13. Scott RM, Smith JL, Robertson RL et al. Long-term outcome in children with moyamoya syndrome after cranial revascularization by pial synangiosis. J Neurosurg 2004 February;100(2 Suppl Pediatrics):142–9

14. Starke RM, Komotar RJ, Hickman ZL, et al. Clinical features, surgical treatment, and long-term outcome in adult patients with moyamoya disease. Clinical article. J Neurosurg 2009;111(5):936–942

15. Kim DS, Huh PW, Kim HS, et al. Surgical treatment of moyamoya disease in adults: combined direct and indirect vs. indirect bypass surgery. Neurol Med Chir (Tokyo) 2012;52(5):333–338

16. Kuroda S, Houkin K. Moyamoya disease: current concepts and future perspectives. Lancet Neurol 2008; 7(11):1056–1066

17. Kuroda S, Houkin K. Bypass surgery for moyamoya disease: concept and essence of sugical techniques. Neurol Med Chir (Tokyo) 2012;52(5):287–294

18. Ikezaki K. Rational approach to treatment of moyamoya disease in childhood. J Child Neurol 2000;15(5): 350–356

19. Matsushima T, Inoue T, Ikezaki K, et al. Multiple combined indirect procedure for the surgical treatment of children with moyamoya disease. A comparison with single indirect anastomosis and direct anastomosis. Neurosurg Focus 1998;5(5):e4

20. Ishikawa T, Kamiyama H, Kuroda S, Yasuda H, Nakayama N, Takizawa K. Simultaneous superficial temporal artery to middle cerebral or anterior cerebral artery bypass with pan-synangiosis for Moyamoya disease covering both anterior and middle cerebral artery territories. Neurol Med Chir (Tokyo) 2006;46(9):462–468

21. Iwama T, Hashimoto N, Miyake H, Yonekawa Y. Direct revascularization to the anterior cerebral artery territory in patients with moyamoya disease: report of five cases. Neurosurgery 1998;42(5):1157–1161, discussion 1161–1162

22. Iwama T, Hashimoto N, Tsukahara T, Miyake H. Superficial temporal artery to anterior cerebral artery direct anastomosis in patients with moyamoya disease. Clin Neurol Neurosurg 1997;99(Suppl 2):S134–S136

23. Kawashima A, Kawamata T, Yamaguchi K, Hori T, Okada Y. Successful superficial temporal artery-anterior cerebral artery direct bypass using a long graft for moyamoya disease: technical note. Neurosurgery 2010 September;67(3 Suppl Operative):ons145-ons149

24. Khan N, Schuknecht B, Boltshauser E, et al. Moyamoya disease and Moyamoya syndrome: experience in Europe; choice of revascularisation procedures. Acta Neurochir (Wien) 2003;145(12):1061–1071, discussion 1071

25. Matsushima T, Aoyagi M, Suzuki R, et al. Dual anastomosis for pediatric moyamoya patients using the anterior and posterior branches of the superficial temporal artery. Nerv Syst Child 1993;18:27–32

26. Suzuki Y, Negoro M, Shibuya M, Yoshida J, Negoro T, Watanabe K. Surgical treatment for pediatric moyamoya disease: use of the superficial temporal artery for both areas supplied by the anterior and middle cerebral arteries. Neurosurgery 1997;40(2):324–329, discussion 329–330

27. Hayashi T, Shirane R, Tominaga T. Additional surgery for postoperative ischemic symptoms in patients with moyamoya disease: the effectiveness of occipital artery-posterior cerebral artery bypass with an indirect procedure: technical case report. Neurosurgery 2009;64(1):E195–E196, discussion E196

28. Ikeda A, Yamamoto I, Sato O, Morota N, Tsuji T, Seguchi T. Revascularization of the calcarine artery in moyamoya disease: OA-cortical PCA anastomosis—case report. Neurol Med Chir (Tokyo) 1991;31(10):658–661

29. Yonekawa Y. Brain revascularization by EC-IC bypass. In: Sindou M, editor. Practical handbook of neurosurgery from leading neurosurgeons. New York: SpringerWien; 2009. p. 355–81.

30. Yonekawa Y, Imhof HG, Taub E, et al. Supracerebellar transtentorial approach to posterior temporomedial structures. J Neurosurg 2001;94(2):339–345

15

Direct and Indirect Bypass Procedures for Posterior Circulation Moyamoya Disease

Reizo Shirane, Toshiaki Hayashi, Tomomi Kimiwada, and
Teiji Tominaga

◆ Introduction

Moyamoya disease is characterized by progressive arterial stenosis or occlusion of the intracranial internal carotid arteries and by the development of extensive collateral vessels.[1,2] It is a cause of stroke and transient ischemic attacks (TIAs) in pediatric and adult patients. Surgery to revascularize the ischemic brain is a recommended treatment option in this patient population.

Several surgical techniques have been used to attempt to revascularize ischemic regions of the brain. Both direct revascularization through a superficial temporal artery (STA)–to–middle cerebral artery (MCA) bypass and various indirect methods have been performed with varying amounts of success.[3–9] Exceptions to this treatment include patients in whom synangiosis fails to perfuse the anterior cerebral artery (ACA) or posterior cerebral artery (PCA) circulation and who require additional revascularization directed at these persistently ischemic areas. Moreover, progression of the disease can require additional revascularization even in patients who at first have no TIAs after they undergo synangiosis. We have performed additional surgery for such lesions using an occipital artery (OA)–to–PCA bypass with indirect revascularization and review the efficacy of the procedure.[10]

◆ Patient Population

Across 15 years, 17 patients underwent additional revascularization for persistent ischemia after revascularization surgery (**Table 15.1**). Three females (mean age at surgery, 23.8 years, age range, 6 to 53 years) with ischemic symptoms underwent the additional revascularization procedure. All 17 patients had undergone indirect and/or direct revascularization surgery for their initial treatment. Bilateral STA-to-MCA anastomosis and encephalogaleomyosynangiosis with dural pedicle insertion,[8] which is the routine surgical procedure for the initial treatment of moyamoya disease in our department, was performed in nine patients. The other eight patients had undergone other indirect procedures such as encephaloduroarteriosynangiosis or STA-to-MCA anastomosis at other facilities.

The most common symptom was a TIA involving the lower extremity with headache. Some patients experienced TIAs with visual impairment. After their first surgery, three patients with headache had intraventricular hemorrhage. The mean time between onset of ischemic symptoms and the previous surgery was 6.4 years (range, 0.9 to 15 years). All patients showed possible progression of their vascular lesion, including narrowing of the PCA (**Figs. 15.1** and **15.2**).

Table 15.1 Clinical Summary of 17 Patients with Moyamoya Disease

Patient	Initial Symptoms	Age/ Sex	Onset (Years)	Age of Initial Surgery/Right	Age of Initial Surgery/Left	Symptoms	Age/Methods of Surgery
1	INF, seizure	8/M	1	1 DIR+IND	1 DIR+IND	TIA, headache	6 FP IND
2	TIA, INF	9/F	3	6 DIR+IND	6 DIR+IND	TIA, seizure	7 R PO IND
3	TIA	20/M	4	4 IND	4 IND	TIA	7 L PTO IND
4	TIA	15/F	5	7 IND	7 IND, 8 DIR	TIA, headache	14 R OA PCA+Fr IND
5	TIA, INF	22/F	5	8 DIR+IND	8 IND	TIA, headache	20 L OA PCA+R IND
6	TIA	27/F	5	9 IND	9 IND	TIA, headache	11 L FT IND
7	TIA	24/F	5	8 IND	11 IND	Headache	11 R PTO IND
8	TIA	16/F	6	9 DIR+IND	9 DIR+IND	TIA, headache	16 R OA PCA+Fr IND
9	TIA, INF	23/F	6	6 IND	6 IND	TIA	21 R OA PCA
10	TIA, INF	16/F	8	15 DIR+IND	14 DIR+IND	TIA, headache	16 L OA PCA
11	TIA, INF	18/F	9		15 DIR+IND	TIA	18 L OA PCA
12	IVH, INF	27/M	10	IND	IND	TIA, headache	27 L IND
13	TIA, INF	32/M	10	18 IND	18 IND	Hemorrhage	20 L OA PCA
14	TIA	21/F	14	18 DIR+IND	16 DIR+IND	Hemorrhage	20 L OA PCA
15	TIA	39/F	22	26 DIR+IND	27 IND	Hemorrhage	34 RL IND
16	TIA	35/F	27		29 IND	TIA	35 L OA PCA
17	INF	53/F	51		51 DIR	TIA	53 R OA PCA+Fr IND

Abbreviations: DIR, direct; F, female; FP, fronto-parietal; Fr, frontal; FT, fronto-temporal; IND, indirect; INF, infarction; IVH, intraventricular hemorrhage; L, left; LOA, left occipital artery; M, male; OA, occipital artery; PCA, posterior cerebral artery; PO, parieto-occipital; PTO, parieto-temporo-occipital; R, right; RL, right and left; TIA, transient ischemic attack.

All patients underwent pre- and post-operative magnetic resonance imaging (MRI) and magnetic resonance angiography (MRA). Pre- and postoperatively, cerebral perfusion was measured in all patients with ^{131}I-iodoamphetamine single photon emission computed tomography (SPECT). Cerebral vasodilatory capacity was also assessed after an intravenous injection of acetazolamide (20 mg/kg; maximum dose, 1 g). All patients underwent clinical and neurological follow-up examinations before and after surgery. MRI and MRA were performed on the seventh postoperative day, 3 to 6 months after surgery, and annually thereafter. All patients underwent SPECT 3 to 6 months after surgery and within 7 days of surgery when neurological symptoms were suspected.

◆ Surgical Technique

After general anesthesia was induced, the patient was placed in the prone position with the head mildly extended on the horseshoe-shaped headrest. After a 1-cm strip of hair was shaved in preparation, a reversed U-shaped occipital skin incision was made (**Fig. 15.3a**). The osteoplastic craniotomy was then performed. The area of craniotomy was 1 cm lateral to the sagittal sinus, posterior to the previous craniotomy (indirect anastomosis), anterior to the transverse sinus, and medial to the mastoid process. The periosteum was left in place on the bone and later dissected to create a periosteal flap preserving the vessels that form the future collateral networks.

As long of a length of the OA as possible (> 5 cm long and > 0.5 mm in diameter) was

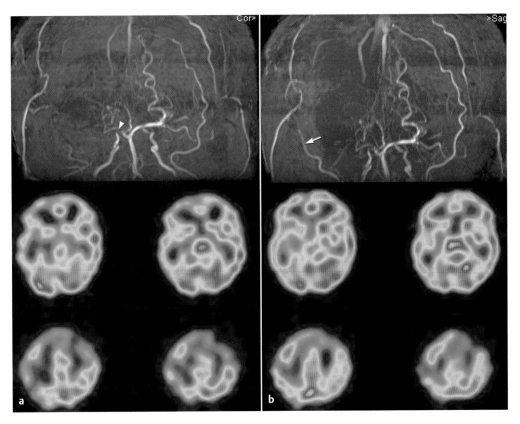

Fig. 15.1a, b (**a**) Magnetic resonance angiography just before the additional surgery showed the steno-occlusive change in the right posterior cerebral artery (*arrowhead*). Images captured with ^{131}I-iodoamphetamine single photon emission computed tomography during acetazolamide challenge showed relative decreased vascular reserve in the right frontal and occipital areas. (**b**) Follow-up studies performed 4 months after additional surgery showed widening of the occipital artery (*arrow*) and increased vascular reserve in the right hemisphere.

dissected from the skin flap using Doppler guidance (**Fig. 15.3b**). The course of the OA meanders and branches; consequently, careful handling under the operative microscope is essential to achieve a satisfactory dissection. The cortical surface was explored via an occipital craniotomy to identify a suitable cortical branch of the PCA (**Fig. 15.3c**). The area anterior to the preoccipital notch was most likely to contain a PCA vessel sufficiently large to be used as a recipient vessel.[11] We usually try to expose PCA branches in the occipital interhemispheric surface. The best recipient has almost the same diameter as the OA. It can be challenging to perform an end-to-side anastomosis between the OA and the cortical branch of the PCA when the diameter of the PCA is smaller than that of the OA.

The dura is incised and inserted in the brain surface around the bone window toward the ischemic region, and the external surface of the dura is attached to the surface of the brain. Then an end-to-side OA-to-PCA anastomosis is performed using 10–0 monofilament nylon suture (**Fig. 15.3d**). The periosteal flap is attached to the surface of the brain and connected to the cut end of the dura with suture. The site of the dural opening where the OA was inserted is loosely sutured without restricting the artery.

The bone flap is replaced and the incision closed. A high-speed drill fitted with a ball-shaped tool is used to make frontal bur holes (1 cm in diameter) in the medial frontal region of each hemisphere beneath a new linear skin incision. The dura is opened through each

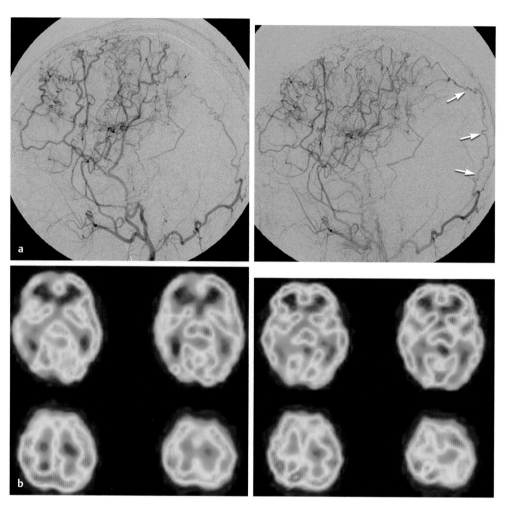

Fig. 15.2a, b (**a**) This patient had transient ischemic attacks in the legs during follow-up for bilateral revascularization. Pre- (*left*) and postoperative (*right*, 3 months after surgery) right external carotid angiography showed newly developed collateral channels (*arrows*) via the right occipital artery toward both the posterior cerebral artery and anterior cerebral artery territories. (**b**) Preoperative (*left*) and postoperative (*right*) single photon emission computed tomography obtained after acetazolamide load revealed marked increase of uptake in the territory of the anterior cerebral artery.

bur hole, and fat tissue (1 cm in diameter) is implanted as autograft.

◆ Clinical and Neuro-radiological Outcomes

All 17 patients showed clinical and radiological improvement. TIAs improved in all three patients. At their recent follow-up examinations, they had no complaints of TIAs. Follow-up MRI showed no additional cerebral infarctions. MRA showed widening of the OA

and the development of peripheral collateral vessels (see **Fig. 15.1**). Postoperative SPECT studies showed a marked increase in the uptake in the territory of both the ACA and the PCA. The patients' cerebral vasodilatory capacity evaluated by acetazolamide testing had also improved markedly (see **Figs. 15.1** and **15.2**).

MRI obtained on postoperative day 7 in one patient showed cerebral edema. During her early postoperative period, she had complained of transient visual impairment on the operated side. The symptom continued 1 month and then improved. When her postoperative cerebral

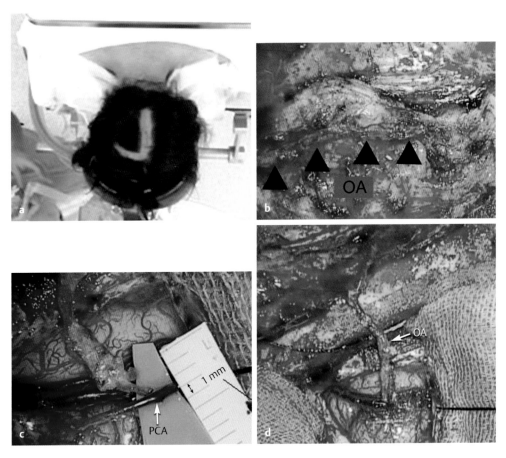

Fig. 15.3a–d (**a**) The patient was placed prone with her head mildly extended on the horseshoe-shaped head-rest. A 1-cm strip of hair was shaved in preparation, and a reversed U-shaped occipital skin incision was made. (**b**) The occipital artery (OA; *arrowheads*) was easily identified and dissected from the skin flap using Doppler guidance. (**c**) The cortical surface was explored via an occipital craniotomy to identify a suitable cortical branch of the posterior cerebral artery (PCA). The best recipient vessel (overlaying the dam) has almost the same diameter as the OA. The dura was incised and inserted in the brain surface around the bone window toward the ischemic region, and the external surface of the dura was attached to the surface of the brain. (**d**) An end-to-side OA-to–posterior cerebral artery anastomosis was performed using 10–0 monofilament nylon suture.

vasodilatory capacity was evaluated by an acetazolamide challenge 4 months after surgery, MRI showed cerebral atrophy, which suggested neural damage adjacent to the anastomotic site. Even in this case, SPECT showed marked increase in the territory of both the ACA and PCA.

◆ Discussion

The symptom of cerebral ischemia associated with moyamoya disease is treated by increasing the blood supply to the ischemic areas of the brain from the external carotid artery system by using several types of vascular reconstructive surgery. Direct revascularization through an STA-to-MCA anastomosis and indirect methods such as encephalomyosynangiosis, encephaloduroarterio-synangiosis, encephalomyoarteriosynangiosis, and encephaloduroarteriomyosynangiosis, and combinations of these procedures have been used to revascularize ischemic regions with various levels of success.[3–9] In such operations, good neovascularization mainly occurs in the MCA territory.

However, some patients, especially those with disease progression, show angiographic and clinical signs of other ischemic territories. Sometimes leg weakness, abnormal mentation, visual field abnormalities, and morning headache related to ischemia[12] in areas supplied mainly by the ACA and PCA do not improve. Given that the PCA is involved in ~30% of patients with moyamoya disease and that the incidence of disease progression in moyamoya disease is relatively high, the ACA and PCA territories are at risk of ischemia.[13–18] Furthermore, given that the PCA plays an important role in providing major collateral circulation in moyamoya disease, the development of additional lesions involving the PCA implies an increased risk for recurrent ischemic stroke (5.6% of our patients showed progression of the PCA lesion after initial surgery). Consequently, additional revascularization surgeries were directed at these persistently or newly developed ischemic areas. Our cases all showed progression of their PCA lesion during follow-up and had a tendency to develop TIAs involving both the ACA and PCA territories.

Considering that the STA and other vascularized flaps such as galea and temporal muscle had already been used in previous procedures, the bur hole procedure or periosteal flap from the occipital and frontal region were the procedures of choice for our patients.[7,19] Sainte-Rose et al reported excellent outcomes associated with bur hole surgery in children undergoing initial treatment for moyamoya disease.[7] Endo et al reported improved blood circulation in the frontal lobe of six children undergoing combined encephalomyosynangiosis with placement of a frontal bur hole.[19] The revascularization occurred no later than that seen after encephalomyosynangiosis and encephaloduroarteriosynangiosis. In cases in which the PCA was severely diseased, occipital bur holes enabled good neovascularization via the OA.

In contrast, Scott et al reported that visible collateral vessels to the brain at the additional bur holes sites could be identified in 57% of the cases but only in 34% could these vessels be termed significant (i.e., filling more than a small focal area at the bur hole site).[20] Three of their patients with late onset frontal lobe ischemia underwent either repeated synangiosis or a wide craniotomy with onlay of a vascularized periosteal flap. One of the patients underwent angiography 1 year after the procedure, but no significant new collateral circulation had been developed after the procedure. Consequently, some cases are refractory to indirect revascularization. Indirect revascularization was considered less effective in the areas with infarction because of the lack of demand for blood supply in those areas. Moreover, the effectiveness of indirect revascularization is limited in adult patients.[10]

To solve this problem, we created anastomoses between the OA and cortical branch of the PCA. Immediate collateral flow was attained by direct revascularization perfusing both the ACA and PCA territories. Considering that the SPECT study performed immediately after surgery showed a marked increase of uptake not only in the PCA territory but also in the ACA territory, the OA-to-PCA bypass could increase the perfusion pressure of the PCA, which also supplies collateral flow to the ACA territory. We believe that progression of the PCA lesion decreased collateral flow to the ACA territories; consequently, symptoms referable to this area occurred. Initial revascularization surgery could have supplied collateral flow to the ischemic areas at the time of the surgery. However, it could not supply enough blood flow to the additional ischemic areas because of the development of the PCA lesion.

Although an OA-to-PCA bypass could supply collateral flow to the ischemic area adjacent to the PCA territory, we did not think that the area far from the watersheds should be supplied by the bypass. Therefore, we performed bur hole procedures in medial frontal regions concomitant with the OA-to-PCA bypass so that further collateralizations could develop in the ACA territory. It has been suggested that a combined technique of direct and indirect surgery may be superior to just one of these options, resulting in better and more extensive revascularization.[19,21]

The combination of procedures should be especially useful for patients with impending stroke and severe and repeated TIAs related to progression of a PCA lesion. Ikeda et al performed an OA-to–cortical PCA anastomosis to prevent impending cortical blindness.[22] In our patients, delayed focal neurological deficit after the procedure resulted in cerebral atrophy on follow-up MRI. T2-weighted MRI performed on the seventh postoperative day showed cerebral edema of the anastomotic site. Fluid-attenuated inversion recovery MRI sequences obtained at the same time showed a high-intensity signal in the meninges, the so-called ivy sign. The lesion was considered to represent the enlargement of the vascular network over the pial surface caused by focal hyperperfusion from the direct anastomosis. Ischemic change was not detected on diffusion-weighted MRI.

Fujimura et al reported a pediatric patient with moyamoya disease who showed focal neurological deficit after undergoing an STA-to-MCA bypass.[23] An early increase in cerebral blood flow was associated with the formation of vasogenic edema at the site of the anastomosis. After performing an STA-to-MCA bypass in a patient with moyamoya disease, Ogasawara et al also reported cerebral hyperperfusion syndrome. The subsequent neural damage was irreversible and caused cognitive impairment.[24] Fortunately, our patient's visual impairment recovered. Further study regarding strategies to decrease the incidence of hyperperfusion after a direct bypass is performed in patients with moyamoya disease is needed.

◆ Conclusion

An OA-to-PCA anastomosis with indirect revascularization was effective treatment for ischemia in patients with moyamoya disease who showed symptoms referable to the ACA and PCA territories after previous surgery. For cases refractory to indirect revascularization or that are at risk for impending stroke or frequent TIAs, this procedure can be considered as a treatment option.

References

1. Suzuki J, Kodama N. Moyamoya disease—a review. Stroke 1983;14(1):104–109
2. Suzuki J, Takaku A. Cerebrovascular "moyamoya" disease. Disease showing abnormal net-like vessels in base of brain. Arch Neurol 1969;20(3):288–299
3. Adelson PD, Scott RM. Pial synangiosis for moyamoya syndrome in children. Pediatr Neurosurg 1995;23(1):26–33
4. Fujita K, Tamaki N, Matsumoto S. Surgical treatment of moyamoya disease in children: which is more effective procedure, EDAS or EMS? Childs Nerv Syst 1986;2(3):134–138
5. Iwama T, Hashimoto N, Miyake H, Yonekawa Y. Direct revascularization to the anterior cerebral artery territory in patients with moyamoya disease: report of five cases. Neurosurgery 1998;42(5):1157–1161, discussion 1161–1162
6. Matsushima T, Fukui M, Kitamura K, Hasuo K, Kuwabara Y, Kurokawa T. Encephalo-duro-arterio-synangiosis in children with moyamoya disease. Acta Neurochir (Wien) 1990;104(3-4):96–102
7. Sainte-Rose C, Oliveira R, Puget S, et al. Multiple bur hole surgery for the treatment of moyamoya disease in children. J Neurosurg 2006;105(6, Suppl)437–443
8. Shirane R, Yoshida Y, Takahashi T, Yoshimoto T. Assessment of encephalo-galeo-myo-synangiosis with dural pedicle insertion in childhood moyamoya disease: characteristics of cerebral blood flow and oxygen metabolism. Clin Neurol Neurosurg 1997;99(Suppl 2):S79–S85
9. Yoshioka N, Tominaga S, Suzuki Y, et al. Vascularized omental graft to brain surface in ischemic cerebrovascular disease. Microsurgery 1995;16(7):455–462
10. Hayashi T, Shirane R, Tominaga T. Additional surgery for postoperative ischemic symptoms in patients with moyamoya disease: the effectiveness of occipital artery-posterior cerebral artery bypass with an indirect procedure: technical case report. Neurosurgery 2009;64(1):E195–E196, discussion E196
11. Zeal AA, Rhoton AL Jr. Microsurgical anatomy of the posterior cerebral artery. J Neurosurg 1978;48(4):534–559
12. Shirane R, Fujimura M. Headache in Moyamoya Disease. In: Cho BK, Tominaga T, eds. Moyamoya Disease Update.Tokyo, Berlin, Heiderberg, New York: Springer; 2010:110–113
13. Kuroda S, Ishikawa T, Houkin K, Nanba R, Hokari M, Iwasaki Y. Incidence and clinical features of disease progression in adult moyamoya disease. Stroke 2005;36(10):2148–2153
14. Miyamoto S, Kikuchi H, Karasawa J, Nagata I, Ihara I, Yamagata S. Study of the posterior circulation in moyamoya disease. Part 2: Visual disturbances and surgical treatment. J Neurosurg 1986;65(4):454–460
15. Mugikura S, Takahashi S, Higano S, Shirane R, Sakurai Y, Yamada S. Predominant involvement of ipsilateral anterior and posterior circulations in moyamoya disease. Stroke 2002;33(6):1497–1500
16. Robertson RL, Burrows PE, Barnes PD, Robson CD, Poussaint TY, Scott RM. Angiographic changes after pial synangiosis in childhood moyamoya disease. AJNR Am J Neuroradiol 1997;18(5):837–845
17. Yamada I, Himeno Y, Suzuki S, Matsushima Y. Posterior circulation in moyamoya disease: angiographic study. Radiology 1995;197(1):239–246
18. Yamada I, Murata Y, Umehara I, Suzuki S, Matsushima Y. SPECT and MRI evaluations of the posterior circulation in moyamoya disease. J Nucl Med 1996;37(10):1613–1617
19. Endo M, Kawano N, Miyaska Y, Yada K. Cranial burr hole for revascularization in moyamoya disease. J Neurosurg 1989;71(2):180–185
20. Scott RM, Smith JL, Robertson RL et al. Long-term outcome in children with moyamoya syndrome after cranial revascularization by pial synangiosis. J Neurosurg 2004 February;100(2 Suppl Pediatrics):142–9
21. Houkin K, Kamiyama H, Takahashi A, Kuroda S, Abe H. Combined revascularization surgery for childhood moyamoya disease: STA-MCA and encephalo-duro-arterio-myo-synangiosis. Childs Nerv Syst 1997;13(1):24–29
22. Ikeda A, Yamamoto I, Sato O, Morota N, Tsuji T, Seguchi T. Revascularization of the calcarine artery in moyamoya disease: OA-cortical PCA anastomosis—case report. Neurol Med Chir (Tokyo) 1991;31(10):658–661
23. Fujimura M, Kaneta T, Shimizu H, Tominaga T. Symptomatic hyperperfusion after superficial temporal artery-middle cerebral artery anastomosis in a child with moyamoya disease. Childs Nerv Syst 2007;23(10):1195–1198
24. Ogasawara K, Komoribayashi N, Kobayashi M, et al. Neural damage caused by cerebral hyperperfusion after arterial bypass surgery in a patient with moyamoya disease: case report. Neurosurgery 2005;56(6):E1380, discussion E1380

15 Direct and Indirect Bypass Procedures for Posterior Circulation Moyamoya Disease

16

Anesthetic and Perioperative Management of Moyamoya Disease

Richard A. Jaffe, Jaime R. López, and Diana G. McGregor

◆ Introduction

Patients with distal occlusion of the internal carotid artery and its proximal branches develop characteristic moyamoya vasculature, and they present special opportunities and unique challenges for perioperative management and monitoring.[1-3] Indeed, appropriate anesthetic management and intraoperative monitoring are essential to achieve successful patient outcomes. This chapter discusses our anesthetic experience with more than 1,000 pediatric and adult revascularization procedures, most commonly direct superficial temporal artery (STA)–to–middle cerebral artery (MCA) bypass surgery.

Given the rarity of this disease, it is not surprising that there are no randomized clinical trials to support a specific anesthetic or monitoring regime. However, the fundamental principles of perioperative management for patients with moyamoya can be based on simple rules of supply and demand. The maintenance of a favorable supply (cerebral blood flow [CBF])–to–demand (cerebral metabolic rate) ratio throughout the perioperative period, the implementation of ischemic protective interventions during cross-clamping of the MCA, along with early detection and prompt remediation of other suboptimal supply-to-demand (CBF:cerebral metabolic rate) states will always be the cornerstones of patient management.

Regional CBF is impaired in patients with moyamoya, and the moyamoya vessels themselves are functionally abnormal. Autoregulation in these vessels may be severely attenuated, making CBF in the affected regions directly pressure dependent. Fortunately, moyamoya vessels do not constrict in response to phenylephrine or ephedrine, and these agents can be used to maintain an appropriate perfusion pressure. Moyamoya vessels appear to be incapable of dilating in response to hypercapnia; however, they may constrict in response to hypocapnia.[4] Thus, in children it is particularly important to avoid crying because the resulting hyperventilation may reduce CBF to critical levels and cause ischemic injury.[3,5,6]

◆ Preoperative Considerations

The patient's preoperative history and physical examination should focus on evidence of unstable cerebral perfusion and characterization of any preexisting neurologic deficits. Patients with moyamoya typically manifest with symptoms and signs of transient ischemic attacks or ischemic stroke.[7] Less commonly, patients become symptomatic with subarachnoid hemorrhage (typically adults), headache, or seizures. Patients with a history of transient ischemic attacks have an increased risk for intraoperative and postoperative ischemic injury,[8] whereas patients with a recent history of intracranial hemorrhage are likely to be at increased risk for subsequent hemorrhage. Both of these groups of patients may benefit from the preoperative placement of an arterial catheter for continuous pressure monitoring during induction of anesthesia. In children, the potential benefit of a preinduction arterial line must be weighed against the risk of procedure-induced stress and pain leading to hyperventilation and consequently decreased CBF.

Moyamoya syndrome has been associated with a variety of coexisting and often contributory medical problems that may affect both anesthetic and postoperative management of these patients (**Table 16.1**). For example,

Table 16.1 Medical Conditions That May Be Associated with Moyamoya Disease[44–46]

Hematologic disorders

  Sickle cell anemia

  Thalassemia

  Fanconi anemia

  Aplastic anemia

  Thrombophilic conditions

Vascular disorders

  Hypertension

  Renal artery stenosis

  Peripheral vascular disease

  Aortic aneurysm

  Cardiomyopathy

  Coarctation of the aorta

  Intracranial arteriolosclerosis

Congenital syndromes

  Neurofibromatosis type 1

  Mitochondrial disorders

  Marfan syndrome

  Down syndrome

  Apert syndrome

Miscellaneous

  Head and neck radiation

  Meningitis

  Nephrotic syndrome

  Pulmonary sarcoidosis

  Hyperthyroidism

  Renal artery stenosis

hematologic disorders may produce anemia that should be corrected preoperatively. Connective tissue changes associated with prior head and neck radiation therapy may make airway management difficult. Airway management also may be affected by several of the associated congenital syndromes. Systemic vascular disorders may make vascular access difficult and also may predispose these patients to perioperative cardiac complications.

Medications for most chronic medical conditions should be continued until the day of surgery. Clopidogrel and other antiplatelet drugs (with the exception of aspirin) should be discontinued 5 to 7 days before surgery. An electrocardiogram should be obtained for all patients with risk factors for cardiac disease. Laboratory studies should include at least a complete blood count, electrolytes, and glucose measurements. Our rules for preoperative fasting permit a light meal up to 8 hours before and clear liquids up to 3 hours before the scheduled time of surgery.

Our patients are counseled on what to expect in the immediate postoperative period, including the need for repeated neurologic testing, the nature and intensity of postoperative pain, effects of residual hypothermia, Foley catheter–related discomfort, and the presence of lines and monitors. Premedication for adults usually consists of 1 to 2 mg of intravenous midazolam before they leave the preoperative holding area. Children often benefit from oral midazolam in flavored syrup (0.5 mg/kg; maximum dose = 20 mg by mouth) 30 to 45 minutes before induction. It is critical to avoid hypotension, respiratory depression, or anxiety-induced hyperventilation in patients of any age with moyamoya.

◆ The Stanford Protocol

Intraoperative Management

Standard Monitors

In addition to the standard monitors approved by the American Society of Anesthesiologists, these patients require invasive arterial pressure monitoring, central venous access, continuous measurement of changes in the QTc interval, a deep esophageal temperature probe, and a Foley catheter for urine output, bladder irrigation, and bladder temperature measurements. Cortical function is monitored using electroencephalography (EEG) and evoked potentials (see following section). Theoretically, near infrared spectroscopy should allow oxygen saturation in cortical tissue to be monitored. In our experience, however, this technique can be difficult to implement (surgical field encroachment) and is unreliable compared with standard electrophysiologic monitoring techniques (EEG, somatosensory evoked potentials [SSEPs], and motor evoked potentials [MEPs]).

Anesthesia Induction

After the patient undergoes thorough preoxygenation (end-tidal oxygen fraction $\geq$ 0.9), anesthesia is induced using fentanyl administered incrementally to a final dose of 7 to 9 mcg/kg combined with thiopental or propofol titrated to loss of consciousness. Muscle relaxation is obtained using rocuronium or vecuronium. Throughout induction, the patient's mean arterial blood pressure (MAP) is maintained at preinduction levels using titrated doses of both ephedrine and phenylephrine. The trachea is intubated, and the position of the endotracheal tube is verified.

Anesthesia Maintenance

Typically, anesthesia is maintained using isoflurane (up to 0.6%) in 50% nitrous oxide and oxygen, supplemented as necessary with an infusion of remifentanil (0.05 to 0.2 mcg/kg/min). If an arterial line has not been placed preoperatively, it is placed at this time.

MAP (measured at head level) continues to be maintained near preoperative levels using titrated doses of ephedrine and phenylephrine. A triple lumen central venous catheter is inserted into a subclavian vein, and venous pressure is transduced from the distal orifice. A bolus dose of remifentanil (2 to 3 mcg/kg) is given through the central line ~60 seconds before placement of the Mayfield head holder to blunt the hemodynamic response to insertion of the skull pins. Most patients eventually require a continuous infusion of phenylephrine through the central line to maintain their MAP near preoperative levels. Ventilation is continuously adjusted to maintain normocarbia throughout the procedure.

The goal of fluid management is to maintain normovolemia and a hematocrit between 30% and 36%. This goal can be accomplished by replacing insensible losses, blood loss, and urine output with a combination of normal saline and 5% albumen. Urine output is an unreliable indicator of volume status in hypothermic patients because of cold-induced diuresis. Arterial blood gas, electrolyte, glucose, and the hematocrit should be measured at regular intervals throughout the case with the goal of maintaining normal values.

Induced Hypothermia

Core temperature, as measured from the distal esophagus, is reduced to ~33°C using either surface cooling or invasive techniques. Patients with a normal body mass index can be cooled adequately and rewarmed using surface techniques. Typically, the patient is sandwiched between two water circulating blankets set at 4°C for cooling and at 42°C for rewarming. Rewarming efforts in these patients often must be supplemented with bladder irrigation using warm (~40°C) saline. Invasive cooling techniques (Innercool™, Philips Medical, Amsterdam, The Netherlands) are reserved for patients with a high body mass index for whom surface cooling, especially surface rewarming techniques, would be too time consuming.

Over the past 15 years, we have made extensive use of induced intraoperative hypothermia with a collective experience that includes more than 1,000 moyamoya revascularization procedures and more than 2,000 other intracranial surgeries. Fortunately, we have observed no increase in adverse events related to hypothermia,[9] including coagulopathy, cardiac dysrhythmias, delayed emergence, or wound infection, in our population of hypothermic neurosurgical patients when compared with our normothermic neurosurgical patient population.

Patient Management during Cross-Clamping

EEG and evoked potential data are evaluated in consultation with the neurophysiologic monitoring team. By combining this information with each patient's pharmocodynamic characteristics, a dose of thiopental or propofol is chosen to produce burst-suppression while preserving the capability of monitoring evoked potentials. At the same time, a dose of ephedrine or phenylephrine that will completely offset the anticipated cardiovascular effects of the thiopental (or propofol) is selected. Immediately before placement of the arterial cross-clamp, the previously determined doses of anesthetic and pressor drugs are administered through the central venous line. Once burst-suppression has been achieved and the MAP is ~10% higher than the preoperative level, the arterial cross-clamp is applied. An elevated MAP is maintained using a phenylephrine or dopamine infusion. Further MAP adjustments are made throughout the cross-clamp period in response to EEG/evoked potential changes and surgical field conditions. Once the arterial cross-clamp has been removed, the MAP is allowed to return to baseline levels.

Intraoperative Neurophysiologic Monitoring

The surgical treatment of moyamoya disease is associated with the risk of intraoperative cerebral ischemia, similar to the operative treatment of other cerebrovascular disorders. Therefore, strategies used to identify and reduce the risk of intraoperative cerebral ischemia should be considered during the surgical treatment of moyamoya disease. This section reviews the neurophysiologic techniques that may be useful and applicable in identifying intraoperative cerebral ischemia, describes the rationale and physiologic basis of their utility, describes our experience in managing these cases using intraoperative neurophysiologic monitoring techniques, and presents clinical examples to highlight the utility of these techniques in the intraoperative management of moyamoya disease.

◆ Neurophysiologic Studies and Cerebral Blood Flow

Cerebral ischemia and possible progression to cerebral infarction are potential complications of the surgical treatment of moyamoya disease. As a result of this risk, different techniques have been studied to determine their utility in identifying and possibly reversing intraoperative cerebral ischemia. The ultimate goals in using these techniques are to prevent intraoperative stroke and to improve patients' postoperative neurologic outcomes. Animal and human clinical studies have shown that SSEPs and EEG can detect changes in the functional state of the brain associated with ischemia. The foundation for these changes is based on the strong correlation between electrophysiologic changes and regional CBF.

Experimental animal studies using SSEPs have demonstrated a predictable pattern of changes in relation to cerebral ischemia. A review of primate studies shows that cortical SSEPs are maintained at levels of regional CBF $\geq$ 16 mL/100 g/min but are absent at levels < 12 mL/100 g/min; at levels between 14 and 16 mL/100 g/min, the amplitude of the evoked response declines sharply, with a 50% reduction in amplitude corresponding to regional CBF of 16 mL/100 g/min.[10–13] Cerebral ischemia also seems to prolong the central conduction time with a regional CBF threshold of < 15 mL/100 g/min, similar to that seen with amplitude reduction.[14,15] These changes in SSEPs occur at regional CBF levels higher than those typically associated with infarction.

In baboon chronic stroke models using an MCA occlusion technique, areas of infarction corresponded to regional CBF levels $\leq$ 10 mL/100 g/min.[13,16] However, in acute stroke primate models, infarcts occurred at higher levels of regional CBF and were only detected in areas where regional CBF was $\leq$ 12 mL/100 g/min.[17,18] These findings suggest that a 50% reduction in the amplitude of cortical SSEPs corresponds to a regional CBF of 14 to 16 mL/100 g/min and is indicative of ischemia, while it is still above the levels associated with cerebral infarction. Thus, these SSEP changes would indicate a potentially reversible cerebral ischemic state that may be corrected by increasing CBF.

EEG has long been known to be altered in a predictable pattern by cerebral ischemia. This point was clearly demonstrated in a series of elegant clinical studies by Sharbrough et al,[19] Sundt et al,[20] and Sundt et al,[21] who reviewed the correlation between CBF measurements and EEG changes in patients undergoing carotid endarterectomy. Major EEG changes occurred when regional CBF was $\leq$ 10 mL/100 g/min. Less severe EEG changes were seen when regional CBF was between 10 to 18 mL/100 g/min. A critical level was defined as 15 mL/100 g/min. As is evident, these EEG changes correlate closely with those seen in SSEP animal models.

Clinical Applications of Intraoperative Neurophysiologic Monitoring in Cerebrovascular Disorders

The utility of intraoperative neurophysiologic monitoring in the surgical treatment of a variety of cerebrovascular diseases has been described for cerebral aneurysm surgery,[22–26] resection of central nervous system arteriovenous malformations,[27] and carotid endarterectomy.[28–30] The usefulness of intraoperative neurophysiologic monitoring has also been described in the endovascular treatment of cerebral aneurysms[31] and arteriovenous malformations.[32] These studies are not reviewed in this chapter, which focuses on moyamoya disease. Instead, the reader is directed to excellent comprehensive reviews of this topic, which can be found in textbooks on intraoperative neurophysiologic monitoring.[33,34]

Moyamoya Disease

In terms of intraoperative neurophysiologic monitoring, it is important to understand what the surgical treatment of moyamoya entails and what pathophysiologic mechanisms may cause cerebral injury. The surgical treatment of this disorder involves direct and indirect revascularization techniques to increase CBF. The more commonly performed direct revascularization procedure requires grafting the STA to a branch of the MCA. In so doing, a portion of the MCA supply may be compromised when the STA-to-MCA anastomosis is actually performed. During this time, a distal segment of the MCA is temporarily occluded; hence, the risk of cerebral ischemia is typically the highest.

Although operative treatment of moyamoya disease is becoming common and is being performed at an increasing number of centers, it is unclear if any methods or techniques are being widely used to identify and monitor for cerebral ischemia. Smith et al[35] suggested that patients undergoing surgical treatment of moyamoya may benefit from intraoperative neurophysiologic monitoring and that intraoperative EEG or near-infrared spectroscopy be considered as methods for identifying cerebral ischemia during general anesthesia. Unfortunately, their publication was not a study of the use of intraoperative neurophysiologic monitoring in moyamoya surgery.

Further review of the literature reveals only one published study, in abstract, on the use of intraoperative neurophysiologic monitoring exclusively during the treatment of moyamoya disease.[36] The Stanford authors reported a series of 700 moyamoya revascularization cases (435 patients) predominantly involving STA-to-MCA anastomosis. Intraoperative neurophysiologic monitoring was performed with bilateral monitoring of SSEPs from the median nerve and with an eight-lead parasagittal scalp EEG. Twenty-nine (4.1%) cases had new strokes detected immediately after recovery from anesthesia; yet, a change correlating with intraoperative neurophysiologic monitoring was present in only four cases. Twenty-three (3.3%) other cases had changes in intraoperative neurophysiologic monitoring. Of these, four had "persistent" changes, and all four had new postoperative events (3 of these strokes are included in the 29 strokes above; one of the four patients had a hemorrhage). "Transient" changes in intraoperative neurophysiologic monitoring correlated with an absence of postoperative events (17 of 19 cases), presumably a result of the intraoperative intervention undertaken to reverse the cerebral ischemia. They concluded that intraoperative neurophysiologic monitoring using upper extremity SSEPs and eight-lead parasagittal scalp EEG was a specific, but insensitive, predictor of postoperative strokes, hemorrhages, or transient neurologic events.

Stanford Intraoperative Neurophysiologic Monitoring Protocol

In addition to understanding the surgical procedure involved, it is also imperative to know and understand the anesthetic regimen being used, because it can significantly affect the results of intraoperative neurophysiologic monitoring. The anesthetic technique described previously in this chapter has only modest effects on the amplitudes of the cortical SSEPs and predictable slowing of the EEG bilaterally. We use the following intraoperative neurophysiologic monitoring techniques in all of our moyamoya surgeries in an attempt to identify and monitor for cortical and subcortical ischemia: EEG, median nerve-generated SSEPs, posterior tibial nerve-generated SSEPs, and transcranial MEPS.

Electroencephalography

A minimum of 8 channels (10 preferred) should be used, with four or five electrodes placed on each side of the head using a parasagittal montage. For example, if eight channels are used, the following sample montage would be useful for monitoring moyamoya surgery: F3/F4, C3′/C4′, P3/P4, T3/T4, referenced to FZ. We have also found it useful to add F7/F8 and/or O1/O2 electrodes to this protocol.

Somatosensory Evoked Potentials

Peripheral Nerve Electrical Stimulation

SSEPs are recorded after bilateral independent median nerve and posterior tibial nerve stimulation using standard surface or subdermal stimulating electrodes at the wrist and ankles, respectively. Stimulation is at a rate of 2 to 5 Hz with a stimulus pulse duration of 0.1 to 0.3 milliseconds. A constant current stimulation intensity of ~50% above the threshold level, sufficient to produce a thumb twitch, is used throughout the case. The ground electrode is placed on the arm proximal to the median nerve–stimulating electrode. An average of 150 to 250 stimulations usually produces adequate and reproducible evoked potentials.

Recommended Recording Montages

1. Median nerve SSEPs
   a. C3′/C4′-FZ (contralateral cortex–midfrontal reference)
   b. Contralateral cortex–ipsilateral cortex
      i. These montages provide recordings of near-field cortical SSEP components (N19, P24, P40, and N45).
   c. Cervical spine, typically C5 or C7, referenced to FZ or contralateral shoulder-FZ. This setup would allow identification of subcortical far-field potentials (P14, N18) and permit monitoring of central conduction time (time interval between

P14 and N19). Central conduction time reflects the intracranial conduction time between the foramen magnum and somatosensory cortex.
   d. Ipsilateral brachial plexus–contralateral brachial plexus
2. Posterior tibial SSEPs
   a. CZ-FZ
   b. CZ′-FZ
   c. C5/C7-FZ
   d. Ipsilateral popliteal fossa–knee reference

Transcranial Motor Evoked Potentials

Stimulation Technique

Transcranial MEPs can be obtained by transcranial electrical stimulation of the motor cortex using standard surface EEG, subdermal needle, or corkscrew electrodes placed on the scalp. The most commonly used stimulation montage, C3-C4, usually generates myogenic MEPs from bilateral upper and lower extremities if stimulated at sufficiently high intensities. A C1-C2 montage also can be used but tends to preferentially generate compound motor action potentials from the lower extremities. Electrical stimulation should be kept at threshold levels that activate the hemisphere of interest. Otherwise, deep subcortical motor pathways may be activated if stimulation levels are too high, which can bypass areas of cortical ischemia.

1. Anodal stimulation is the key to obtaining MEPs. Therefore, the electrode corresponding to the motor cortex of interest should be connected to the anode on the stimulator. On occasion, we use a montage that isolates the hemisphere of interest, such as C3/C4-CZ or C3/C4-FZ, to obtain myogenic MEPs from the contralateral limbs.

2. Specific stimulation parameters partially depend on the equipment being used and the anesthetic regimen. However, the following stimulation settings usually produce reproducible transcranial MEPs recorded from muscle: pulse duration of 50 μsec, stimulus train of 3 to 6, interstimulus interval of 1.5 to 3.0 milliseconds, and a maximum intensity of 500 V. Appropriate stimulation settings need to be established for each case and can vary widely among patients.

3. An understanding of the possible complications and contraindications of transcranial MEP electrical stimulation is critical before this technique is used. The most common complication is tongue biting due to direct electrical activation of the masseter and temporalis muscles. Thus, an adequate bite-blocking device must be in place before obtaining transcranial MEPs. Detailed review of other possible complications associated with transcranial MEPs is beyond the scope of this review, and the reader is again referred to the previously mentioned textbooks on intraoperative neurophysiologic monitoring.

Recording Technique

Compound motor action potentials can be recorded using surface or subdermal needle electrodes. Our preferred method is to use needle electrodes, which are easy to place, require no electrolyte contact gel, and tend to be more secure. The needle electrodes often penetrate muscle and then effectively become intramuscular recording electrodes. We record from a minimum of six muscles, with compound motor action potentials typically recorded from the following bilateral muscles: abductor pollicus brevis, first dorsal interosseus, tibialis anterior, and abductor hallucis.

Case Example

A 5-year-old boy with history of bilateral hemispheric transient ischemic attacks related to moyamoya disease was surgically treated with a left STA–to–left MCA bypass. Soon thereafter, severe slowing in the left hemisphere EEG (C: traces 1 to 4) was detected, without corresponding changes in the left (A) or right median (B) nerve cortical SSEP. The slowing was persistent and failed to correct after mean arterial pressure was increased. Postoperatively, the patient developed right hemiparesis (**Fig. 16.1**).

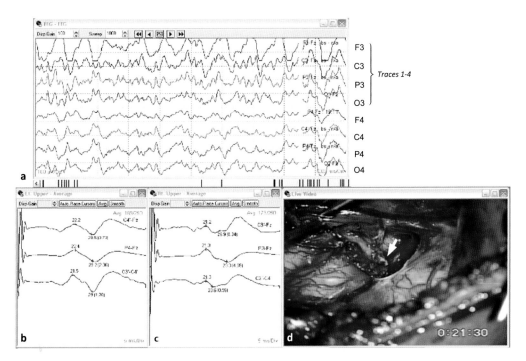

Fig. 16.1a–d Example of intraoperative neurophysiologic monitoring of cerebral function using multimodality electroencephalography (**a**) and somatosensory evoked potentials of the left (**b**) and right (**c**) median nerves in a 5-year-old boy with moyamoya disease and a history of bilateral hemispheric translent ischemic attacks during surgical treatment with a left superficial temporal artery–to–left middle cerebral artery bypass procedure. After the anastomosis was performed (**d**, arrow), slow-wave electroencephalographic activity was seen on the left hemisphere (**a:** traces 1–4), without corresponding changes in the somatosensory evoked potentials (**b, c**). Postoperatively, the patient developed hemiparesis on the right.

◆ Postoperative Considerations

Emergence from Anesthesia

Antiemetics (e.g., intravenous ondansetron 4 to 8 mg) are administered during dural closure. After surgery is concluded, inhaled anesthetics are discontinued while the patient is maintained on a low-dose infusion of remifentanil (typically 0.05 mcg/kg/min). Following the return of spontaneous ventilation and protective airway reflexes, the patient's trachea is extubated and the remifentanil infusion is discontinued. MAP is maintained near preoperative levels. Doing so typically requires labetalol in combination with esmolol and sodium nitroprusside infusions. Temperature criteria for extubation vary from patient to patient depending on coexisting medical concerns. However, most patients can be extubated safely once their core temperature, as measured in the distal esophagus, reaches 35°C.

Soon after extubation and while still in the operating room, the patient is examined neurologically to verify the return of normal motor, sensory, and command functions. If necessary, pain is controlled and shivering is suppressed with a low dose of meperidine (15 to 25 mg) administered intravenously. The patient is transported with full monitoring to the intensive care unit, and care is transferred to the intensive care unit team. Routine postoperative orders include a chest X-ray to verify central venous catheter placement and implementation of arterial blood pressure management parameters derived from the patient's intraoperative pressure requirements. MAP should continue to be monitored at head level to avoid iatrogenic intracranial hypotension that could occur when the head of the bed is placed in a more upright position while leaving the arterial transducer at heart level.

Typical Complications and Risk Factors

Intraoperative ischemic injuries detected by persistent changes in neurophysiologic monitoring or by neurologic examination in the immediate postoperative period are extremely rare. A small number of patients ($<4\%$) develop an ischemic or hemorrhagic injury, typically on postoperative day 1 or 2. Almost all of these patients have bilateral disease with the complication occurring after successful treatment of the first side. So far, correlation analysis has failed to identify likely causative factors.

Mild Hypothermia Controversy

Unfortunately, the use of intraoperative hypothermia remains controversial. The well-publicized risks of mild hypothermia include a tripling of the incidence of surgical wound infections and adverse cardiac events along with significant increases in intraoperative blood loss and duration of hospitalization.[9] Hypothermia advocates cite the extensive laboratory data demonstrating that mild hypothermia is remarkably protective against ischemic injury in a variety of experimental models and across many animal species.[37] These laboratory studies have been supported clinically by the demonstrated beneficial effects of hypothermia during cardiac bypass and, more recently, in postmyocardial infarction studies.[38–41] What seems clear from all these studies is that mild hypothermia is most effective when it has been established at or very near the time of the ischemic insult and preferably maintained during the postischemic period when reperfusion injury is likely to occur.

Detractors of mild hypothermia cite the second Intraoperative Hypothermia for Aneurysm Surgery Trial (IHAST 2) study[42] (disclosure: R.A.J. and D.G.M. were coinvestigators in the IHAST2 study). IHAST 2 failed to demonstrate any beneficial effect of mild hypothermia during surgery for aneurysm clipping, when that surgery occurred as long as 2 weeks after aneurysmal rupture. In the IHAST 2 study, injury that occurred at the time of aneurysm rupture or as a result of subsequent vasospasm was not treated with mild hypothermia because hypothermia was induced only briefly during surgery 1 to 14 days after rupture. Furthermore, the occurrence of intraoperative ischemic events that could have benefited from mild hypothermia were uncommon in this study because temporary arterial clipping either was not used or was of very limited duration in $>94\%$ of the patients. To address this issue, data from IHAST 2 patients with long total temporary clip times were analyzed separately.[43] Again, no outcome differences between hypothermic and normothermic patients were detected when total temporary clip time was $\geq$ 20 minutes.

The absence of effect in the IHAST study in general and specifically for those patients with prolonged total temporary clip times may be the result of confounding by the variable effects of injury occurring at the time of and immediately after aneurysm rupture. While the subset of IHAST patients with long total temporary clip times should have been the most likely to benefit from intraoperative hypothermia, data analysis from this group was complicated by the fact that total clip time was defined as the sum of shorter clip times separated by reperfusion intervals of undocumented length. This group of patients also had a significantly worse preoperative neurologic status as assessed on the National Institutes of Health Stroke and Glasgow Coma Scales. This group also had a significantly higher incidence of postoperative meningitis and ventriculitis compared with the IHAST 2 subjects with shorter total clip times. These preexisting injuries and postoperative complications, combined with unknown reperfusion intervals, could have obscured any beneficial effect of hypothermia.

Although IHAST 2 was designed as well as it could be given the constraints imposed by the nature of clinical studies and good clinical care, its design precludes conclusions regarding the efficacy of mild hypothermia during deliberate temporary ischemia in cortical areas already known to be marginally perfused as is the case in patients with moyamoya disease. To suggest that the absence of beneficial effect in the IHAST 2 study negates the positive results of the many carefully controlled laboratory and clinical studies and thereby justifies withholding this potentially beneficial treatment from patients with moyamoya seems ill advised.

References

1. Baykan N, Ozgen S, Ustalar ZS, Dagçinar A, Ozek MM. Moyamoya disease and anesthesia. Paediatr Anaesth 2005;15(12):1111–1115
2. Henderson MA, Irwin MG. Anaesthesia and moyamoya disease. Anaesth Intensive Care 1995;23(4):503–506
3. Nomura S, Kashiwagi S, Uetsuka S, Uchida T, Kubota H, Ito H. Perioperative management protocols for children with moyamoya disease. Childs Nerv Syst 2001;17(4-5):270–274
4. Yusa T, Yamashiro K. Local cortical cerebral blood flow and response to carbon dioxide during anesthesia in patients with moyamoya disease. J Anesth 1999;13(3):131–135
5. Kansha M, Irita K, Takahashi S, Matsushima T. Anesthetic management of children with moyamoya disease. Clin Neurol Neurosurg 1997;99(Suppl 2):S110–S113
6. Soriano SG, Sethna NF, Scott RM. Anesthetic management of children with moyamoya syndrome. Anesth Analg 1993;77(5):1066–1070
7. Scott RM, Smith ER. Moyamoya disease and moyamoya syndrome. N Engl J Med 2009;360(12):1226–1237
8. Iwama T, Hashimoto N, Yonekawa Y. The relevance of hemodynamic factors to perioperative ischemic complications in childhood moyamoya disease. Neurosurgery 1996;38(6):1120–1125, discussion 1125–1126
9. Sessler DI. Complications and treatment of mild hypothermia. Anesthesiology 2001;95(2):531–543
10. Branston NM, Symon L, Crockard HA, Pasztor E. Relationship between the cortical evoked potential and local cortical blood flow following acute middle cerebral artery occlusion in the baboon. Exp Neurol 1974;45(2):195–208
11. Branston NM, Strong AJ, Symon L. Extracellular potassium activity, evoked potential and tissue blood flow. Relationships during progressive ischaemia in baboon cerebral cortex. J Neurol Sci 1977;32(3):305–321
12. Branston NM, Ladds A, Symon L, Wang AD. Comparison of the effects of ischaemia on early components of the somatosensory evoked potential in brainstem, thalamus, and cerebral cortex. J Cereb Blood Flow Metab 1984;4(1):68–81
13. Symon L. The relationship between CBF, evoked potentials and the clinical features in cerebral ischaemia. Acta Neurol Scand Suppl 1980;78:175–190
14. Hargadine JR, Branston NM, Symon L. Central conduction time in primate brain ischemia — a study in baboons. Stroke 1980;11(6):637–642
15. Lesnick JE, Michele JJ, Simeone FA, DeFeo S, Welsh FA. Alteration of somatosensory evoked potentials in response to global ischemia. J Neurosurg 1984;60(3):490–494
16. Symon L, Crockard HA, Dorsch NW, Branston NM, Juhasz J. Local cerebral blood flow and vascular reactivity in a chronic stable stroke in baboons. Stroke 1975;6(5):482–492
17. Jones TH, Morawetz RB, Crowell RM, et al. Thresholds of focal cerebral ischemia in awake monkeys. J Neurosurg 1981;54(6):773–782
18. Morawetz RB, DeGirolami U, Ojemann RG, Marcoux FW, Crowell RM. Cerebral blood flow determined by hydrogen clearance during middle cerebral artery occlusion in unanesthetized monkeys. Stroke 1978;9(2):143–149
19. Sharbrough FW, Messick JM Jr, Sundt TM Jr. Correlation of continuous electroencephalograms with cerebral blood flow measurements during carotid endarterectomy. Stroke 1973;4(4):674–683
20. Sundt TM Jr, Sharbrough FW, Anderson RE, Michenfelder JD. Cerebral blood flow measurements and electroencephalograms during carotid endarterectomy. J Neurosurg 1974;41(3):310–320
21. Sundt TM Jr, Sharbrough FW, Piepgras DG, Kearns TP, Messick JM Jr, O'Fallon WM. Correlation of cerebral blood flow and electroencephalographic changes during carotid endarterectomy: with results of surgery and hemodynamics of cerebral ischemia. Mayo Clin Proc 1981;56(9):533–543
22. Friedman WA, Kaplan BL, Day AL, Sypert GW, Curran MT. Evoked potential monitoring during aneurysm operation: observations after fifty cases. Neurosurgery 1987;20(5):678–687

23. Schramm J, Koht A, Schmidt G, Pechstein U, Taniguchi M, Fahlbusch R. Surgical and electrophysiological observations during clipping of 134 aneurysms with evoked potential monitoring. Neurosurgery 1990; 26(1):61–70

24. Friedman WA, Chadwick GM, Verhoeven FJ, Mahla M, Day AL. Monitoring of somatosensory evoked potentials during surgery for middle cerebral artery aneurysms. Neurosurgery 1991;29(1):83–88

25. Palatinsky E, DiScenna A, McDonald H, Whittingham T, Selman W. SSEP and Baep monitoring of temporary clip application and induced hypotension during cerebrovascular surgery. In: Loftus CM, Traynelis VC, editors. Intraoperative monitoring techniques in neurosurgery. New York: McGraw-Hill; 1994:61–71

26. Lopéz JR, Chang SD, Steinberg GK. The use of electrophysiological monitoring in the intraoperative management of intracranial aneurysms. J Neurol Neurosurg Psychiatry 1999;66(2):189–196

27. Chang SD, Lopez JR, Steinberg GK. The usefulness of electrophysiological monitoring during resection of central nervous system vascular malformations. J Stroke Cerebrovasc Dis 1999;8(6):412–422

28. Pedrini L, Tarantini S, Cirelli MR, Ballester A, Cifiello BI, D'Addato M. Intraoperative assessment of cerebral ischaemia during carotid surgery. Int Angiol 1998;17(1):10–14

29. Manninen PH, Tan TK, Sarjeant RM. Somatosensory evoked potential monitoring during carotid endarterectomy in patients with a stroke. Anesth Analg 2001;93(1):39–44

30. Lam AM, Manninen PH, Ferguson GG, Nantau W. Monitoring electrophysiologic function during carotid endarterectomy: a comparison of somatosensory evoked potentials and conventional electroencephalogram. Anesthesiology 1991;75(1):15–21

31. Liu AY, Lopez JR, Do HM, Steinberg GK, Cockroft K, Marks MP. Neurophysiological monitoring in the endovascular therapy of aneurysms. AJNR Am J Neuroradiol 2003;24(8):1520–1527

32. Paulsen RD, Steinberg GK, Norbash AM, Marcellus ML, Lopez JR, Marks MP. Embolization of rolandic cortex arteriovenous malformations. Neurosurgery 1999;44(3):479–484, discussion 484–486

33. Nuwer MR. Intraoperative monitoring of neural function. In: Nuwer MR, editor. Handbook of Clinical Neurophysiology. 2008.

34. Galloway GM, Nuwer MR, Lopez JR, Zamel KM. Intraoperative Neurophysiologic Monitoring. Cambridge: Cambridge University Press; 2010

35. Smith ER, Butler WE, Ogilvy CS. Surgical approaches to vascular anomalies of the child's brain. Curr Opin Neurol 2002;15(2):165–171

36. Nguyen V, Khan N, Steinberg G, Cho S, López J. Intraoperative neurophysiologic monitoring in the surgical management of moyamoya disease. Poster presented at: American Academy of Neurology; 2011 April; Honolulu, HI

37. Dietrich WD, Atkins CM, Bramlett HM. Protection in animal models of brain and spinal cord injury with mild to moderate hypothermia. J Neurotrauma 2009;26(3):301–312

38. Arrich J, Holzer M, Herkner H, Müllner M. Hypothermia for neuroprotection in adults after cardiopulmonary resuscitation. Cochrane Database Syst Rev 2009; (4):CD004128

39. Bernard SA, Gray TW, Buist MD, et al. Treatment of comatose survivors of out-of-hospital cardiac arrest with induced hypothermia. N Engl J Med 2002;346(8):557–563

40. Hypothermia after Cardiac Arrest Study Group. Mild therapeutic hypothermia to improve the neurologic outcome after cardiac arrest. N Engl J Med 2002;346(8):549–556

41. Holzer M, Bernard SA, Hachimi-Idrissi S, Roine RO, Sterz F, Müllner M; Collaborative Group on Induced Hypothermia for Neuroprotection After Cardiac Arrest. Hypothermia for neuroprotection after cardiac arrest: systematic review and individual patient data meta-analysis. Crit Care Med 2005;33(2):414–418

42. Todd MM, Hindman BJ, Clarke WR, Torner JC; Intraoperative Hypothermia for Aneurysm Surgery Trial (IHAST) Investigators. Mild intraoperative hypothermia during surgery for intracranial aneurysm. N Engl J Med 2005;352(2):135–145

43. Hindman BJ, Bayman EO, Pfisterer WK, Torner JC, Todd MM; IHAST Investigators. No association between intraoperative hypothermia or supplemental protective drug and neurologic outcomes in patients undergoing temporary clipping during cerebral aneurysm surgery: findings from the Intraoperative Hypothermia for Aneurysm Surgery Trial. Anesthesiology 2010;112(1):86–101

44. Hervé D, Touraine P, Verloes A, et al. A hereditary moyamoya syndrome with multisystemic manifestations. Neurology 2010;75(3):259–264

45. Kikuta K, Takagi Y, Nozaki K, et al. Effects of intravenous anesthesia with propofol on regional cortical blood flow and intracranial pressure in surgery for moyamoya disease. Surg Neurol 2007;68(4):421–424

46. Parray T, Martin TW, Siddiqui S. Moyamoya disease: a review of the disease and anesthetic management. J Neurosurg Anesthesiol 2011;23(2):100–109

III

Regional Long-term Experience with Cerebral Revascularization

17

Long-term Results after Cerebral Revascularization in Adult Moyamoya

Ramon L. Navarro, Terry C. Burns, Peter A. Gooderham, and
Gary K. Steinberg

◆ Introduction

Our current knowledge of long-term outcomes for moyamoya disease is limited by the lack of prospective randomized data that can test the natural history of the disease against medical and surgical treatment. The Research Committee on Spontaneous Occlusion of the Circle of Willis (Moyamoya Disease) of the Ministry of Health and Welfare, Japan, has established guidelines for the treatment of moyamoya disease. These guidelines recommend treatment for ischemic cases that fail medical management, but the management of hemorrhagic cases remains unclear.[1]

However, abundant data, mostly from Asian centers, suggest that surgical revascularization improves the course of moyamoya disease. In analyzing outcomes for adult patients with moyamoya disease, we have become aware of the following contributory variables: ethnicity, unilateral versus bilateral disease, cerebrovascular hemodynamics, type of clinical presentation, medical versus surgical treatment, and type of surgical intervention.

Analysis of Long-term Results

Different temporal patterns have been observed in Asian and non-Asian patients with moyamoya disease: the onset is more delayed in the latter. Nonetheless, the disease is progressive in both Asian and non-Asian patients, especially among women.[2] In Asian patients, there are two peaks of presentation: in childhood with ischemic symptoms and in adults with a higher incidence of hemorrhage than occurs in children. This statement may not be true for non-Asians, who may have a later onset of the disease during young adulthood with principally ischemic symptoms as well as a less advanced stage of the disease. However, two recent papers based on Chinese and Korean populations with moyamoya disease found that these two nationalities had more similarities with non-Asian patients than with their Japanese counterparts.[3,4] Different natural histories may therefore exist for different phenotypes of moyamoya disease. However, moyamoya disease also may now be diagnosed at earlier stages in adulthood, especially when ischemia might be the predominant manifestation, because advanced imaging techniques are more widely available than in the past.

Sex also might be a prognostic factor. We have found differences in presentation with females more likely to suffer preoperative transient ischemic attacks than males. We recently analyzed 307 females and 123 males undergoing 717 revascularization surgeries. All patients significantly improved after treatment as measured on the modified Rankin Scale (mRS). However, the 5-year significant cumulative risk of adverse postoperative events, despite successful revascularization, was 11.4% in females compared with 5.3% in males.[5]

Once the disease manifests, additional differences such as laterality, cerebrovascular reactivity, and other symptoms can be seen. True unilateral moyamoya disease, especially if asymptomatic, seems to have the most benign course. Its rate of progression to bilateral disease is between 7% and 30%.[2,6–8] Alternatively, the chance of unilateral moyamoya disease associated with equivocal or mild involvement of the contralateral side progressing to bilateral disease can be as high as 40%.[9] Headache is present in most adult patients with moyamoya disease, but headache does not appear to be a prognostic factor.[10,11] The origin of headache is thought to be borderline ischemia in patients with impaired cerebrovascular reserve, nociception related to collateral formation, or both.

The outcome of the hemorrhagic form of moyamoya disease is usually worse than that of the ischemic form, and surgical treatment for patients with intracranial bleeding is controversial. In contrast to ischemia, where progressive stenosis of the supraclinoidal internal carotid arteries, M1 segment of the middle cerebral arteries (MCAs), or A1 segment of the anterior cerebral arteries is involved and can be treated successfully with revascularization, the source of hemorrhage is not always clear. It may be caused by rupture of dilated, fragile moyamoya vessels under hemodynamic stress, by rupture of a saccular aneurysm primarily in the posterior circulation, or by rupture of dilated collateral arteries on the surface of the brain.[12] Not all of these causes may respond equally to revascularization.

The status of a patient's cerebral hemodynamics and cerebrovascular reserve also may affect prognosis. Patients with impaired cerebrovascular reserve and signs of misery perfusion may benefit the most from cerebral revascularization because ischemia is the main driving force for neovascularization.[13] Zipfel et al studied the oxygen extraction fraction as a predictor of stroke in adults with moyamoya disease.[14] Other studies have shown that more events occur during the first 2 years after initial presentation than thereafter.[6,15] Theoretically, during that early period the discrepancy between oxygen demand and blood flow supplied to the brain is greater. The disease also may be more active at that time. A subgroup of patients, young adults with bilateral moyamoya disease who become symptomatic with headaches and ischemic symptoms, may therefore benefit the most from an effective treatment.

In both Asian and non-Asian populations, there is a clear risk of disease progression, and currently there is no effective medical treatment for moyamoya disease. Antiplatelet agents, calcium-channel blockers, vasoconstrictors, and other rheological drugs have no significant effect on the disease. On a recent questionnaire, more non-Asian neurologists and neurosurgeons responded that they were likely to use antiplatelet agents to treat patients with moyamoya disease than their Asian colleagues.[16] In a Japanese study, the per-year risk of stroke in nonsurgically treated hemispheres was 3.2%,[17] and the rate of recurrent bleeding in patients with hemorrhagic moyamoya disease was 7%.[18] North American and European studies suggest an even higher 5-year cumulative risk of stroke ranging from 40 to 80%, especially if patients have impaired hemodynamic reserve.[6,15,19]

Several studies have demonstrated that revascularization substantially decreases the subsequent rate of ischemic stroke and improves clinical outcomes compared with conservative management. The 5-year Kaplan-Meier risk of stroke has ranged from 5 to 17% compared with 65% with medical treatment alone.[3,6,10] However, Chiu et al failed to demonstrate a benefit from surgery,[15] probably due to a high perioperative rate of complications. From a radiographic perspective, angiographic progression of the disease is faster after revascularization. Surgery also appears to have a beneficial effect on cerebral hemodynamics with improvement of cerebrovascular reserve. Although some data conflict, this improvement may not only involve the revascularized hemisphere but may also extend to the contralateral hemisphere.[20–24]

The effect of revascularization in patients who become symptomatic with hemorrhage is controversial.[4,7,25–29] In contrast to ischemia, surgery may have a more modest impact on rates of rehemorrhage. Furthermore, rebleeding often has a devastating effect on clinical outcome. The incidence of a second hemorrhage has ranged between 14% and 18% after surgical revascularization with a mean follow-up of 4 and 6 years, respectively,[4,7,26] from the estimated occurrence of 30 to 65% over more than 5 years.[4,18,25,29]

Revascularization reduces moyamoya vessels, which, however, are only one cause of hemorrhage.[26,27,30] At our institution, about half of our patients are non-Asian adults who manifest with ischemic or hemorrhagic symptoms. After treating 417 patients, our late hemorrhage rate (range 1 month to 13 years after surgery, mean 9 years) is 1.4%. On angiography, these patients had prominent choroidal vessels (unpublished data). Our preliminary analysis of 60 patients with hemorrhage suggests a rehemorrhage rate of ~10% based on more than 2 years of follow-up (unpublished data). Headache, another prominent symptom, improves in as many as 80% of patients undergoing revascularization.[10] This improvement is attributed to improved perfusion pressure and cerebral circulation.[30]

Scant data are available on the neuropsychological performance of patients with moyamoya disease. We studied 30 patients with moyamoya disease but without strokes. Almost a fourth of these patients were impaired significantly in terms of their executive function, mental efficiency, and word-finding ability, whereas their memory was relatively intact. Furthermore, 37% of these patients had significant emotional distress (depression/anxiety). This finding raises the question of whether earlier surgical revascularization can prevent cognitive impairment and possibly ameliorate emotional distress.[31]

Another area of debate is the choice among different types of revascularization surgery, primarily direct versus indirect bypass. Unfortunately, no randomized study on efficacy of treatment is available. A literature review failed to demonstrate superiority of or increased safety associated with either treatment. There is a trend toward using direct superficial temporal artery (STA)-to-MCA anastomosis in adults rather than indirect procedures such as encephaloduroarteriosynangiosis, encephalomyosynangiosis, multiple bur holes, and omental transposition. Indirect procedures are more commonly performed in pediatric populations. The outcomes of long-term clinical revascularization may be similar after both direct and indirect treatment,[3,6,10,13] but the reduction in the size and number of moyamoya vessels seems to be higher with direct bypass.[26,27,30]

An ongoing randomized prospective Japanese study may clarify some aspects of the natural history and treatment of hemorrhagic moyamoya disease.[32]

Recently, Bang et al showed that angiographic revascularization and perfusion as measured by single photon emission computed tomography improved most in adult patients with moyamoya after combined direct plus indirect STA-to-MCA bypass; perfusion improved least after encephaloduroarteriosynangiosis only. Nevertheless, there was no difference in the stroke rate 6 months after either treatment.[33] A recent large Chinese series of mostly adult patients with moyamoya disease primarily treated with encephaloduroarteriosynangiosis reported very satisfactory results for prevention of stroke (comparable to direct bypass).[3] Another study of Korean patients with moyamoya disease, however, suggested that patients may fare worse after an indirect bypass and that combined techniques may achieve the best results.[4]

Our preferred revascularization method is direct STA-to-MCA bypass when feasible. Its main advantage is immediate revascularization. Its disadvantages include technical difficulty and abrupt alteration of cerebral hemodynamics, which can induce acute complications such as hemorrhage and ischemia. In 450 revascularization surgeries, our postoperative ($\leq$ 30 day) morbidity and mortality rates were 2.8% and 4.5%, respectively, and 0.7% and 1.1% per procedure/patient, respectively. We performed direct STA-to-MCA anastomoses in 95% of our adult patients with durable results, as also reported in other American series.[34] In our series,[10] quality of life improved significantly in 90% of the patients who had an mRS score of 0 to 2 (mean follow-up 4.1 years). The strongest predictor of good outcome was a low preoperative mRS score. During the first postoperative month, the transient ischemic attack rate was 15%; it decreased to 8.8% after the first year. Two recent series using indirect revascularization procedures to treat adults with moyamoya disease reported similar outcomes with decreased stroke rates and excellent outcomes with a median follow-up of 14 to 41 months.[13,35] Some North American studies, however, have failed to demonstrate differences in functional outcomes between surgically and medically treated patients.[6,15,36]

We also recently reported outcomes of repeat revascularization surgery after unsuccessful indirect bypass procedures. The addition of direct bypass if adequate donor and recipient vessels were available or an additional indirect procedure such as encephalomyosynangiosis or omental transposition improved clinical outcomes in five of the six adult patients who failed their initial revascularization surgery.[37]

◆ Conclusion

Regardless of the revascularization method of choice, treating patients with moyamoya disease involves close multidisciplinary collaboration in specialized centers, because these patients often have unstable hemodynamics that place them at high risk for perioperative events. To reduce the number of complications and to ensure the best long-term outcome possible, we carefully control perioperative blood pressure in these patients. Intraoperatively, we use electrophysiological and hemodynamic monitoring and mild hypothermia.

To date, surgical revascularization is the only treatment that improves the natural clinical history of moyamoya disease. Long-term outcomes are better in young adults who present with ischemic symptoms and a good preoperative mRS score compared with patients who present with hemorrhage. We believe that the surgical techniques used to treat moyamoya disease should be performed in specialized centers to minimize complications. Although randomized studies are difficult to perform due to the rarity of moyamoya disease, we look forward to such investigations to help resolve the many outstanding questions regarding its treatment and outcome.

◆ Acknowledgments

We thank Cindy H. Samos for editorial assistance and Stuart Minami for assistance with video production.

This chapter was supported in part by the Edward G. Hills Fund, Russell and Elizabeth Siegelman, Bernard and Ronni Lacroute, and the William Randolph Hearst Foundation (to Dr. Steinberg).

References

1. Fukui M. Guidelines for the diagnosis and treatment of spontaneous occlusion of the circle of Willis ('moyamoya' disease). Research Committee on Spontaneous Occlusion of the Circle of Willis (Moyamoya Disease) of the Ministry of Health and Welfare, Japan. Clin Neurol Neurosurg 1997;99(Suppl 2):S238–S240

2. Kuroda S, Ishikawa T, Houkin K, Nanba R, Hokari M, Iwasaki Y. Incidence and clinical features of disease progression in adult moyamoya disease. Stroke 2005;36(10):2148–2153

3. Duan L, Bao XY, Yang WZ, et al. Moyamoya disease in China: its clinical features and outcomes. Stroke 2012;43(1):56–60

4. Lee SB, Kim DS, Huh PW, Yoo DS, Lee TG, Cho KS. Long-term follow-up results in 142 adult patients with moyamoya disease according to management modality. Acta Neurochir (Wien) 2012;154(7):1179–1187

5. Khan N, Achrol AS, Guzman R, et al. Sex differences in clinical presentation and treatment outcomes in Moyamoya disease. Neurosurgery 2012;71(3):587–593, discussion 593

6. Hallemeier CL, Rich KM, Grubb RL Jr, et al. Clinical features and outcome in North American adults with moyamoya phenomenon. Stroke 2006;37(6):1490–1496

7. Ikezaki K, Inamura T, Kawano T, Fukui M. Clinical features of probable moyamoya disease in Japan. Clin Neurol Neurosurg 1997;99(Suppl 2):S173–S177

8. Ogata T, Yasaka M, Inoue T, et al. The clinical features of adult unilateral moyamoya disease: does it have the same clinical characteristics as typical moyamoya disease? Cerebrovasc Dis 2008;26(3):244–249

9. Kelly ME, Bell-Stephens TE, Marks MP, Do HM, Steinberg GK. Progression of unilateral moyamoya disease: A clinical series. Cerebrovasc Dis 2006;22(2-3):109–115

10. Guzman R, Lee M, Achrol A, et al. Clinical outcome after 450 revascularization procedures for moyamoya disease. Clinical article. J Neurosurg 2009;111(5):927–935

11. Okada Y, Kawamata T, Kawashima A, Yamaguchi K, Ono Y, Hori T. The efficacy of superficial temporal artery-middle cerebral artery anastomosis in patients with moyamoya disease complaining of severe headache. J Neurosurg 2012;116(3):672–679

12. Kuroda S, Houkin K. Moyamoya disease: current concepts and future perspectives. Lancet Neurol 2008;7(11):1056–1066

13. Starke RM, Komotar RJ, Hickman ZL, et al. Clinical features, surgical treatment, and long-term outcome in adult patients with moyamoya disease. Clinical article. J Neurosurg 2009;111(5):936–942

14. Zipfel GJ, Sagar J, Miller JP, et al. Cerebral hemodynamics as a predictor of stroke in adult patients with moyamoya disease: a prospective observational study. Neurosurg Focus 2009;26(4):E6

15. Chiu D, Shedden P, Bratina P, Grotta JC. Clinical features of moyamoya disease in the United States. Stroke 1998;29(7):1347–1351

16. Kraemer M, Berlit P, Diesner F, Khan N. What is the expert's opinion on antiplatelet therapy in moyamoya disease? Results of a worldwide Survey. Eur J Neurol 2012;19(1):163–167

17. Kuroda S, Hashimoto N, Yoshimoto T, Iwasaki Y; Research Committee on Moyamoya Disease in Japan. Radiological findings, clinical course, and outcome

in asymptomatic moyamoya disease: results of multicenter survey in Japan. Stroke 2007;38(5): 1430–1435

18. Kobayashi E, Saeki N, Oishi H, Hirai S, Yamaura A. Long-term natural history of hemorrhagic moyamoya disease in 42 patients. J Neurosurg 2000;93(6): 976–980

19. Kraemer M, Heienbrok W, Berlit P. Moyamoya disease in Europeans. Stroke 2008;39(12):3193–3200

20. Bacigaluppi S, Dehdashti AR, Agid R, Krings T, Tymianski M, Mikulis DJ. The contribution of imaging in diagnosis, preoperative assessment, and follow-up of moyamoya disease: a review. Neurosurg Focus 2009;26(4):E3

21. Esposito G, Fierstra J, Kronenburg A, Regli L. A comment on "Contralateral cerebral hemodynamic changes after unilateral direct revascularization in patients with moyamoya disease". Neurosurg Rev 2012;35(1): 141–143, author reply 143

22. Han JS, Abou-Hamden A, Mandell DM, et al. Impact of extracranial-intracranial bypass on cerebrovascular reactivity and clinical outcome in patients with symptomatic moyamoya vasculopathy. Stroke 2011;42(11):3047–3054

23. Ma Y, Li M, Jiao LQ, Zhang HQ, Ling F. Contralateral cerebral hemodynamic changes after unilateral direct revascularization in patients with moyamoya disease. Neurosurg Rev 2011;34(3):347–353, discussion 353–354

24. Nair AK, Drazin D, Yamamoto J, Boulos AS. Computed tomographic perfusion in assessing postoperative revascularization in moyamoya disease. World Neurosurg 2010;73(2):93–99, discussion e13

25. Fujii K, Ikezaki K, Irikura K, Miyasaka Y, Fukui M. The efficacy of bypass surgery for the patients with hemorrhagic moyamoya disease. Clin Neurol Neurosurg 1997;99(Suppl 2):S194–S195

26. Houkin K, Kamiyama H, Abe H, Takahashi A, Kuroda S. Surgical therapy for adult moyamoya disease. Can surgical revascularization prevent the recurrence of intracerebral hemorrhage? Stroke 1996;27(8): 1342–1346

27. Kawaguchi S, Okuno S, Sakaki T. Effect of direct arterial bypass on the prevention of future stroke in patients with the hemorrhagic variety of moyamoya disease. J Neurosurg 2000;93(3):397–401

28. Wanifuchi H, Takeshita M, Izawa M, Aoki N, Kagawa M. Management of adult moyamoya disease. Neurol Med Chir (Tokyo) 1993;33(5):300–305

29. Yoshida Y, Yoshimoto T, Shirane R, Sakurai Y. Clinical course, surgical management, and long-term outcome of moyamoya patients with rebleeding after an episode of intracerebral hemorrhage: An extensive follow-Up study. Stroke 1999;30(11):2272–2276

30. Okada Y, Shima T, Nishida M, Yamane K, Yamada T, Yamanaka C. Effectiveness of superficial temporal artery-middle cerebral artery anastomosis in adult moyamoya disease: cerebral hemodynamics and clinical course in ischemic and hemorrhagic varieties. Stroke 1998;29(3):625–630

31. Karzmark P, Zeifert PD, Bell-Stephens TE, Steinberg GK, Dorfman LJ. Neurocognitive impairment in adults with moyamoya disease without stroke. Neurosurgery 2012;70(3):634–638

32. Miyamoto S; Japan Adult Moyamoya Trial Group. Study design for a prospective randomized trial of extracranial-intracranial bypass surgery for adults with moyamoya disease and hemorrhagic onset—the Japan Adult Moyamoya Trial Group. Neurol Med Chir (Tokyo) 2004;44(4):218–219

33. Bang JS, Kwon OK, Kim JE, et al. Quantitative angiographic comparison with the OSIRIS program between the direct and indirect revascularization modalities in adult moyamoya disease. Neurosurgery 2012;70(3):625–632, discussion 632–633

34. Mesiwala AH, Sviri G, Fatemi N, Britz GW, Newell DW. Long-term outcome of superficial temporal artery-middle cerebral artery bypass for patients with moyamoya disease in the US. Neurosurg Focus 2008;24(2):E15

35. Dusick JR, Gonzalez NR, Martin NA. Clinical and angiographic outcomes from indirect revascularization surgery for Moyamoya disease in adults and children: a review of 63 procedures. Neurosurgery 2011;68(1):34–43, discussion 43

36. Yilmaz EY, Pritz MB, Bruno A, Lopez-Yunez A, Biller J. Moyamoya: Indiana University Medical Center experience. Arch Neurol 2001;58(8):1274–1278

37. Pandey P, Steinberg GK. Outcome of repeat revascularization surgery for moyamoya disease after an unsuccessful indirect revascularization. Clinical article. J Neurosurg 2011;115(2):328–336

18

Japanese Experience: Long-term Results after Cerebral Revascularization

Toshio Higashi, Hiroshi Abe, Tooru Inoue, and Kiyonobu Ikezaki

◆ Introduction

Moyamoya is a Japanese word meaning "hazy" (like a puff of smoke) and was first used to describe the angiographic appearance of this unusual vascular network.[1] The term is now used throughout the world to describe this condition. Because there is no effective medical therapy for moyamoya disease, surgical revascularization is considered to be the most effective treatment for improving cerebral hemodynamics and for reducing the risk of subsequent stroke.[2–4] A consensus on this issue was announced in recently published guidelines.[5] In pediatric cases, a direct or indirect bypass procedure is effective at improving hemodynamic impairment. In adult cases, a direct bypass procedure, with or without indirect bypass, is effective; an indirect bypass procedure alone is not recommended.[5] This chapter summarizes the Japanese experience with surgical treatment for the prevention of stroke associated with moyamoya disease based on the available literature on revascularization surgery for this vasculopathy.

◆ Surgical Treatment for Moyamoya Disease

According to published studies, surgical revascularization is considered to be a standard treatment for improving cerebral hemodynamics and reducing the incidence of subsequent ischemic stroke in both pediatric and adult patients with moyamoya disease. These surgical procedures can be classified into three categories: direct bypass, indirect bypass, and combined bypass.[2–4] In 1994, among the registered cases of the Japanese study group (Research Committee on Spontaneous Occlusion of the Circle of Willis [Moyamoya Disease] of the Ministry of Health and Welfare, Japan), direct bypass was performed in 21%, indirect bypass in 36%, combined bypass in 20%, and conservative treatment in 23% of cases.[6] Superficial temporal artery (STA)–to–middle cerebral artery (MCA) anastomosis is most frequently used for direct revascularization.[7] Direct bypass is effective for improving cerebral hemodynamics and resolving ischemic symptoms immediately after the procedure (**Figs. 18.1a, b** and **18.2a**). Perioperative ischemic events are less frequently observed after direct or combined bypass than after indirect bypass.[8]

Spontaneous angiogenesis between the brain surface and the vascularized donor tissues is elicited by indirect bypass surgery (**Figs. 18.1c** and **18.2b**). Various methods of indirect bypass have been developed in Japan, including encephalomyosynangiosis (EMS), encephaloduroarteriosynangiosis (EDAS), encephaloduroarteriomyosynangiosis, and multiple bur hole surgery, using the superficial temporal artery, dura mater, temporal muscle, galeal tissue, and omentum as the pediculate

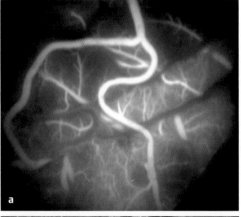

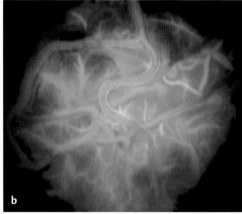

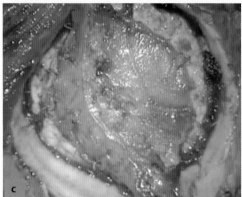

Fig. 18.1a–c Revascularization surgery for moya-moya disease. (**a**) Near-infrared indocyanine green (ICG) video angiography after a double superficial temporal artery–to–middle cerebral artery anastomosis. Real-time bypass patency was confirmed during the operation. (**b**) ICG video angiography shown as a continuous color map using the FLOW800 system (Carl Zeiss Meditec AG, Jena, Germany). This integrated software compiles ICG video sequences into color visual maps and provides information on vascular blood flow dynamics. Perfusion areas from the direct bypass are clearly observed as the yellow-to-orange color. (**c**) Encephaloduroarteriosynangiosis. The authors routinely prepare a wide galeal strip around the superficial temporal artery so that the flap can cover a larger area of the brain surface to improve revascularization.

donor tissues (**Fig. 18.1c**).[9–16] Indirect bypass is specific for moyamoya disease and is widely used because direct bypass surgery can be technically challenging in pediatric patients with small and fragile cortical branches.[4] The effects of indirect bypass are not observed immediately, because surgical collaterals require several months to develop.[17,18] Combined direct and indirect bypass surgery offers the benefits of both and has been used at many centers.[8,19,20]

◆ Surgical Treatment for Pediatric Ischemic-type Moyamoya Disease

In conservatively treated pediatric patients, transient ischemic attacks (TIAs) are most frequently observed during the first 4 years after disease onset; thereafter, the occurrence decreases.[21] In contrast, in most pediatric patients the incidence of ischemic events promptly decreases or disappears after revascularization surgery.[8,22,23]

Direct Bypass with or without Indirect Bypass

Karasawa et al treated 104 pediatric patients with STA-to-MCA bypass, EMS, or both, and demonstrated a marked decrease in ischemic events at a mean follow-up of 9.6 years.[22] They concluded that a major stroke before surgery was the primary factor in poor outcomes, especially in patients under the age of 3 years. Miyamoto et al also reported the results of STA-to-MCA bypass, EMS, or both in 113 patients. At a mean follow-up of 14.4 years, they obtained complete remission of TIAs in 110 cases (97.3%).[23]

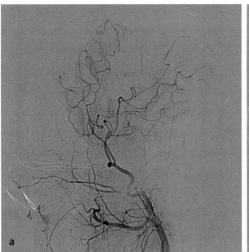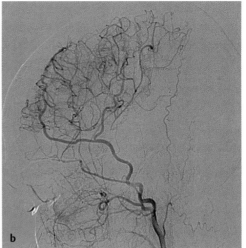

Fig. 18.2a, b External carotid artery angiogram after extracranial-to-intracranial bypass surgery. (**a**) Right external carotid artery angiogram 18 days after surgical treatment of an 18-year-old man with repeated transient ischemic attacks involving his left lower extremity. The right cerebral angiogram indicated stage 3 moyamoya disease based on Suzuki's classification.[1] After undergoing right superficial temporal artery–to–middle cerebral artery bypass surgery, the patient's transient ischemic attacks disappeared completely. (**b**) Right external carotid artery angiogram 3 years after surgical treatment in a 49-year-old woman with moyamoya disease who experienced intraventricular hemorrhage. After conservative treatment, bilateral indirect revascularization surgeries were performed to improve her hemodynamic compromise. The angiogram shows prominent revascularization from frontal encephaloduroarteriosynangiosis and parietal encephaloduroarteriomyosynangiosis. She experienced no hemorrhagic episodes after the treatment.

Indirect Bypass

Yoshiharu Matsushima and coworkers demonstrated the efficacy of EDAS for eliminating ischemic episodes over a long-term period in 65 pediatric patients.[24] The ischemic attacks disappeared after a mean postoperative period of 239 days. Since then, however, some reports have suggested that indirect bypass alone is insufficient for resolving ischemic symptoms. Miyamoto et al reported that 11 cases refractory to EDAS or EMS subsequently required additional treatment by STA-to-MCA bypass with EMS or an omentum graft.[25] Multiple combined indirect procedures can be associated with the development of collateral formations in the distributions of the anterior cerebral artery (ACA) and MCA. Toshio Matsushima and colleagues showed the efficacy of multiple indirect bypass procedures for covering a large area and reducing ischemic symptoms compared with a single indirect bypass.[26,27]

Combined Bypass

To increase the efficacy of collateral revascularization, combined bypass surgery has been used increasingly to improve the elimination of ischemic episodes. Toshio Matsushima and coworkers reported complete resolution of symptoms in 7 of 7 cases after STA-to-MCA bypass plus EMS and in 3 of 13 cases (23%) after EDAS ($p < 0.01$).[19] Ishikawa et al also showed that the incidence of postoperative ischemic events was reduced significantly in a combined-treatment group (10% of the pretreatment level) compared with an indirect-bypass group (56% of the pretreatment level, $p < 0.01$).[28] The STA also can be anastomosed to the branch of the ACA in patients who have hemodynamic compromise involving that region.[8,29] Kuroda et al developed a combined procedure: STA-to-MCA anastomosis and encephaloduromyoarteriopericraniosynangiosis using a frontal pericranial flap to supply blood flow over a wide surface of the brain, especially in the ACA territory.[20] Among

75 patients, including 28 pediatric and 47 adult patients, the overall rates of mortality and morbidity were 0% and 5.7%, respectively. The annual risk of cerebrovascular events during the mean follow-up of 12.5 years was 0% in the pediatric and 0.4% in the adult patients.

Even after remission of ischemic symptoms by surgical revascularization, more than 20% of pediatric patients could not maintain an independent social life due to intellectual impairment.[23,28,30,31] In pediatric patients, intelligence is often diminished compared with the general population.[21,30,32] Earlier studies demonstrated that poor intellectual outcome correlated with early onset (age < 5 years) of moyamoya disease, completed stroke, cerebral infarction, or a longer disease period.[31,33] Surgical revascularization has the beneficial effect for slowing cognitive decline in pediatric patients with moyamoya disease.[24,31,34] Yoshiharu Matsushima and colleagues evaluated cognitive function after EDAS in 65 pediatric patients.[24] Although cognitive decline halted after EDAS, this procedure alone did not improve the impaired function. However, they also found that patients with a preoperative Full-Scale IQ > 70 had normal intelligence levels 9.5 years after surgery.[35] Multivariate analyses have demonstrated that completed stroke and small craniotomy surgery are independent predictors of poor intellectual outcomes in pediatric patients who have undergone surgical revascularization.[32]

◆ Surgical Treatment for Adult Ischemic-type Moyamoya Disease

Increasing evidence suggests that a significant number of the patients with adult-onset moyamoya disease also present with progressive steno-occlusive lesions.[36,37] Based on a nationwide questionnaire survey of 2,193 definite cases of moyamoya disease in Japan, 33 (1.5%) cases were asymptomatic. Of these 33 patients, 7 (21.2%) became symptomatic during a mean follow-up period of 3.7 years.[38] Kuroda et al reported that occlusive lesions in the major intracranial arteries progressed in 15 of 86 affected hemispheres (17.4%) or in 15 of 63 patients (23.8%) during follow-up (mean 12.1 years). Of the 15 patients, 8 developed ischemic or hemorrhagic events in relation to disease progression.[36] Narisawa et al also reported that among

47 hemispheres conservatively followed after initial diagnosis (mean 2.1 years), 6 hemispheres (12.8%) in four patients showed apparent progression of steno-occlusive lesions and were treated with revascularization surgery.[37] In patients with adult-onset moyamoya disease, the direct bypass is considered to be effective for preventing subsequent ischemic stroke[17,39]; indirect bypass alone is less effective.[40] Surgical indications proposed for adult-onset ischemic patients are as follows: (1) presence of ischemic symptoms, (2) apparent blood flow compromise on single photon emission computed tomography (SPECT), (3) independent activity of daily life, and (4) absence of major cerebral infarction.[37]

◆ Surgical Treatment for Hemorrhagic-type Moyamoya Disease

The most significant factor affecting poor outcome is hemorrhagic manifestations of moyamoya disease.[41] The annual rebleeding rate is reported to be 7.09%[42]; thus, the management of the hemorrhagic type of this disease is crucial. Bleeding develops primarily in the thalamus and basal ganglia with frequent perforation to the ventricles. Chronic hemodynamic stress may lead to some pathological changes in the moyamoya vessels and eventually evoke the rupture of fragile moyamoya vessels, microaneurysms, and saccular aneurysms.[43]

Revascularization surgery has been performed based on the hypothesis that reducing hemodynamic stress will prevent recurrent bleeding. Some reports have demonstrated the efficacy of direct bypass for hemorrhagic-type moyamoya disease.[44,45] Other reports, however, have found no significant effect on rebleeding rates.[46–48] The recent guideline states that revascularization surgery may be considered for the hemorrhagic type of moyamoya disease, but there is no scientific evidence to support this recommendation.[5] To address this issue, the Japan Adult Moyamoya trial began in 2001. The goal of this multicenter prospective randomized trial is to determine whether direct bypass surgery reduces the rate of recurrent bleeding attacks. Registration was closed in June 2008, and the results will be disclosed in 2013.[43,49]

Literature reviews of studies on outcomes of revascularization surgery are listed in **Table 18.1**. Surgical revascularization remarkably

Table 18.1 Literature Reviews of Studies on Outcomes of Revascularization Surgery

Reference	Revascularization Surgery	No. of Patients (No. of Hemispheres)	Patient Population	Outcome	Mean Follow-up
Mainly pediatric					
Matsushima Y. et al 1991[24]	EDAS	65(NA)	Pediatric	Ischemic attacks disappeared a mean of 239 days after operation	6 y 5 mo
Matsushima T. et al 1992[19]	STA-to-MCA+ EMS or EDAS alone	16(20)	Pediatric	Complete resolution of symptoms in 100% after STA-to-MCA+EMS and in 23% after EDAS (hemispheres)	6–12 mo
Kinugasa et al 1993[14]	EDAMS	17(28)	13 pediatric 4 adult	Neurological deficits recovered completely and TIA disappeared in 47% Neurological deficits improved and TIA markedly reduced in 29% (patients)	3 y 2 mo
Kashiwagi et al 1996[15]	EDAS+split dura	18(25)	Pediatric	All patients symptom free 1.5 years after surgery 81% able to lead normal lives at follow-up (patients)	6.5 y
Kawaguchi et al 1996[16]	Multiple bur holes	10(18)	Adult	TIA disappeared in 100% (6/6), neurological symptoms improved in 100% (2/2) with CI and in 100% (2/2) with IVH	34.7 mo
Ishikawa et al 1997[28]	STA-to-MCA+ EDAMS or EDAS alone	34(64)	Pediatric	Incidence of postoperative ischemic events significantly reduced in combined (10%) and indirect bypass (56%) group (pretreatment level, hemispheres)	6.6 y
Matsushima T. et al 1997[26]	EMAS+EDAS+ EMS or EDAS alone	12(16)	Pediatric	Ischemic symptoms disappeared or improved in 94% in combined and in 76% in EDAS group (hemispheres)	>1 y
Iwama et al 1997[29]	STA-to-ACA and/ or STA-to-MCA	5(NA)	Mean age, 19.0 years (range, 5–35yrs)	No ischemic attack in 80%, frequency of TIA markedly decreased in 20% (patients)	2.5 to 8 y
Miyamoto et al 1998[23]	STA-to-MCA and/ or EMS	113(NA)	Pediatric	Complete resolution of TIA in 97.3%, independent lifestyle achieved in 88.5% (patients)	14.4 y
Kuroda et al 2010[20,a]	STA-to-MCA+ EDMAPS	28(47)	Pediatric	Complete resolution of TIA in 96.4%, no cerebrovascular event in 100% (patients), morbidity 4.3%, mortality 0% (3 mo)	72.8 mo

(Continued on page 180)

Table 18.1 *(Continued)* Literature Reviews of Studies on Outcomes of Revascularization Surgery

Reference	Revascularization Surgery	No. of Patients (No. of Hemispheres)	Patient Population	Outcome	Mean Follow-up
Mainly adult					
Mizoi et al 1996[40]	STA-to-MCA+ EMS or STA-to-MCA+EDAS	23(NA)	7 pediatric 16 adult	All pediatric patients showed good or moderate development of collaterals through indirect bypass while 56% older than 30 years had opposite outcome (patients)	3.4 y
Houkin et al 1996[44]	STA-to-MCA+ EDAMS	35	Adult	16% of hemorrhagic and 18% of ischemic patients had hemorrhage after revascularization surgery (overall, 14.3%)	6.4 y
Okada et al 1998[39]	STA-to-MCA	30	Adult 15 ischemic 15 hemorrhagic	86% in ischemic group recovered without neurological deficits, 67% in hemorrhagic group had good recoveries, 6.7% in ischemic group had perioperative fatal ICH, perioperative ICH (6.7%) and fatal ICH (20%) during follow-up in hemorrhagic group	Ischemic, 67 mo Hemorrhagic, 94 mo
Kawaguchi et al 2000[45]	STA-to-MCA or EDAS or conservative	22	Adult hemorrhagic	41% of patients presented with an ischemic or rebleeding event, incidence of stroke event after STA-to-MCA was significantly lower than that in patients treated conservatively or with EDAS	8 y
Kuroda et al 2010[20,a]	STA-to-MCA+ EDMAPS	47(76)	Adult	No cerebrovascular event in 97.9% (patients), morbidity 6.6%, mortality 0% (3 mo)	63.1 mo

[a]Report from Kuroda et al[20] is divided to pediatric and adult group as it has enough and detailed data.

Abbreviations: ACA, anterior cerebral artery; CI, cerebral infarction; EDAMS, encephaloduroarteriomyosynangiosis; EDAS, encephaloduroarteriosynangiosis; EDMAPS, encephaloduromyoarteriopericraniosynangiosis; EDS, encephalodurosynangiosis; EMAS, encephalomyoarteriosynangiosis; EMS, encephalomyosynangiosis; ICH, intracerebral hemorrhage; IVH, intraventricular hemorrhage; MCA, middle cerebral artery; NA, not available; STA, superficial temporal artery; TIA, transient ischemic attack.

decreases the incidence of TIAs and the risk of subsequent ischemic stroke, especially in pediatric patients, although its efficacy for preventing rebleeding needs to be clarified. Several clinical factors help predict long-term outcomes, including age of onset, procedure for surgical revascularization, and postoperative cerebral hemodynamics.[4] Early diagnosis and appropriate timing for cerebral revascularization are crucial to improve long-term outcomes.

◆ Perioperative Complications

Although cerebral revascularization procedures are well established and can be performed safely, perioperative management is essential for patients with moyamoya disease. Revascularization surgery for moyamoya disease is associated with a higher risk of perioperative ischemic events compared with other occlusive diseases.[40] The reported incidence of perioperative ischemic complications has ranged from 7.4 to 22.2%.[28,50-52] Iwama et al demonstrated the relevance of preoperative hemodynamic factors (incidence of TIAs) to perioperative ischemic complications in pediatric patients.[50] During surgery, respiratory and hemodynamic factors such as hypercapnia, hypocapnia, and hypotension can increase the risk of perioperative complications. Normocapnic control during general anesthesia with sufficient hydration is essential to avoid perioperative ischemic complications.[50,51,53,54]

Patients with poor cerebrovascular reactivity are known to be at a high risk for hyperperfusion syndrome.[55] Intracerebral hemorrhage after revascularization surgery in patients with moyamoya disease also has been reported, with an incidence ranging from 3.3 to 6.6%.[20,39,56] Recent studies suggest that after a direct bypass procedure is performed for moyamoya disease, focal cerebral hyperperfusion causes potential complications such as transient neurological deterioration or delayed intracerebral hemorrhage.[56,57] The incidence of transient neurological deterioration caused by hyperperfusion has been reported to range from 16.7 to 28.1%.[58] The vulnerability of the blood–brain barrier in patients subjected to chronic ischemia is considered to be one of the reasons for cerebral hyperperfusion.[55] Preoperative and postoperative evaluations of cerebral hemodynamics are necessary to prevent serious complications related to postoperative hyperperfusion.[58,59] Fujimura et al reported that patients with symptomatic hyperperfusion were treated with intensive control of blood pressure and that no patients suffered from permanent neurological deficits resulting from cerebral hyperperfusion.[58]

◆ Surgical Indications and Novel Approaches for the Surgical Treatment of Moyamoya Disease

Since the late 1980s, cerebral hemodynamics and metabolism in moyamoya disease have been extensively studied using SPECT, positron emission tomography, and xenon computed tomography.[60-70] Recently, less invasive measures such as perfusion computed tomography or magnetic resonance imaging have superseded radioactive tracer studies.[71-73] All these results suggest that the perfusion reserve capacity is markedly decreased in both pediatric and adult patients with moyamoya disease, when measured by transit time or cerebrovascular response to hypercapnia, and that the reserve improves after bypass surgery.

Kikuta et al reported on the "target bypass" technique, which uses a neuronavigation system with topographical (3-Tesla magnetic resonance imaging) and regional cerebral blood flow (SPECT) data to select the most appropriate recipient cortical artery for functionally effective bypass surgery.[74] The technique of microscope-integrated near-infrared indocyanine green video angiography has recently advanced strikingly, especially in cerebrovascular surgery.[75,76] It has been accepted as a less invasive, simple, real-time technique (**Fig. 18.1c, d**). Awano et al compared this technique for monitoring blood flow through STA-to-MCA bypasses in patients with moyamoya disease and in those with nonmoyamoya ischemic stroke.[77] The bypass supplied blood flow to a greater extent in patients with moyamoya disease than in those with nonmoyamoya diseases, probably reflecting a larger pressure gradient between the anastomosed STA and recipient vessels in patients with moyamoya disease. Awano et al also promoted awareness regarding cerebral hyperperfusion syndrome.[77] The role of the neuroendoscope is increasing for the treatment of intraventricular hemorrhage and intracerebral hemorrhage. This procedure improves safety and accuracy, especially when intraventricular hematomas are removed, even in the third ventricle, aqueduct of Sylvius, and fourth ventricle (**Fig. 18.3a–d**).[78] Less invasive treatments, such as endovascular surgery, have also been

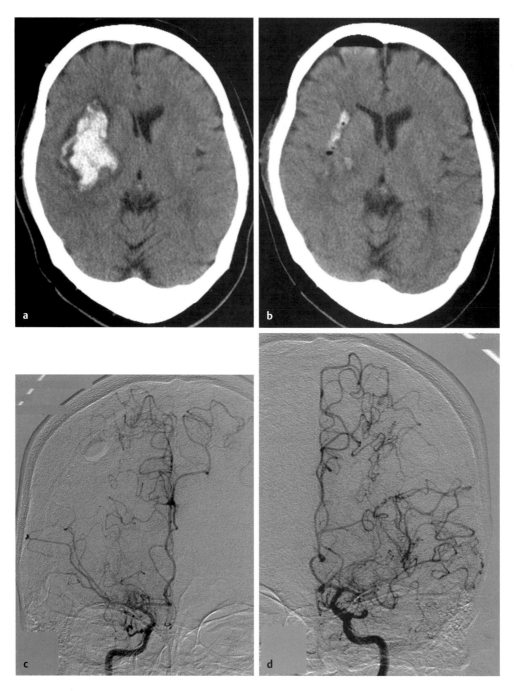

Fig. 18.3a–d Less invasive treatment for hemorrhagic moyamoya disease in a 41-year-old woman who developed left motor weakness from a right putaminal hemorrhage. On the day of onset, the intracerebral hematoma was evacuated using a neuroendoscope. She was diagnosed with stage 3 moyamoya disease based on Suzuki's classification[1] in both the right and left hemispheres. An unruptured aneurysm at the basilar bifurcation was treated by endovascular coil embolization after rehabilitation 1 year after onset. (**a**) Computed tomography scan at admission shows the right putaminal hemorrhage. (**b**) Computed tomography scan obtained one day after endoscopic evacuation of the hematoma. Right (**c**) and left (**d**) carotid artery angiograms, anteroposterior views, show moyamoya changes at the bifurcation of the internal carotid artery on both sides.   *(Continued)*

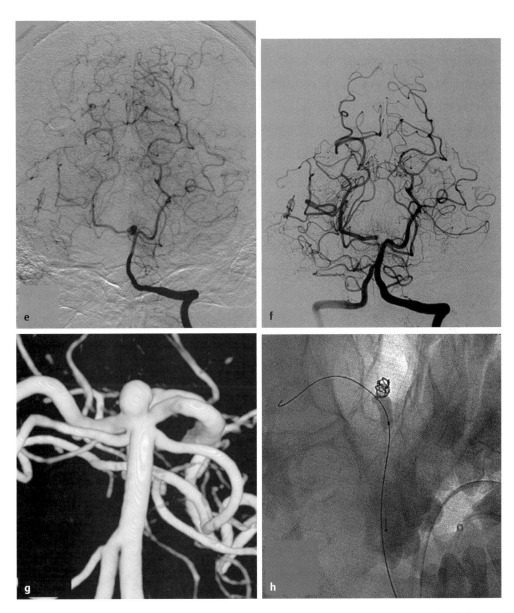

Fig. 18.3e–h *(Continued)* Left vertebral angiograms, Towne's view, before (**e**) and after (**f**) coil embolization of the basilar bifurcation aneurysm. (**g**) Three-dimensional rotational angiogram shows basilar bifurcation aneurysm with a 4-mm diameter. (**h**) Plain X-ray photogram shows coil embolization using the balloon-assist technique.

used in the management of vascular pathology related to moyamoya disease (**Fig. 18.3e–h**).

◆ Conclusion

Since moyamoya disease was first recognized in the 1960s, Japanese neurosurgeons have directed constant effort toward improving clinical outcomes for patients with ischemic and hemorrhagic strokes caused by the distinct and characteristic vasculopathy of this disease. However, numerous issues remain unresolved regarding revascularization surgery for moyamoya disease, such as the appropriate indication for ischemic manifestation, prevention of recurrent bleeding, and preservation of cognitive function. Continuing efforts are necessary to answer these questions.

References

1. Suzuki J, Takaku A. Cerebrovascular "moyamoya" disease. Disease showing abnormal net-like vessels in base of brain. Arch Neurol 1969;20(3):288–299

2. Houkin K. Management strategies part 2: Selection of surgical procedures, outcome, ischemic versus hemorrhagic forms, adults versus children. In: Ikezaki K, Loftus ML, editors. Moyamoya Disease. New York: Thieme; 2001:127–136

3. Matsushima T. Part X surgical technique. In: Cho BK, Tominaga T, editors. Moyamoya Disease Update. New York: Springer; 2010. p. 227–33.

4. Kuroda S, Houkin K. Moyamoya disease: current concepts and future perspectives. Lancet Neurol 2008; 7(11):1056–1066

5. Research committee on the pathology and treatment of spontaneous occlusion of the circle of Willis; Health labour sciences research grant for research on measures for intractable diseases. Guidelines for diagnosis and treatment of moyamoya disease. Neurol Med Chir (Tokyo) 2012;52(5):245–266

6. Fukui M. Current state of study on moyamoya disease in Japan. Surg Neurol 1997;47(2):138–143

7. Karasawa J, Kikuchi H, Furuse S, Kawamura J, Sakaki T. Treatment of moyamoya disease with STA-MCA anastomosis. J Neurosurg 1978;49(5):679–688

8. Ishikawa T, Kamiyama H, Kuroda S, Yasuda H, Nakayama N, Takizawa K. Simultaneous superficial temporal artery to middle cerebral or anterior cerebral artery bypass with pan-synangiosis for Moyamoya disease covering both anterior and middle cerebral artery territories. Neurol Med Chir (Tokyo) 2006;46(9):462–468

9. Karasawa J, Kikuchi H, Furuse S, Sakaki T, Yoshida Y. A surgical treatment of "moyamoya" disease "encephalo-myo synangiosis". Neurol Med Chir (Tokyo) 1977; 17(1 Pt 1):29–37

10. Karasawa J, Kikuchi H, Kawamura J, Sakai T. Intracranial transplantation of the omentum for cerebrovascular moyamoya disease: a two-year follow-up study. Surg Neurol 1980;14(6):444–449

11. Matsushima Y, Fukai N, Tanaka K, et al. A new surgical treatment of moyamoya disease in children: a preliminary report. Surg Neurol 1981;15(4):313–320

12. Matsushima Y, Inaba Y. Moyamoya disease in children and its surgical treatment. Introduction of a new surgical procedure and its follow-up angiograms. Childs Brain 1984;11(3):155–170

13. Ishii R. [Surgical treatment of moyamoya disease]. No Shinkei Geka 1986;14(9):1059–1068

14. Kinugasa K, Mandai S, Kamata I, Sugiu K, Ohmoto T. Surgical treatment of moyamoya disease: operative technique for encephalo-duro-arterio-myo-synangiosis, its follow-up, clinical results, and angiograms. Neurosurgery 1993;32(4):527–531

15. Kashiwagi S, Kato S, Yasuhara S, Wakuta Y, Yamashita T, Ito H. Use of a split dura for revascularization of ischemic hemispheres in moyamoya disease. J Neurosurg 1996;85(3):380–383

16. Kawaguchi T, Fujita S, Hosoda K, et al. Multiple burr-hole operation for adult moyamoya disease. J Neurosurg 1996;84(3):468–476

17. Houkin K, Kuroda S, Ishikawa T, Abe H. Neovascularization (angiogenesis) after revascularization in moyamoya disease. Which technique is most useful for moyamoya disease? Acta Neurochir (Wien) 2000;142(3):269–276

18. Houkin K, Nakayama N, Kuroda S, Ishikawa T, Nonaka T. How does angiogenesis develop in pediatric moyamoya disease after surgery? A prospective study with MR angiography. Childs Nerv Syst 2004;20(10): 734–741

19. Matsushima T, Inoue T, Suzuki SO, Fujii K, Fukui M, Hasuo K. Surgical treatment of moyamoya disease in pediatric patients—comparison between the results of indirect and direct revascularization procedures. Neurosurgery 1992;31(3):401–405

20. Kuroda S, Houkin K, Ishikawa T, Nakayama N, Iwasaki Y. Novel bypass surgery for moyamoya disease using pericranial flap: its impacts on cerebral hemodynamics and long-term outcome. Neurosurgery 2010;66(6):1093–1101, discussion 1101

21. Kurokawa T, Tomita S, Ueda K, et al. Prognosis of occlusive disease of the circle of Willis (moyamoya disease) in children. Pediatr Neurol 1985;1(5):274–277

22. Karasawa J, Touho H, Ohnishi H, Miyamoto S, Kikuchi H. Long-term follow-up study after extracranial-intracranial bypass surgery for anterior circulation ischemia in childhood moyamoya disease. J Neurosurg 1992;77(1):84–89

23. Miyamoto S, Akiyama Y, Nagata I, et al. Long-term outcome after STA-MCA anastomosis for moyamoya disease. Neurosurg Focus 1998;5(5):e5

24. Matsushima Y, Aoyagi M, Koumo Y, et al. Effects of encephalo-duro-arterio-synangiosis on childhood moyamoya patients—swift disappearance of ischemic attacks and maintenance of mental capacity. Neurol Med Chir (Tokyo) 1991;31(11):708–714

25. Miyamoto S, Kikuchi H, Karasawa J, Nagata I, Yamazoe N, Akiyama Y. Pitfalls in the surgical treatment of moyamoya disease. Operative techniques for refractory cases. J Neurosurg 1988;68(4):537–543

26. Matsushima T, Inoue TK, Suzuki SO, et al. Surgical techniques and the results of a fronto-temporo-parietal combined indirect bypass procedure for children with moyamoya disease: a comparison with the results of encephalo-duro-arterio-synangiosis alone. Clin Neurol Neurosurg 1997;99(Suppl 2):S123–S127

27. Matsushima T, Inoue T, Ikezaki K, et al. Multiple combined indirect procedure for the surgical treatment of children with moyamoya disease. A comparison with single indirect anastomosis and direct anastomosis. Neurosurg Focus 1998;5(5):e4

28. Ishikawa T, Houkin K, Kamiyama H, Abe H. Effects of surgical revascularization on outcome of patients with pediatric moyamoya disease. Stroke 1997;28(6): 1170–1173

29. Iwama T, Hashimoto N, Tsukahara T, Miyake H. Superficial temporal artery to anterior cerebral artery direct anastomosis in patients with moyamoya disease. Clin Neurol Neurosurg 1997;99(Suppl 2):S134–S136

30. Imaizumi C, Imaizumi T, Osawa M, Fukuyama Y, Takeshita M. Serial intelligence test scores in pediatric moyamoya disease. Neuropediatrics 1999;30(6): 294–299

31. Matsushima Y, Aoyagi M, Masaoka H, Suzuki R, Ohno K. Mental outcome following encephaloduroarteriosynangiosis in children with moyamoya disease with the onset earlier than 5 years of age. Childs Nerv Syst 1990;6(8):440–443

32. Kuroda S, Houkin K, Ishikawa T, et al. Determinants of intellectual outcome after surgical revascularization in pediatric moyamoya disease: a multivariate analysis. Childs Nerv Syst 2004;20(5):302–308

33. Fukuyama Y, Umezu R. Clinical and cerebral angiographic evolutions of idiopathic progressive occlusive

disease of the circle of Willis ("moyamoya" disease) in children. Brain Dev 1985;7(1):21–37

34. Imaizumi T, Hayashi K, Saito K, Osawa M, Fukuyama Y. Long-term outcomes of pediatric moyamoya disease monitored to adulthood. Pediatr Neurol 1998;18(4): 321–325

35. Matsushima Y, Aoyagi M, Nariai T, Takada Y, Hirakawa K. Long-term intelligence outcome of post-encephalo-duro-arterio-synangiosis childhood moyamoya patients. Clin Neurol Neurosurg 1997;99(Suppl 2): S147–S150

36. Kuroda S, Ishikawa T, Houkin K, Nanba R, Hokari M, Iwasaki Y. Incidence and clinical features of disease progression in adult moyamoya disease. Stroke 2005;36(10):2148–2153

37. Narisawa A, Fujimura M, Tominaga T. Efficacy of the revascularization surgery for adult-onset moyamoya disease with the progression of cerebrovascular lesions. Clin Neurol Neurosurg 2009;111(2):123–126

38. Yamada M, Fujii K, Fukui M. [Clinical features and outcomes in patients with asymptomatic moyamoya disease—from the results of nation-wide questionnaire survey]. No Shinkei Geka 2005;33(4):337–342

39. Okada Y, Shima T, Nishida M, Yamane K, Yamada T, Yamanaka C. Effectiveness of superficial temporal artery-middle cerebral artery anastomosis in adult moyamoya disease: cerebral hemodynamics and clinical course in ischemic and hemorrhagic varieties. Stroke 1998;29(3):625–630

40. Mizoi K, Kayama T, Yoshimoto T, Nagamine Y. Indirect revascularization for moyamoya disease: is there a beneficial effect for adult patients? Surg Neurol 1996;45(6):541–548, discussion 548–549

41. Han DH, Kwon OK, Byun BJ, et al; Korean Society for Cerebrovascular Disease. A co-operative study: clinical characteristics of 334 Korean patients with moyamoya disease treated at neurosurgical institutes (1976-1994). Acta Neurochir (Wien) 2000;142(11): 1263–1273, discussion 1273–1274

42. Kobayashi E, Saeki N, Oishi H, Hirai S, Yamaura A. Long-term natural history of hemorrhagic moyamoya disease in 42 patients. J Neurosurg 2000;93(6): 976–980

43. Takahashi JC, Miyamoto S. Moyamoya disease: recent progress and outlook. Neurol Med Chir (Tokyo) 2010;50(9):824–832

44. Houkin K, Kamiyama H, Abe H, Takahashi A, Kuroda S. Surgical therapy for adult moyamoya disease. Can surgical revascularization prevent the recurrence of intracerebral hemorrhage? Stroke 1996;27(8): 1342–1346

45. Kawaguchi S, Okuno S, Sakaki T. Effect of direct arterial bypass on the prevention of future stroke in patients with the hemorrhagic variety of moyamoya disease. J Neurosurg 2000;93(3):397–401

46. Ikezaki K, Fukui M, Inamura T, Kinukawa N, Wakai K, Ono Y. The current status of the treatment for hemorrhagic type moyamoya disease based on a 1995 nationwide survey in Japan. Clin Neurol Neurosurg 1997;99(Suppl 2):S183–S186

47. Fujii K, Ikezaki K, Irikura K, Miyasaka Y, Fukui M. The efficacy of bypass surgery for the patients with hemorrhagic moyamoya disease. Clin Neurol Neurosurg 1997;99(Suppl 2):S194–S195

48. Yoshida Y, Yoshimoto T, Shirane R, Sakurai Y. Clinical course, surgical management, and long-term outcome of moyamoya patients with rebleeding after an episode of intracerebral hemorrhage: An extensive follow-Up study. Stroke 1999;30(11):2272–2276

49. Miyamoto S; Japan Adult Moyamoya Trial Group. Study design for a prospective randomized trial of extracranial-intracranial bypass surgery for adults with moyamoya disease and hemorrhagic onset—the Japan Adult Moyamoya Trial Group. Neurol Med Chir (Tokyo) 2004;44(4):218–219

50. Iwama T, Hashimoto N, Yonekawa Y. The relevance of hemodynamic factors to perioperative ischemic complications in childhood moyamoya disease. Neurosurgery 1996;38(6):1120–1125, discussion 1125–1126

51. Sato K, Shirane R, Yoshimoto T. Perioperative factors related to the development of ischemic complications in patients with moyamoya disease. Childs Nerv Syst 1997;13(2):68–72

52. Matsushima Y, Aoyagi M, Suzuki R, Tabata H, Ohno K. Perioperative complications of encephalo-duro-arterio-synangiosis: prevention and treatment. Surg Neurol 1991;36(5):343–353

53. Nomura S, Kashiwagi S, Uetsuka S, Uchida T, Kubota H, Ito H. Perioperative management protocols for children with moyamoya disease. Childs Nerv Syst 2001; 17(4-5):270–274

54. Sakamoto T, Kawaguchi M, Kurehara K, Kitaguchi K, Furuya H, Karasawa J. Risk factors for neurologic deterioration after revascularization surgery in patients with moyamoya disease. Anesth Analg 1997;85(5): 1060–1065

55. van Mook WN, Rennenberg RJ, Schurink GW, et al. Cerebral hyperperfusion syndrome. Lancet Neurol 2005;4(12):877–888

56. Fujimura M, Shimizu H, Mugikura S, Tominaga T. Delayed intracerebral hemorrhage after superficial temporal artery-middle cerebral artery anastomosis in a patient with moyamoya disease: possible involvement of cerebral hyperperfusion and increased vascular permeability. Surg Neurol 2009;71(2):223–227, discussion 227

57. Fujimura M, Mugikura S, Kaneta T, Shimizu H, Tominaga T. Incidence and risk factors for symptomatic cerebral hyperperfusion after superficial temporal artery-middle cerebral artery anastomosis in patients with moyamoya disease. Surg Neurol 2009;71(4): 442–447

58. Fujimura M, Shimizu H, Inoue T, Mugikura S, Saito A, Tominaga T. Significance of focal cerebral hyperperfusion as a cause of transient neurologic deterioration after extracranial-intracranial bypass for moyamoya disease: comparative study with non-moyamoya patients using N-isopropyl-p-[(123)I]iodoamphetamine single-photon emission computed tomography. Neurosurgery 2011;68(4):957–964, discussion 964–965

59. Fujimura M, Kaneta T, Mugikura S, Shimizu H, Tominaga T. Temporary neurologic deterioration due to cerebral hyperperfusion after superficial temporal artery-middle cerebral artery anastomosis in patients with adult-onset moyamoya disease. Surg Neurol 2007;67(3):273–282

60. Tomura N, Kanno I, Shishido F, et al. [Vascular responses in cerebrovascular "Moyamoya" disease—evaluated by positron emission tomography]. No To Shinkei 1989;41(9):895–904

61. Kuwabara Y, Ichiya Y, Otsuka M, et al. Cerebral hemodynamic change in the child and the adult with moyamoya disease. Stroke 1990;21(2):272–277

62. Ogawa A, Yoshimoto T, Suzuki J, Sakurai Y. Cerebral blood flow in moyamoya disease. Part 1: Correlation with age and regional distribution. Acta Neurochir (Wien) 1990;105(1-2):30–34

63. Ogawa A, Nakamura N, Yoshimoto T, Suzuki J. Cerebral blood flow in moyamoya disease. Part 2: Autoregulation

and CO2 response. Acta Neurochir (Wien) 1990;105 (3-4):107–111

64. Kuroda S, Kamiyama H, Abe H, et al. Cerebral blood flow in children with spontaneous occlusion of the circle of Willis (moyamoya disease): comparison with healthy children and evaluation of annual changes. Neurol Med Chir (Tokyo) 1993;33(7):434–438

65. Ikezaki K, Matsushima T, Kuwabara Y, Suzuki SO, Nomura T, Fukui M. Cerebral circulation and oxygen metabolism in childhood moyamoya disease: a perioperative positron emission tomography study. J Neurosurg 1994;81(6):843–850

66. Kuroda S, Kamiyama H, Isobe M, Houkin K, Abe H, Mitsumori K. Cerebral hemodynamics and "re-build-up" phenomenon on electroencephalogram in children with moyamoya disease. Childs Nerv Syst 1995;11(4):214–219

67. Kuroda S, Houkin K, Kamiyama H, Abe H, Mitsumori K. Regional cerebral hemodynamics in childhood moyamoya disease. Childs Nerv Syst 1995;11(10): 584–590

68. Kuwabara Y, Ichiya Y, Sasaki M, et al. Cerebral hemodynamics and metabolism in moyamoya disease—a positron emission tomography study. Clin Neurol Neurosurg 1997;99(Suppl 2):S74–S78

69. Shirane R, Yoshida Y, Takahashi T, Yoshimoto T. Assessment of encephalo-galeo-myo-synangiosis with dural pedicle insertion in childhood moyamoya disease: characteristics of cerebral blood flow and oxygen metabolism. Clin Neurol Neurosurg 1997;99(Suppl 2):S79–S85

70. Ikezaki K. Rational approach to treatment of moyamoya disease in childhood. J Child Neurol 2000;15(5): 350–356

71. Sakamoto S, Ohba S, Shibukawa M, Kiura Y, Arita K, Kurisu K. CT perfusion imaging for childhood moyamoya disease before and after surgical revascular-

ization. Acta Neurochir (Wien) 2006;148(1):77–81, discussion 81

72. Tanaka Y, Nariai T, Nagaoka T, et al. Quantitative evaluation of cerebral hemodynamics in patients with moyamoya disease by dynamic susceptibility contrast magnetic resonance imaging—comparison with positron emission tomography. J Cereb Blood Flow Metab 2006;26(2):291–300

73. Togao O, Mihara F, Yoshiura T, et al. Cerebral hemodynamics in Moyamoya disease: correlation between perfusion-weighted MR imaging and cerebral angiography. AJNR Am J Neuroradiol 2006;27(2): 391–397

74. Kikuta K, Takagi Y, Fushimi Y, et al. "Target bypass": a method for preoperative targeting of a recipient artery in superficial temporal artery-to-middle cerebral artery anastomoses. Neurosurgery 2008; 62(6, Suppl 3)1434–1441

75. Raabe A, Beck J, Gerlach R, Zimmermann M, Seifert V. Near-infrared indocyanine green video angiography: a new method for intraoperative assessment of vascular flow. Neurosurgery 2003;52(1):132–139, discussion 139

76. Raabe A, Nakaji P, Beck J, et al. Prospective evaluation of surgical microscope-integrated intraoperative near-infrared indocyanine green videoangiography during aneurysm surgery. J Neurosurg 2005;103(6):982–989

77. Awano T, Sakatani K, Yokose N, et al. Intraoperative EC-IC bypass blood flow assessment with indocyanine green angiography in moyamoya and non-moyamoya ischemic stroke. World Neurosurg 2010;73(6): 668–674

78. Hamada H, Hayashi N, Kurimoto M, et al. Neuroendoscopic removal of intraventricular hemorrhage combined with hydrocephalus. Minim Invasive Neurosurg 2008;51(6):345–349

19

Moyamoya Angiopathy in Korea

Hyoung Kyun Rha

◆ Introduction

Moyamoya disease is characterized by a chronic and progressive steno-occlusive change of the distal internal carotid artery and abnormal development of a fine vascular network (moyamoya vessels) at the base of the brain. The disease was first reported in 1957.[1] A subsequent report coined the name "moyamoya" (the Japanese word for "puff of smoke").[2,3]

◆ Epidemiology

Initially thought to be endemic to Japan, the global scope of moyamoya disease has since been recognized.[4] The frequency of this disease is greatest in Japan, followed by China and Korea. The incidence in each of these three nations is markedly higher than in other countries. In Japan, the prevalence and incidence rates per 100,000 persons were 3.16 and 0.35, respectively, in 1994, and 6.03 and 0.54, respectively, in 2003.[5] The near doubling of the prevalence rate in just under 10 years likely reflects both an increased incidence of the disease and more accurate diagnostic techniques.[5]

Moyamoya disease was first reported in Korea in 1969 and has since been recognized with increasing frequency.[6] Based on National Health Insurance Corporation data, 2,539 patients with moyamoya disease were treated in Korea in 2004, representing a prevalence of 5.2 per 100,000 people. The overall prevalence was 2,987 in 2005, 3,429 in 2006, 4,051 in 2007, and 4,517 in 2008. The prevalence rates per 100,000 were 6.3% in 2005, 7% in 2006, 8.6% in 2007, and 9.1% in 2008. These figures represent an average increase of 15% per year (**Figs. 19.1** and **19.2**). As noted, this increase likely reflects both an increase in new cases as well as improved detection of existing cases. In 2008, 466 people were newly diagnosed with moyamoya disease, representing an incidence of 1 per 100,000 persons.

In 2008, 4,517 patients were treated in Korea: 1,547 males (34%) and 2,970 females (66%), or a 1.94 higher incidence in females. A bimodal age–related distribution was evident, with peak occurrences in teenagers and in adults 40 to 49 years old (**Fig. 19.3**).

◆ Surgical Treatment in Korea

In the 17 years from 1969 to 1986, 33 hospitals in Korea participated in a cooperative study of moyamoya disease. These studies involved 289 cases (130 males and 159 females). Of these 289 patients, 97 were younger than 20 years old. Cerebral infarcts or transient ischemic attacks were the most common presentation (186 cases), followed by hemorrhage (103 cases). Surgical bypass procedures were performed in 36 cases (12.5%). There were 12 cases of direct anastomosis via a superficial temporal

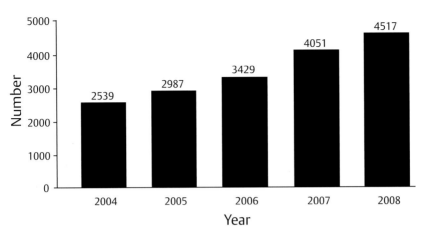

Fig. 19.1 Numbers of patients diagnosed with moyamoya disease in Korea 2004 to 2008.

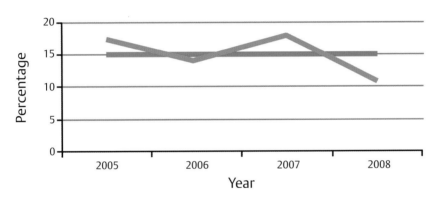

Fig. 19.2 Increasing percentage of newly diagnosed cases of moyamoya disease in Korea.

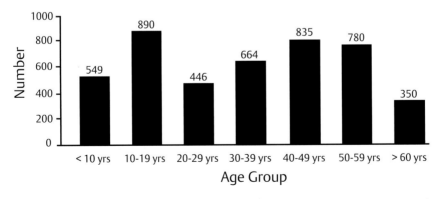

Fig. 19.3 Age distribution of Korean patients diagnosed with moyamoya disease in 2008. (These data were presented by the author at The 10th Korean and Japanese Friendship Conference on Surgery for Cerebral Stroke, held in Nagasaki, Japan, 2010.)

artery–to–middle cerebral artery bypass, 21 cases of indirect anastomosis, and 3 cases of combined direct-indirect anastomosis.

Han et al reviewed 334 cases of moyamoya disease reported from 26 Korean hospitals from 1976 to 1994.[7] These cases most often involved individuals aged 6 to 15 years and 31 to 40 years. Hemorrhagic and ischemic moyamoya disease involved 43% and 57% of these patients, respectively. In adults, the primary manifestation was hemorrhage (62.4%), while 61.2% of children presented with ischemia. About 38% of patients underwent surgery (62% of children, 24% of adults), with 53% of the surgeries performed bilaterally. The frequency of surgery was related to presentation. Revascularization procedures were performed in 25.7% of patients presenting with hemorrhage and in 53.9% of those with ischemic symptoms. Of the indirect bypass procedures, 82% involved encephaloduroarteriosynangiosis and encephalomyosynangiosis. Nine cases were treated with direct bypass alone, and 15 cases were treated with combined direct and indirect bypass procedures. A good outcome was reported in 73% of the cases. Subsequently, the incidence of the disease increased, and additional studies were initiated in Korea.[2,8-10] Surgical treatment has become more common in the management of these patients.

The author reviewed the surgical management of moyamoya disease at 19 hospitals in Korea from 2004 to 2008 in a presentation at The 10th Korean and Japanese Friendship Conference on Surgery for Cerebral Stroke held in Nagasaki, Japan, in 2010. Altogether, 473 surgical cases were identified. Moyamoya disease was most frequent in individuals aged 40 to 49 years (107 cases), followed by those aged 30 to 39 years (104 cases), 20 to 29 years (71 cases), 13 to 19 years (62 cases), 50 to 59 years (45 cases), and 60+ years (13 cases). Females ($n = 322$) were more commonly affected than males ($n = 151$). Of the 473 cases studied, 83 were operated on using direct bypass, 261 using indirect bypass, and 129 using combined direct-indirect procedures. A total of 78 patients (16%) experienced complications, including transient ischemic attacks and cerebral infarcts in 38 patients, intracranial hemorrhage in 23 patients, seizures in 8 patients, wound infections in 7 patients, and other symptoms in 2 patients. During the average follow-up period of 29.17 ± 17.15 months (range, 1 to 67 months), symptoms recurred in

105 cases (22%). Of these, recurrent ischemic symptoms were the most common ($n = 77$) followed by hemorrhage ($n = 13$), epileptic seizures ($n = 8$), and other symptoms ($n = 7$). Clinical outcome was assessed using the Karnofsky Performance Scale with a mean of 88.97 ± 15.13 points.

Surgical management of patients with moyamoya disease has gradually shifted to the more frequent use of direct revascularization techniques. In the earlier review of surgical treatment of moyamoya disease conducted in 26 hospitals in Korea from 1976 to 1994, indirect techniques accounted for ~82% of revascularization procedures. In comparison, in the study evaluating surgical cases from 19 hospitals in Korea from 2004 to 2008, direct anastomosis and combined direct-indirect bypass procedures accounted for 45% of cases, whereas the indirect approach accounted for 55%. These later results compare favorably with those from Japan.[11]

◆ Conclusion

The incidence of moyamoya disease in Korea approaches that in Japan. In recent studies, direct and combined direct-indirect bypasses have accounted for 45% of the revascularization procedures performed to treat these patients in Korea.

References

1. Takeuchi K, Shimizu K. Hypoplasia of the bilateral internal carotid arteries. No To Shinkei 1957;9:37–43
2. Suzuki J, Takaku A, Asahi M. Etiological consideration of Moyamoya disease. In: Kudo T, editor. A disease with abnormal intracranial vascular networks. Spontaneous occlusion of the Circle of Willis. Tokyo: Igaku Shoin; 1967:73–75
3. Suzuki J, Takaku A. Cerebrovascular "moyamoya" disease. Disease showing abnormal net-like vessels in base of brain. Arch Neurol 1969;20(3):288–299
4. Kudo T. Spontaneous occlusion of the circle of Willis. A disease apparently confined to Japanese. Neurology 1968;18(5):485–496
5. Kuriyama S, Kusaka Y, Fujimura M, et al. Prevalence and clinicoepidemiological features of moyamoya disease in Japan: findings from a nationwide epidemiological survey. Stroke 2008;39(1):42–47
6. Choi KS. Moyamoya disease in Korea: A cooperative study. In: Suzuki J, editor. Advance in surgery for cerebral stroke.Tokyo: Springer-Verlag; 1988:107–109
7. Han DH, Kwon OK, Byun BJ, et al; Korean Society for Cerebrovascular Disease. A co-operative study: clinical characteristics of 334 Korean patients with moyamoya disease treated at neurosurgical institutes (1976-1994). Acta Neurochir (Wien) 2000;142(11):1263–1273, discussion 1273–1274

8. Choi JU, Kim DS, Kim EY, Lee KC. Natural history of moyamoya disease: comparison of activity of daily living in surgery and non surgery groups. Clin Neurol Neurosurg 1997;99(Suppl 2):S11–S18

9. Kim DS, Kang SG, Yoo DS, Huh PW, Cho KS, Park CK. Surgical results in pediatric moyamoya disease: angiographic revascularization and the clinical results. Clin Neurol Neurosurg 2007;109(2):125–131

10. Kim H, Kim YW, Joo WI, et al. Effect of direct bypass on the prevention of hemorrhage in patients with the hemorrhagic type of Moyamoya disease. Korean J Cerebrovascular Surg 2007;9(1):14–19

11. Ikezaki K, Han DH, Kawano T, Kinukawa N, Fukui M. A clinical comparison of definite moyamoya disease between South Korea and Japan. Stroke 1997; 28(12):2513–2517

Index

Note: Page numbers followed by *f* and *t* indicate figures and tables, respectively.

Index

Index

Index

Index

W

WAIS. *See* Wechsler Adult Intelligence Scale
WCST. *See* Wisconsin Card Sorting Test
Wechsler Adult Intelligence Scale (WAIS), 64, 70*t*
Wechsler Preschool and Primary Scale of
    Intelligence (WPPSI), 70*t*
Williams syndrome, moyamoya syndrome
    associated with, 7*t*
Wilms tumor, moyamoya syndrome associated
    with, 7*t*

Wisconsin Card Sorting Test (WCST), 70*t*
WPPSI. *See* Wechsler Preschool and Primary Scale
    of Intelligence

X

xenon computed tomography, 20, 22*f*
    CVRC assessed with, 57–59

Z

Zurich experience, 144–145